Neuroanatomy

Basic and clinical

Third Edition

M. J. T. FitzGerald MD, PhD, DSc, MRIA

Emeritus Professor, Department of Anatomy, University College, Galway, Ireland

W.B. SAUNDERS COMPANY LTD

London   Philadelphia   Toronto   Sydney   Tokyo

W.B. Saunders Company Ltd   24–28 Oval Road
London NW1 7DX

The Curtis Center
Independence Square West
Philadelphia, PA 19106-3399, USA

Harcourt Brace & Company
55 Horner Avenue
Toronto, Ontario M8Z 4X6, Canada

Harcourt Brace & Company, Australia
30–52 Smidmore Street
Marrickville, NSW 2204, Australia

Harcourt Brace & Company, Japan
Ichibancho Central Building, 22-1 Ichibancho
Chiyoda-ku, Tokyo 102, Japan

First Edition 1985
Reprinted 1985 and 1990
Second Edition 1992
Reprinted three times, final reprint 1995.

A catalogue record for this book is available from the British Library

ISBN 0-7020-1994-1

Typeset by Selwood Systems, Midsomer Norton.

Printed in Great Britain by Bath Press Colour Books, Glasgow.

Neuroanatomy
Basic and Clinical

CONTENTS

Preface xiii

1   Embryology 1
    Spinal cord 1
        Neurulation 1
        Spinal nerves 1
    Brain 1
        Brain vesicles 1
        Ventricular system and choroid plexuses 2
        Cranial nerves 4
        Cerebral hemispheres..4

2   Cerebral topography...8
    Surface features..8
        Lobes 8
        Diencephalon...11
    Internal anatomy of the cerebrum...12
        Thalamus, caudate and lentiform nuclei, internal capsule 12
        Hippocampus and fornix...15
        Association and commissural fibers 17
        Lateral and third ventricles 20

3   Midbrain, hindbrain, spinal cord 25
    Brainstem 25
        Ventral view 25
        Dorsal view 26
        Sectional views 26
    Cerebellum 28
    Spinal cord 29
        General features..29
        Internal anatomy 29

4   Meninges 32
    Cranial meninges 32
        Dura mater 32
        Meningeal arteries 32
        Arachnoid mater 32
        Pia mater 32
        Subarachnoid cisterns 36
        Sheath of the optic nerve 36
    Spinal meninges 37
    Circulation of cerebrospinal fluid 37

CLINICAL PANELS
    Extradural/subdural hematomas 35
    Hydrocephalus 38

5   Blood supply of the brain 42
Arterial supply of the forebrain 42
    Anterior cerebral artery 43
    Middle cerebral artery 43
    Posterior cerebral artery 45
Blood supply of the brainstem 45
    Vertebral branches 45
    Basilar branches 45
Venous drainage of the brain 46
    Superficial veins 47
    Deep veins 47
Regulation of blood flow 48
    Blood–brain barrier 49
    Functions of the blood–brain barrier 50
CLINICAL PANEL
    Blood–brain barrier pathology 50

6   Neurons and neuroglia 53
Neurons 53
    Internal structure of neurons 53
Synapses 55
    Chemical synapses 55
    Receptor activation 56
    Electrical synapses 57
Neuroglial cells of the CNS 58
    Astrocytes 58
    Oligodendrocytes 59
    Microglia 60
    Ependyma 60
CLINICAL PANELS
    Clinical relevance of neuronal transport 56
    Gliomas 60
    Multiple sclerosis 61

7   Peripheral nerves 63
General features 63
Microscopic structure 63
    Myelin formation 64
Degeneration and regeneration 65
    Wallerian degeneration of peripheral nerves 65
    Regeneration of peripheral nerves 65
    Degeneration in the CNS 67
    Regeneration in the CNS 68

8   Innervation of muscles and joints 70
Motor innervation of skeletal muscle 70
    Motor end plates 71
    Motor units in old age 71
Sensory innervation of skeletal muscle 72
    Neuromuscular spindles 72

Tendon endings 74
Free nerve endings 74
Innervation of joints 75
CLINICAL PANEL
Myasthenia gravis 72

9   Innervation of skin 77
Sensory units...77
Nerve endings 78
Free nerve endings 78
Follicular nerve endings 78
Merkel cell–neurite complexes 78
Encapsulated nerve endings 78
CLINICAL PANELS
Axon reflex 79
Peripheral neuropathies 80

10   Autonomic nervous system and visceral afferents 83
Components of the autonomic nervous system...83
Sympathetic nervous system 84
Parasympathetic nervous system 86
Cranial parasympathetic system 86
Sacral parasympathetic system..86
Neurotransmission in the autonomic system...87
Ganglionic transmission 87
Junctional transmission 87
Other types of neuron 89
Interaction of the autonomic and immune systems 91
Visceral afferents..91
Visceral pain 91
Tenderness 92
Pain and the mind 92
CLINICAL PANELS
Sympathetic interruption 85
Drugs and the sympathetic system...89
Drugs and the parasympathetic system 90

11   Nerve roots...95
Development of the spinal cord 95
Cellular differentiation 95
Ascent of the cord 96
Neural arches 97
Adult anatomy 97
Distribution of spinal nerves...98
Segmental sensory distribution 99
Segmental motor distribution 99
Nerve root compression syndromes..101
Lumbar puncture...101
Anesthetic procedures 101
Anesthesia and childbirth 103
CLINICAL PANELS
Spina bifida 98
Nerve root compression..102

Contents

12 Spinal cord: ascending pathways 105
  General features 105
     Types of spinal neurons 105
     Spinal ganglia 107
  Ascending sensory pathways 108
     Categories of sensation 108
     Sensory testing 108
  Somatic sensory pathways 109
     Posterior column-medial lemniscal pathway 110
     Spinothalamic pathway 111
     Spinoreticular tracts 113
     Spinocerebellar pathways 114
     Other ascending pathways 115
  CLINICAL PANEL
     Syringomyelia 113

13 Spinal cord: descending pathways 117
  Anatomy of the anterior gray horn 117
     Cell columns 117
     Cell types 117
  Descending motor pathways 119
     Corticospinal tract 119
     Upper and lower motor neurons 122
     Reticulospinal tracts 122
     Tectospinal tract 125
     Vestibulospinal tract 125
     Raphespinal tract 125
     Aminergic pathways 126
     Central autonomic pathways 126
  Blood supply of the spinal cord 128
     Arteries 128
     Veins 128
  CLINICAL PANELS
     Strychnine poisoning 119
     Upper motor neuron disease 124
     Lower motor neuron disease 126
     Spinal cord injury 127

14 Brainstem 131
  Spinomedullary junction 131
  Middle of medulla oblongata 131
  Upper part of medulla oblongata 133
  Pons 135
  Isthmus 136
  Midbrain 136
  Orientation of brainstem 'slices' in MR images 138

15 The last four cranial nerves 141
  General arrangement of the cranial nerves 141
     Cell columns in the Medulla oblongata 142
  Hypoglossal nerve 143
     Motor supply to the hypoglossal nucleus 144
  Spinal accessory nerve 144
  Glossopharyngeal, vagus, and cranial accessory nerves 147

Nucleus solitarius 147
Nucleus ambiguus 148
Glossopharyngeal nerve 148
Vagus and cranial accessory nerves 149
CLINICAL PANELS
Supranuclear lesions of IX, X, and XI cranial nerves 145
Nuclear lesions of X, XI, and XII cranial nerves 145
Infranuclear lesions of the last four cranial nerves........................... 146

16 **Vestibulocochlear nerve** 152
Introduction 152
Vestibular system 152
Static labyrinth: anatomy and actions 153
Kinetic labyrinth: anatomy and actions 154
Auditory system 157
The cochlea 157
Cochlear nerve 159
Central auditory pathways 159
Descending auditory pathways 161
Deafness 162
CLINICAL PANELS
Vestibular disorders 155
Lateral medullary syndrome 157
Two kinds of deafness 161

17 **Trigeminal and facial nerves** 164
Trigeminal nerve 164
Motor nucleus of the V nerve 164
Sensory nuclei of the V nerve 164
Innervation of the teeth 167
Innervation of the cerebral arteries 168
Trigeminothalamic tract 169
Mastication 169
Facial nerve.. 170
Facial nerve proper 170
Nervus intermedius 171
CLINICAL PANELS
Trigeminal neuralgia 165
Referred pain in diseases of the head and neck 167
Lesions of the facial nerve 172
Syndromes of the cerebellopontine angle....................................... 173

18 **Ocular motor nerves** 176
The nerves 176
Oculomotor nerve 177
Trochlear nerve 177
Abducens nerve 178
Nerve endings... 178
Motor endings 178
Sensory endings 178
Pupillary light reflex 178
Accommodation 179
The near response 179
The far response 179

Contents

Notes on the sympathetic pathway to the eye..180
    Occular palsies 182
Control of eye movements 182
    Scanning 182
    Tracking 183
CLINICAL PANEL
    Ocular palsies 180

19 Reticular formation 186
Introduction 186
Organization..186
    Aminergic neurons of the brainstem 187
Functional anatomy 189
    Pattern generators 189
    Bladder control 189
    Respiratory control 190
    Cardiovascular control 191
    Sleeping and wakefulness...191
    Sensory modulation 192

20 Cerebellum 196
Introduction 196
Functional anatomy 196
Microscopic anatomy 197
    Spatial effects of mossy fiber activity..198
Representation of body parts 199
Afferent pathways..199
    Olivocerebellar tract 200
Efferent pathways 200
The cerebellum and higher brain function 201
Clinical disorders of the cerebellum 202
    Posturography 203
CLINICAL PANELS
    Midline lesions: truncal ataxia...201
    Anterior lobe lesions: gait ataxia 202
    Neocerebellar lesions: incoordination of voluntary movement 202

21 Hypothalamus 205
Introduction 205
Gross anatomy 205
    Boundaries...205
    Subdivisions and nuclei 205
Functions 206
    Hypothalamic control of the pituitary gland 206
    Other hypothalamic connections and functions............................210
CLINICAL PANELS
    Hypothalamic disorders..208
    Major depression...209

22 Thalamus, epithalamus...213
Thalamus 213
    Thalamic nuclei 213
    Thalamic peduncles 216
Epithalamus 216
    Pineal gland 217

23 **Visual system** 219
   Introduction 219
   Retina 219
   Structure of the retina 220
   Central visual pathways 222
      Optic nerve, optic tract 222
      Geniculocalcarine tract and primary visual cortex................................224
   CLINICAL PANEL
      Lesions of the visual pathways 224

24 **Cerebral cortex** 228
   Structure 228
      Laminar organization 228
   Cortical areas 231
      Sensory areas 231
      Motor areas 235
      Prefrontal cortex 236
   Hemispheric asymmetries 236
      Handedness and language 236
      Cognitive style 238
      Parietal lobe...239
   CLINICAL PANELS
      Frontal lobe dysfunction 237
      The aphasias 240
      Developmental dyslexia 241
      Schizophrenia 242
      Parietal lobe dysfunction 243

25 **Basal ganglia**...247
   Introduction 247
   Basic circuits 247
      Motor loop 247
      Cognitive loop 252
      Limbic loop 252
      Oculomotor loop..253
   CLINICAL PANELS
      Hypokinesia: Parkinson's disease 251
      Hyperkinesia 252

26 **Olfactory and limbic systems** 256
   Olfactory system..256
      Olfactory epithelium 256
      Olfactory bulb..257
   Limbic system 258
      Parahippocampal gyrus 258
      Hippocampal formation 260
      Insula..262
      Cingulate cortex and posterior parahippocampal gyrus 262
      Septal area 264
      Amygdala 265
      Basal forebrain 266

Contents

CLINICAL PANELS
Olfactory disturbance 258
Temporal lobe seizures 259
Alzheimer's disease 263

27 Cerebrovascular disease 270
Introduction 270
Anterior versus posterior circulation 274
Occlusions within the anterior circulation 275
Transient ischemic attacks 275
Aneurysms 277
CLINICAL PANELS
Anterior cerebral artery occlusion 271
Middle cerebral artery occlusion 272
Internal carotid artery occlusion 275
Posterior cerebral artery occlusion 276
Subarachnoid hemorrhage 277

Glossary 279

Index 284

Answers to self-test questions 294

PREFACE

This, third edition has the same fundamental objective as before: to provide a short account of functional neuroanatomy, in the general context of practical clinical neurology.

The overall design of the second edition received widespread approval, and the structure is retained, with one exception. The blood supply of the brain is now treated in two chapters rather than one: the basic anatomy joins the early, topographic chapters and the clinical applications are described in a new final chapter devoted to cerebrovascular disease.

Notable additions to this edition are:

- an expanded use of color in order to enhance the general appearance and to facilitate interpretation of the illustrations;
- introduction of Study Guidelines at the beginning of each chapter, and a synopsis of Core Information at the end;
- a Self Test set of Multiple Choice questions for each chapter; and
- a Glossary of Neuroanatomical/Neurological terms, including reference to the main chapters where they occur.

I am grateful to colleagues for constructive advice: notably, to my wife, Dr. Maeve FitzGerald for assistance with the Study Guidelines; to Drs Estomih Mtui and Dana Brooks of The New York Hospital-Cornell Medical Center, and Dr A.K. Afifi of the Departments of Anatomy and Pediatrics at the University of Iowa College of Medicine, for general comments arising from the second edition; to Professor Brian Leonard here at UCG, for an update concerning the Clinical Panels related to psychiatry; to Dr J. Paul Finn, Director, MR Research and Development, Siemens Medical Systems, Inc., Iselin, New Jersey for provision of original MR images, and to Drs Michael T. Modic and Cormac O'Donovan of the Cleveland Clinic Foundation, Ohio for provision of angiograms. Diane Keen at the UK headquarters of the ISI at Uxbridge, Kent ensured regular delivery of the invaluable Neuroscience Citation Index CD-ROMs from Philadelphia.

The final four chapters are the most clinically oriented. For his nuanced commentaries on these, I am privileged to acknowledge Dr Hugh Staunton of the Department of Neurology, Baumont Hospital, Dublin.

As always, my colleagues at W.B. Saunders Co. Ltd. London have been thoroughly helpful and supportive during the preparation of the new edition.

Turlough FitzGerald

1

EMBRYOLOGY

Chapter Summary

Spinal cord
Neurulation
Spinal nerves

Brain
Brain vesicles
Ventricular system and choroid
   plexuses
Cranial nerves
Cerebral hemispheres

Study Guidelines

1 This chapter aims to give you sufficient insight into development to be able to account for the arrangement of structures in the mature nervous system. If you are not already familiar with the basic anatomy of the mature nervous system, you should review this chapter after studying Chapters 2 and 3.
2 For descriptive purposes, the human embryo is in the prone (face down) position. The terms *ventral* and *dorsal* correspond to the adult *anterior* and *posterior*. The terms *rostral* and *caudal* correspond to *superior* and *inferior*.

SPINAL CORD

NEURULATION

The entire nervous system originates from the **neural plate,** an ectodermal thickening in the floor of the amniotic sac (*Figure 1.1*). During the third week after fertilization the plate forms paired **neural folds,** which unite to create the **neural tube** and **neural canal.** Union of the folds commences in the future neck region of the embryo and proceeds rostrally and caudally from there. The open ends of the tube, the **neuropores,** are closed off before the end of the fourth week. The process of formation of the neural tube from the ectoderm is known as *neurulation.*

Cells at the edge of each neural fold escape from the line of union and form the **neural crest** alongside the tube. Cell types derived from the neural crest include spinal and autonomic ganglion cells and the Schwann cells of peripheral nerves.

SPINAL NERVES

The dorsal part of the neural tube is called the **alar plate;** the ventral part is the **basal plate** (*Figure 1.2*). Neurons developing in the alar plate are predominantly sensory in function and receive dorsal nerve roots growing in from the spinal ganglia. Neurons in the basal plate are predominantly motor and give rise to ventral nerve roots. At appropriate levels of the spinal cord the ventral roots also contain autonomic fibers. The dorsal and ventral roots unite to form the spinal nerves, which emerge from the vertebral canal in the interval between the neural arches being formed by the mesenchymal vertebrae.

The cells of the spinal (dorsal root) ganglia are initially bipolar. They become unipolar by the coalescence of their two processes at one side of the parent cells.

BRAIN

BRAIN VESICLES

Rostrally, the closed neural tube expands in the form of three brain vesicles: the **prosencephalon** or forebrain, the **mesencephalon** or midbrain, and the **rhombencephalon** or hindbrain (*Figure 1.3A*).

The alar plate of the prosencephalon expands on each side to form the **telencephalon,** or cerebral hemispheres. The basal plate remains in place

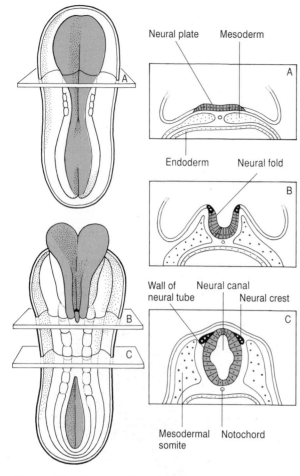

Figure 1.1 Cross-section A is from a 3-somite (20-day) embryo. Cross-sections B and C are from an 8-somite (22-day) embryo.

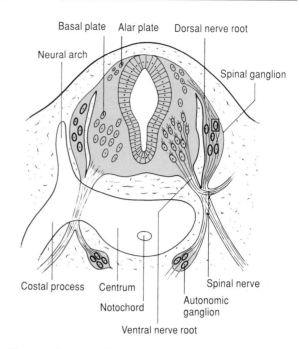

Figure 1.2 Neural tube, spinal nerve, and mesenchymal vertebra of an embryo at 6 weeks.

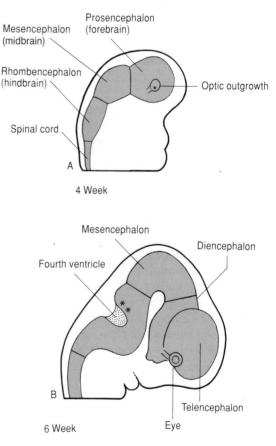

Figure 1.3 Brain vesicles, seen from the right side. Asterisks indicate the site of initial development of the cerebellum.

here, as the **diencephalon.** Finally, an **optic outgrowth** from the diencephalon is the forerunner of the retina and optic nerve.

The diencephalon, mesencephalon and rhombencephalon constitute the embryonic brainstem.

The brainstem buckles as development proceeds. As a result, the mesencephalon is carried to the summit of the brain. The rhombencephalon folds upon itself, causing the alar plates to flare and creating the rhomboid (diamond-shaped) fourth ventricle of the brain. The rostral part of the rhombencephalon gives rise to the pons and cerebellum. The caudal part gives rise to the medulla oblongata (*Table 1.1*).

VENTRICULAR SYSTEM AND CHOROID PLEXUSES

The neural canal dilates within the cerebral hemi-

Table 1.1 Some derivatives of the brain vesicles

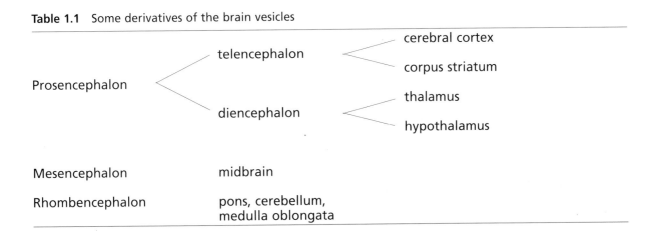

Prosencephalon	telencephalon	cerebral cortex
		corpus striatum
	diencephalon	thalamus
		hypothalamus
Mesencephalon	midbrain	
Rhombencephalon	pons, cerebellum, medulla oblongata	

spheres, forming the lateral ventricles; these communicate with the third ventricle contained within the diencephalon. The third and fourth ventricles communicate through the aqueduct of the midbrain (*Figure 1.4*).

The thin roofs of the forebrain and hindbrain are invaginated by tufts of capillaries which form the choroid plexuses of the four ventricles. The

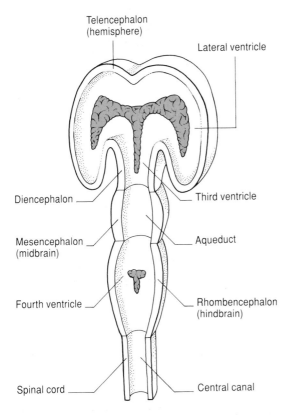

Figure 1.4 Diagram of the developing ventricular system. Choroid plexuses are shown in red.

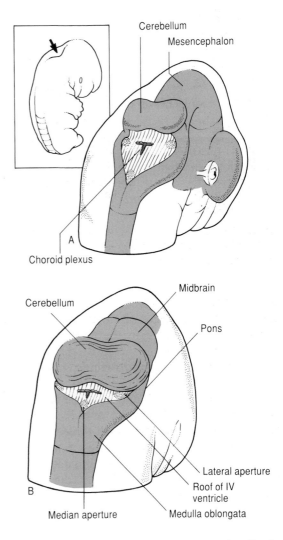

Figure 1.5 Dorsal views of the developing hindbrain (see arrow in inset). **(A)** At 6 weeks, the cerebellum is emerging through the roof of the fourth ventricle. **(B)** At 10 weeks, the ventricle is being covered over by the cerebellum.

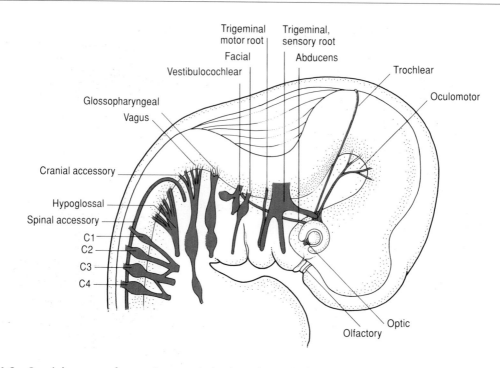

Figure 1.6 Cranial nerves of an embryo early in the 6th week. (Adapted from Bossy *et al.*, 1990.)

choroid plexuses secrete cerebrospinal fluid which flows through the ventricular system. The fluid leaves the fourth ventricle through three apertures in its roof (*Figure 1.5*).

CRANIAL NERVES

Figure 1.6 illustrates the state of development of the cranial nerves during the sixth week after fertilization.

- The olfactory nerve (I) forms from bipolar neurons developing in the epithelium lining the olfactory pit.
- The optic nerve (II) is growing centrally from the retina.
- The oculomotor (III) and trochlear (IV) nerves arise from the midbrain, and the abducens (VI) arises from the pons; all three will supply extrinsic muscles of the eye.
- The three divisions of the trigeminal (V) nerve will be sensory to the skin of the face and scalp, to the mucous membranes of the oronasal cavity, and to the teeth. A motor root will supply the muscles of mastication (chewing).
- The facial (VII) nerve will supply the muscles of facial expression. The vestibulocochlear (VIII) nerve will supply the organs of hearing and balance, which develop from the otocyst.

- The glossopharyngeal (IX) nerve is composite. Most of its fibers will be sensory to the oropharynx. The vagus (X) nerve is also composite; it contains a large sensory element for the supply of the mucous membranes of the digestive system, and a large motor (parasympathetic) element for the supply of the heart and gastrointestinal tract.
- The cranial accessory (XIc) nerve will be distributed by the vagus to the muscles of the larynx and pharynx.
- The spinal accessory (XIs) nerve will supply the sternomastoid and trapezius muscles. The hypoglossal (XII) nerve will supply the muscles of the tongue.

CEREBRAL HEMISPHERES

In the telencephalon, mitotic activity takes place in the **ventricular zone,** just outside the lateral ventricle. Daughter cells migrate to the outer surface of the expanding hemisphere and form the cerebral cortex.

Expansion of the cerebral hemispheres is not uniform. A region on the lateral surface, the insula, is relatively quiescent and forms a pivot around which the expanding hemisphere rotates. Frontal, parietal, occipital and temporal lobes can be identified at 14 weeks' gestational age (*Figure 1.7*).

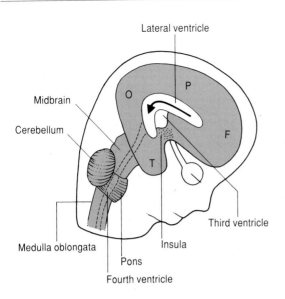

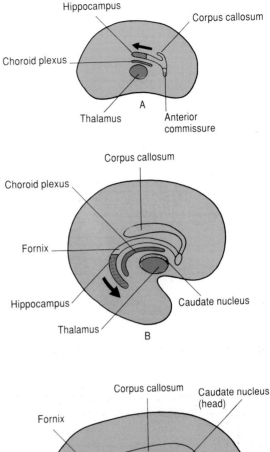

Figure 1.7 Fetal brain at 14 weeks. The arrow indicates the C-shaped growth of the hemisphere around the insula. F, P, O, T, frontal, parietal, occipital, temporal lobes.

On the medial surface of the hemisphere, a patch of cerebral cortex, the hippocampus, belongs to a fifth, limbic lobe of the brain. The hippocampus is drawn into the temporal lobe, leaving in its wake a strand of fibers called the fornix. Within the concavity of this arc is the choroid fissure, through which the choroid plexus invaginates into the lateral ventricle (*Figure 1.8*).

The anterior commissure develops as a connection linking olfactory (smell) regions of the left and right sides. Above this, a much larger commissure, the corpus callosum links matching areas of the cerebral cortex of the two sides. It extends backward above the fornix.

Coronal sections of the telencephalon reveal a mass of gray matter in the base of each hemisphere which is the forerunner of the corpus striatum. Beside the third ventricle the diencephalon gives rise to the thalamus and hypothalamus (*Figure 1.9*).

The expanding cerebral hemispheres come into contact with the diencephalon and they fuse with it (see 'site of fusion' in Figure 1.9A). One consequence is that the term 'brainstem' is restricted thereafter to the remaining, free parts: midbrain, pons, and medulla oblongata. A second consequence is that the cerebral cortex is able to project fibers direct to the brainstem. Together with fibers projecting from thalamus to cortex, they

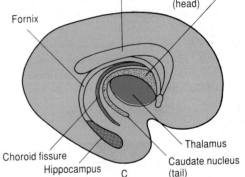

Figure 1.8 Medial aspect of developing left hemisphere. The hippocampus, initially dorsal to the thalamus, migrates into the temporal lobe (arrows in **A** and **B**), leaving the fornix in its wake. The concavity of the arch so formed contains the choroid fissure (the line of insertion of the choroid plexus into the lateral ventricle) and the tail of the caudate nucleus.

split the corpus striatum into caudate and lentiform nuclei (*Figure 1.9B*).

By the 28th week of development, several sulci (fissures) have appeared on the surface of the brain, notably the lateral, central, and calcarine sulci (*Figure 1.10*).

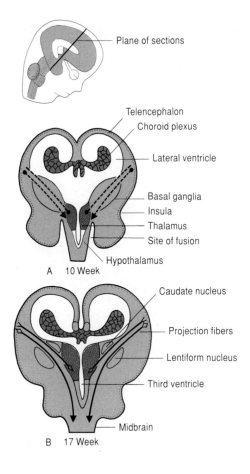

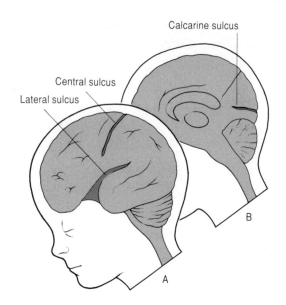

Figure 1.10 Three major cortical sulci in a fetus of 28 weeks. **(A)** Lateral surface of hemisphere; **(B)** medial surface of hemisphere.

Figure 1.9 Coronal sections of the developing cerebrum. The corpus striatum is cleft by fibers projecting to and from the cerebral cortex. See text for other details.

CORE INFORMATION

The nervous system takes the initial form of a cellular neural tube derived from the ectoderm and enclosing a neural canal. A ribbon of cells escapes along each side of the tube to form the neural crest. The more caudal part of the tube forms the spinal cord. The neural crest forms spinal ganglion cells that send dorsal nerve roots into the sensory, alar plate of the cord. The basal plate of the cord contains motor neurons that emit ventral roots to complete the spinal nerves by joining the dorsal roots.

The more rostral part of the tube forms three brain vesicles. Of these, the prosencephalon (forebrain) gives rise to the cerebral hemispheres (telencephalon) dorsally and the diencephalon ventrally; the mesencephalon becomes the midbrain; and the rhombencephalon

becomes the hindbrain (pons, medulla oblongata, cerebellum).

The neural tube expands rostrally to create the ventricular system of the brain. Cerebrospinal fluid is secreted by a choroid capillary plexuses that invaginate the roof plates of the ventricles.

The cerebral hemispheres develop frontal, parietal, temporal, occipital and limbic lobes. The hemispheres are cross-linked by the corpus callosum and anterior commissure. Gray matter in the base of each hemisphere is the forerunner of the corpus striatum. The hemispheres fuse with the side walls of the diencephalon, whereupon the mesencephalon and rhombencephalon are all that remain of the embryonic brainstem.

SELF TEST

Select the best response:

1 Which of the following cell types are derived from neural crest epithelium:

A Schwann cells
B Spinal ganglion cells
C Autonomic ganglion cells
D All of the above
E A and B only

2 Spinal ganglion cells:

A Are multipolar
B Are mesodermal in origin
C Are motor in function
D Form posterior nerve roots
E Project into the basal plate

3 Which of the following is/are derived from the rhombencephalon:

A Medulla oblongata
B Pons
C Cerebellum
D All of the above
E A and B only

4 The mesencephalon is the embryonic:

A Forebrain
B Midbrain
C Hindbrain
D Cerebellum
E None of the above

5 Develop(s) from the embryonic telencephalon:

A Cerebral hemispheres
B Prosencephalon
C Diencephalon
D All of the above
E A and B only

6 The caudate and lentiform nuclei belong to the:

A Corpus thalami
B Corpus callosum
C Corpus striatum
D Corpus pontis
E None of the above

7 Which of the following cranial nerves is attached to the midbrain?:

A Olfactory
B Optic
C Trigeminal
D Abducens
E None of the above

8 The only cranial nerve to emerge from the dorsal aspect of the brainstem is the:

A Oculomotor
B Trochlear
C Abducens
D Trigeminal
E Vagus

9 The sensory nerve to the orofacial epithelia is the:

A Trigeminal
B Facial
C Glossopharyngeal
D Vagus
E Accessory

REFERENCES

Bossy, J., O'Rahilly, R. and Müller, F. (1990) Ontogenese du systeme nerveux. In *Anatomie Clinique: Neuroanatomie* (Bossy, J., ed.), pp. 357–388. Paris: Springer-Verlag.

Cabana, T. (1993) Development of the nervous system. In *Neuroscience for Rehabilitation* (Cohen, M., ed.), pp. 357–387. Philadelphia: Lippincott.

FitzGerald, M.J.T. and FitzGerald, M. (1994) *Human Embryology*. London: Ballière Tindall.

Larsen, W.J. (1993) *Human Embryology*. New York: Churchill Livingstone.

O'Rahilly, R. and Gardner, E. (1979) *The initial development of the human brain*. Acta Anat. **104:** 123–133.

O'Rahilly, R. and Müller, F. (1987) The developmental anatomy and histology of the human central nervous system. In *Handbook of Clinical Neurology,* Vol. 6, Malformations (Myrianthopoulos, N.C., ed.), pp. 1–17. Amsterdam: Elsevier.

Sadler, T.W. (1990) *Langman's Medical Embryology,* 6th edn. Baltimore: Williams & Wilkins.

2

CEREBRAL TOPOGRAPHY

Chapter Summary

Surface features
Lobes
Diencephalon

Internal anatomy of the cerebrum
Thalamus, caudate and lentiform nuclei, internal capsule
Hippocampus and fornix
Association and commissural fibers
Lateral and third ventricles

Study Guidelines

1 Become familiar enough with the 6 macrophotographs to be able to sing out the names of structures at the tips of the pointers without looking at the labels. Then see how well you do with the MR images.
2 Try to get the nomenclature of the basal ganglia into long-term memory.
3 Be quite clear about the position of the internal capsule and its named parts.
4 Appreciate the continuity of corona radiata, internal capsule, crus cerebri.

SURFACE FEATURES

LOBES

The surfaces of the two cerebral hemispheres are furrowed by **sulci,** the intervening ridges being called **gyri.** Most of the cerebral cortex is concealed from view in the walls of the sulci. Although the patterns of the various sulci vary from brain to brain, some are sufficiently constant to serve as descriptive landmarks.

The deepest sulci are the **lateral sulcus** (*Sylvian fissure*) and the **central sulcus** (*Rolandic fissure*) (*Figure 2.1A*). These two serve to divide the hemisphere into four **lobes,** with the aid of two imaginary lines: one line extends back from the lateral sulcus; the other reaches from the upper end of the **parieto-occipital sulcus** (*Figure 2.1B*) to a blunt **pre-occipital notch** at the lower border of the hemisphere. The lobes are called **frontal, parietal, occipital** and **temporal.**

The blunt tips of the frontal, occipital and temporal lobes are the respective **poles** of the brain.

The lips (**opercula**) of the lateral sulcus can be pulled apart to expose the **insula** (*Figure 2.2*). The insula was mentioned in Chapter 1 as being

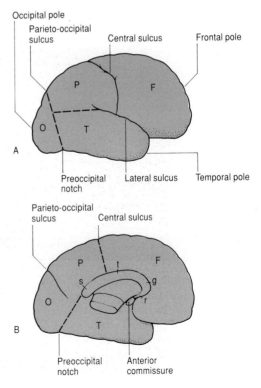

Figure 2.1 Boundaries of the frontal (F), parietal (L), occipital (O), and temporal (T) lobes. s, Splenium; t, trunk; g, genu; r, rostrum of corpus callosum.

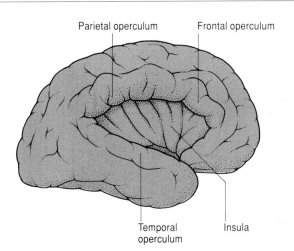

Figure 2.2 Insula, seen upon retraction of the opercula.

relatively quiescent during prenatal expansion of the telencephalon.

The medial surface of the hemisphere is exposed by cutting the **corpus callosum,** a massive band of white matter connecting matching areas of the cortex of the two hemispheres. The corpus callosum consists of a main part or **trunk,** a posterior end or **splenium,** an anterior end or **genu** ('knee'), and a narrow **rostrum** reaching from the genu to the **anterior commissure** (*Figure 2.1B*). The frontal lobe lies anterior to a line drawn from the upper end of the central sulcus to the trunk of the corpus callosum (*Figure 2.1B*). The parietal lobe lies behind this line, and it is separated from the occipital lobe by the parieto-occipital sulcus. The temporal lobe lies in front of a line drawn from the preoccipital notch to the splenium.

Figures 2.3 to *2.6* should be consulted along with the following description of surface features of the lobes of the brain.

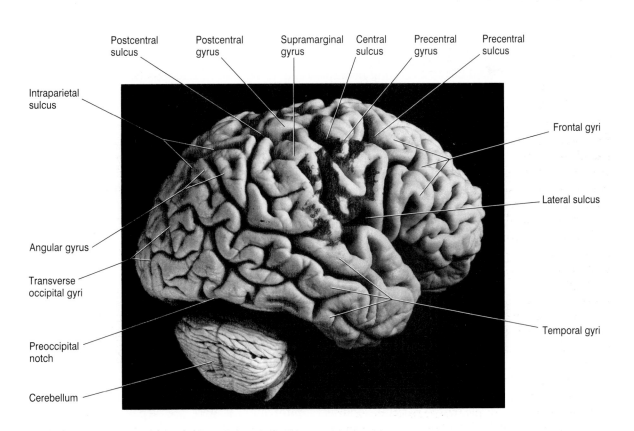

Figure 2.3 Lateral view of right cerebral hemisphere. (Photograph reproduced from Gluhbegovic and Williams (1980) with kind permission of the authors and of J.B. Lippincott, Inc.)

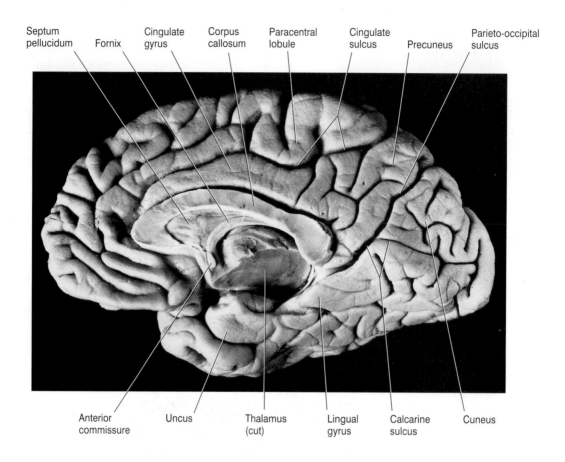

Septum pellucidum | Fornix | Cingulate gyrus | Corpus callosum | Paracentral lobule | Cingulate sulcus | Precuneus | Parieto-occipital sulcus

Anterior commissure | Uncus | Thalamus (cut) | Lingual gyrus | Calcarine sulcus | Cuneus

Figure 2.4 Medial view of right cerebral hemisphere. (Photograph reproduced from Gluhbegovic and Williams (1980) with kind permission of the authors and of J.B. Lippincott, Inc.)

Frontal lobe

The lateral surface of the **frontal lobe** contains the **precentral gyrus** bounded in front by the **precentral sulcus**. Further forward, **superior, middle** and **inferior frontal gyri** are separated by **superior** and **inferior frontal sulci**. On the medial surface, the superior frontal gyrus is separated from the **cingulate gyrus** by the **cingulate sulcus**. The inferior or orbital surface is marked by several **orbital gyri**. In contact with this surface are the **olfactory bulb** and **olfactory tract**.

Parietal lobe

The anterior part of the parietal lobe contains the **postcentral gyrus** bounded behind by the **postcentral sulcus**. The posterior parietal lobe is divided into **superior** and **inferior parietal lobules** by an **intra-parietal sulcus**. The inferior parietal lobule shows a **supramarginal gyrus**, capping the

upturned end of the lateral sulcus, and an **angular gyrus** capping the superior temporal sulcus. The medial surface contains the posterior part of the **paracentral lobule** and, behind this, the **precuneus**. The paracentral lobule (partly contained in the frontal lobe) is so called because of its relationship to the central sulcus.

Occipital lobe

The lateral surface of the occipital lobe is marked by several **lateral occipital gyri**. The medial surface contains the **cuneus** ('wedge') between the parieto-occipital sulcus and the important **calcarine sulcus**. The inferior surface shows three gyri and three sulci. The **lateral** and **medial occipitotemporal gyri** are separated by the **occipitotemporal sulcus**. The **lingual gyrus** lies between the collateral sulcus and the anterior end of the calcarine sulcus.

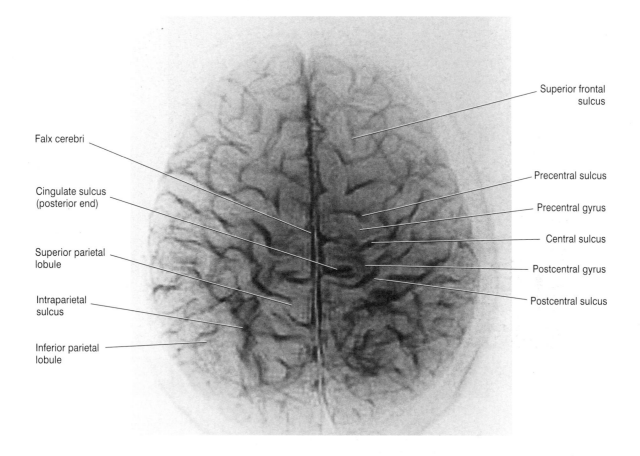

Falx cerebri

Cingulate sulcus
(posterior end)

Superior parietal
lobule

Intraparietal
sulcus

Inferior parietal
lobule

Superior frontal
sulcus

Precentral sulcus

Precentral gyrus

Central sulcus

Postcentral gyrus

Postcentral sulcus

Figure 2.5 'Thick slice' surface anatomy brain MR scan from a healthy volunteer. (Reproduced from Neuroradiology (1990) 32: 439—448 with kind permission of Professor K. Katada and of the Publishers.)

Temporal lobe

The lateral surface of the temporal lobe displays **superior, middle,** and **inferior temporal gyri** separated by **superior** and **inferior temporal sulci.** The inferior surface shows the anterior parts of the occipitotemporal gyri. The lingual gyrus continues forward as the **parahippocampal gyrus** which ends in a blunt medial projection, the **uncus.** As will be seen later in views of the sectioned brain, the parahippocampal gyrus underlies a rolled-in part of the cortex, the **hippocampus.**

Limbic lobe

A fifth, **limbic lobe** of the brain surrounds the medial margin of the hemisphere. Surface contributors to the limbic lobe include the cingulate and parahippocampal gyri. It is more usual to speak of the *limbic system,* which includes the hippocampus, fornix, amygdala and other elements (Chapter 26).

DIENCEPHALON

The largest components of the diencephalon are

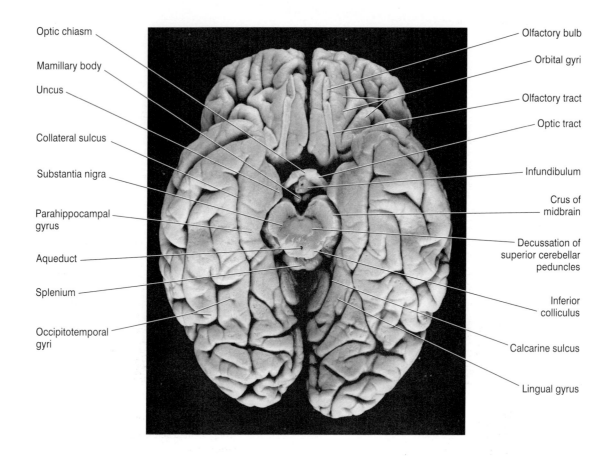

Figure 2.6 Cerebrum, viewed from below. (Photograph reproduced from Gluhbegovic and Williams (1980) with kind permission of the authors and of J.B. Lippincott, Inc.)

the **thalamus** and the **hypothalamus** (*Figure 2.7*) These nuclear groups form the side walls of the third ventricle. Between them is a shallow **hypothalamic sulcus,** which represents the rostral limit of the embryonic sulcus limitans. The hypothalamus forms the floor of the third ventricle as well.

The MRI picture in *Figure 2.8* should be examined in conjunction with *Figures 2.4* and *2.7*.

INTERNAL ANATOMY OF THE CEREBRUM

The arrangement of the following structures will now be described: thalamus, caudate and lentiform nuclei, internal capsule; hippocampus and fornix; association and commissural fibers; lateral and third ventricles.

THALAMUS, CAUDATE AND LENTIFORM NUCLEI, INTERNAL CAPSULE

The two thalami face one another across the slot-like third ventricle. More often than not, they kiss, creating an **interthalamic adhesion** (*Figure 2.9*). In *Figure 2.10* the thalamus, caudate nucleus, internal capsule, lentiform nucleus and internal capsule are assembled piecemeal. In contact with the upper surface of the thalamus are the **head** and **body** of the **caudate nucleus**. The **tail** of the caudate nucleus passes forward below the thalamus, but not in contact with it.

The thalamus is separated from the lentiform

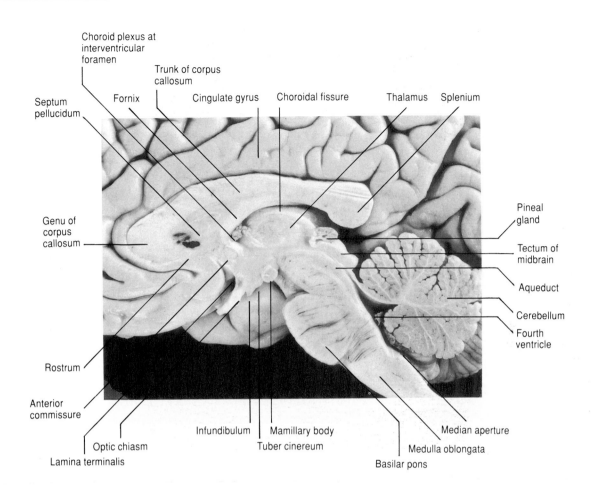

Choroid plexus at interventricular foramen

Trunk of corpus callosum

Septum pellucidum

Fornix

Cingulate gyrus

Choroidal fissure

Thalamus

Splenium

Genu of corpus callosum

Pineal gland

Tectum of midbrain

Aqueduct

Cerebellum

Fourth ventricle

Rostrum

Anterior commissure

Optic chiasm

Lamina terminalis

Infundibulum

Tuber cinereum

Mamillary body

Median aperture

Medulla oblongata

Basilar pons

Figure 2.7 Median sagittal section of fixed brain. Note that in the living state, the orientation of the brainstem is more vertical (cf. Figure 2.8). (Photograph reproduced from Gluhbegovic and Williams (1980) by kind permission of the authors and of J.B. Lippincott, Inc.)

nucleus by the **internal capsule,** which is a common site for a *stroke* resulting from local arterial hemorrhage. The internal capsule contains fibers running from thalamus to cortex and from cortex to thalamus, brainstem and spinal cord. In the interval between cortex and internal capsule, these ascending and descending fibers form the **corona radiata.** Below the internal capsule, the **crus** of the midbrain receives descending fibers continuing into the brainstem.

The lens-shaped **lentiform nucleus** is composed of two parts, **putamen** and **globus pallidus.** The putamen and caudate nucleus are of similar structure and their anterior ends are fused. Behind this they are linked by strands of gray matter which traverse the internal capsule: hence the term **corpus striatum** (or, simply, **striatum**) used to include the putamen and caudate nuc-

leus. The term **pallidum** refers to the globus pallidus.

The caudate and lentiform nuclei belong to the **basal ganglia,** a term originally applied to a half-dozen masses of gray matter located near the base of the hemisphere. In current usage the term designates four nuclei known to be involved in motor control: the caudate and lentiform nuclei, the subthalamic nucleus in the diencephalon, and the substantia nigra in the midbrain (*Table 2.1*).

In horizontal section, the internal capsule has a dog-leg shape (see photograph of a fixed-brain section in *Figure 2.11,* and living-brain MR 'slice' in *Figure 2.12*). The internal capsule has four named parts in horizontal sections:

1 the **anterior limb,** between the lentiform nucleus and the head of the caudate nucleus;

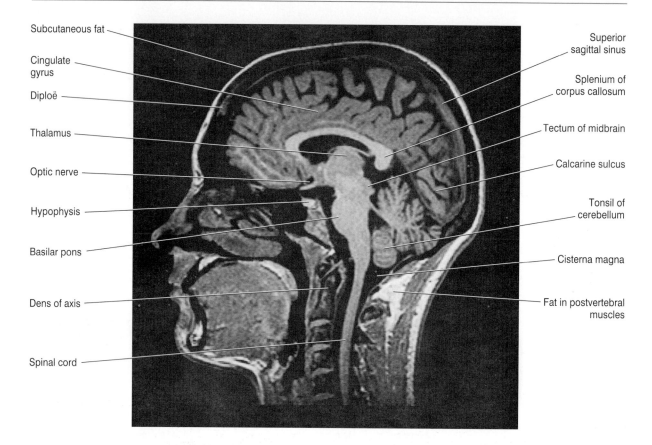

Subcutaneous fat

Cingulate gyrus

Diploë

Thalamus

Optic nerve

Hypophysis

Basilar pons

Dens of axis

Spinal cord

Superior sagittal sinus

Splenium of corpus callosum

Tectum of midbrain

Calcarine sulcus

Tonsil of cerebellum

Cisterna magna

Fat in postvertebral muscles

Figure 2.8 Sagittal MRI 'slice' of the living brain. (From a series kindly provided by Dr. J. Paul Finn, Director, MR Research and Development, Siemens Medical Systems Inc., Iselin, New Jersey) (*Note:* Lipid-rich tissues are especially enhanced, e.g. CNS myelin, subcutaneous fat, lipid in muscle and bone marrow.)

2 the **genu;**
3 the **posterior limb,** between the lentiform nucleus and the thalamus;
4 the **retrolentiform part,** behind the lentiform nucleus and lateral to the thalamus.

The **corticospinal tract** descends in the posterior limb of the internal capsule. It is also called the **pyramidal tract,** a *tract* being a bundle of fibers

serving a common function. The corticospinal tract originates mainly from the *motor cortex* within the precentral gyrus. It descends through the corona radiata, internal capsule, and crus of midbrain and continues to the lower end of the brainstem before crossing to the opposite side of the spinal cord.

From a clinical standpoint, *the corticospinal tract is the most important pathway in the entire*

Table 2.1 Nomenclature of basal ganglia*

Caudate nucleus ———————————————————————————

                                      Corpus striatum

                      Putamen

Lentiform nucleus

                      Globus pallidus

Subthalamic nucleus

Substantia nigra
                Striatum = caudate + putamen
                Pallidum = globus pallidus

*For further details, see Chapter 25

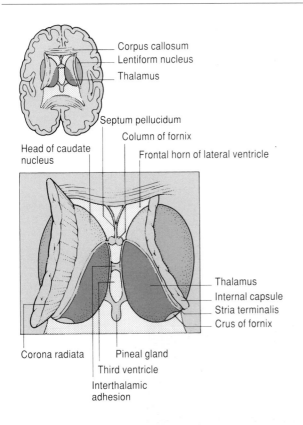

Figure 2.9 Thalamus and corpus striatum, seen upon removal of the trunk of the corpus callosum and the body of the fornix.

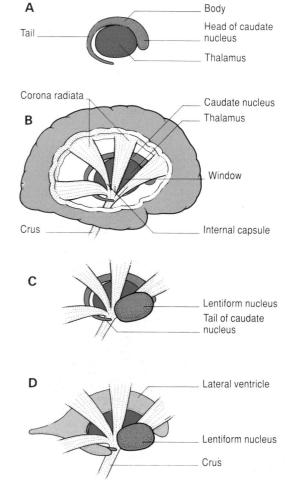

Figure 2.10 Diagrammatic reconstruction of corpus striatum and related structures (right side, lateral view). **(A)** Caudate nucleus and thalamus. **(B)** Addition of projections from cerebral cortex to brainstem. Three windows have been made in the corona radiata. **(C)** Addition of lentiform nucleus. **(D)** Addition of lateral ventricle.

CNS, for two reasons. First, it mediates voluntary movements of all kinds, and interruption of the tract by disease leads to motor weakness (called *paresis*) or motor paralysis. Secondly, it extends the entire vertical length of the CNS, rendering it vulnerable to disease or trauma in the cerebral hemisphere or brainstem on one side, and to spinal cord disease or trauma on the other side.

A coronal section through the anterior limb is represented in *Figure 2.13*; a corresponding MR image is shown in *Figure 2.14*. A coronal section through the posterior limb from a fixed brain is shown in *Figure 2.15*; a corresponding MR 'slice' is shown in *Figure 2.16*.

Lateral to the lentiform nucleus are the **external capsule, claustrum,** and **extreme capsule.**

HIPPOCAMPUS AND FORNIX

The **hippocampus** is first seen in embryonic life above the corpus callosum (Chapter 1). The bulk of it remains in that position in lower mammals, including rodents. In primates it retreats into the temporal lobe as this develops, leaving a tract of white matter, the **fornix,** in its wake. The mature hippocampus stretches the full length of the floor of the inferior (temporal) horn of the lateral ventricle (*Figure 2.17*). The mature fornix comprises a **body,** beneath the trunk of the corpus callosum, a **crus** which enters it from each hippocampus, and two **pillars** (**columns**) which leave it to enter the diencephalon. Intimately related to the crus and body is the **choroid fissure,** through which the choroid plexus is inserted into the lateral ventricle.

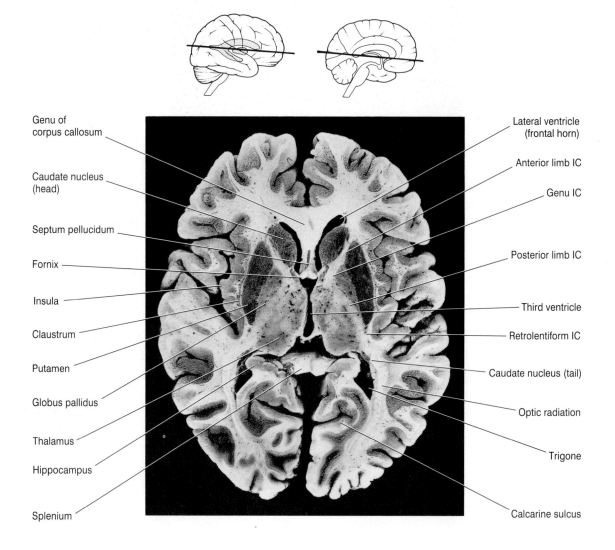

Genu of
corpus callosum

Caudate nucleus
(head)

Septum pellucidum

Fornix

Insula

Claustrum

Putamen

Globus pallidus

Thalamus

Hippocampus

Splenium

Lateral ventricle
(frontal horn)

Anterior limb IC

Genu IC

Posterior limb IC

Third ventricle

Retrolentiform IC

Caudate nucleus (tail)

Optic radiation

Trigone

Calcarine sulcus

Figure 2.11 Horizontal section of fixed brain in the plane indicated at top. IC, internal capsule. (Photograph reproduced from Gluhbecovic and Williams (1980) with kind permission of the authors and of J.B. Lippincott, Inc.)

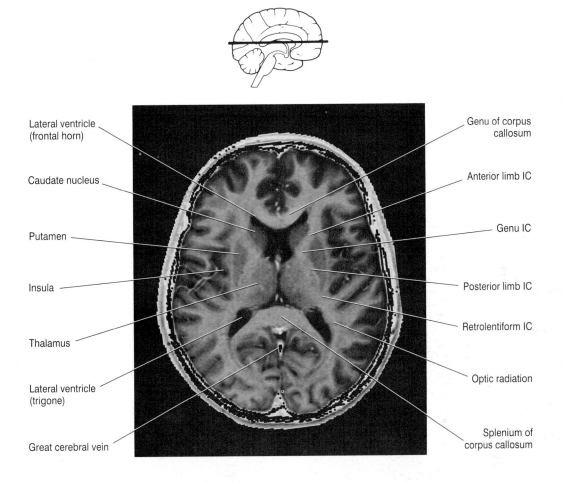

Figure 2.12 Horizontal MRI 'slice' at the level indicated at top. IC, internal capsule. (From a series kindly provided by Dr. J. Paul Finn, Director, MR Research and Development, Siemens Medical Systems Inc., Iselin, New Jersey.)
Note: Horizontal 'slices' are viewed from below.

ASSOCIATION AND COMMISSURAL FIBERS

Fibers leaving the cerebral cortex fall into three groups:

- **association fibers,** which pass from one part of a single hemisphere to another;
- **commissural fibers,** which link matching areas of the two hemispheres;
- **projection fibers,** which run to subcortical nuclei in the cerebral hemisphere, brainstem, and spinal cord.

Association fibers

Short association fibers pass from one gyrus to another within a lobe (Figure 2.18). **Long association fibers** link one lobe with another. Bundles of long association fibers include:

- the **superior longitudinal fasciculus,** linking the frontal and occipital lobes;
- the **inferior longitudinal fasciculus,** linking the occipital and temporal lobes;

- the **arcuate fasciculus,** linking the frontal lobe with the occipitotemporal cortex;
- the **uncinate fasciculus,** linking the frontal and anterior temporal lobes; and
- the **cingulum,** underlying the cortex of the cingulate gyrus.

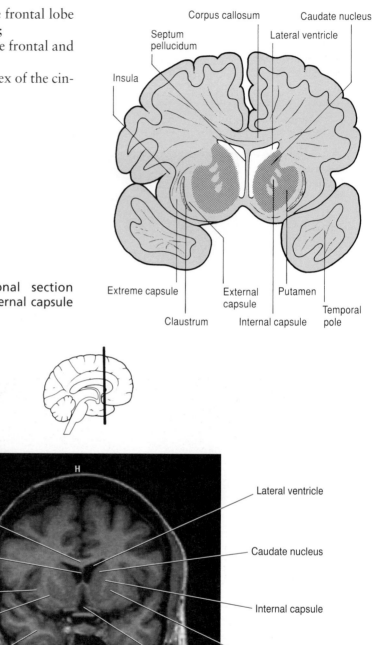

Figure 2.13 Drawing of a coronal section through the anterior limb of the internal capsule (cf. Figure 2.14).

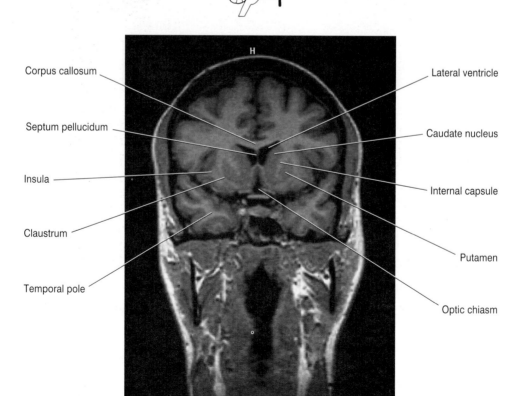

Figure 2.14 Coronal MRI 'slice' at the level indicated at top. (Courtesy of Dr. J. Paul Finn, Director, MR Research and Development, Siemens Medical Systems Inc., Iselin, New Jersey) *Note:* Coronal 'slices' are viewed from the front.

Cerebral commissures

Corpus Callosum

The **corpus callosum** is much the largest of the commissures linking matching areas of the left and right cerebral cortex (*Figure 2.19*). From the **trunk (body)**, some fibers pass laterally and upward, intersecting the corona radiata. Other fibers pass laterally and then bend downward as the **tapetum** to reach the lower parts of the temporal and occipital lobes. Fibers traveling to the medial wall of the occipital lobe emerge from the splenium on each side and form the **occipital (major) forceps**. The **frontal (minor) forceps** emerges from each side of the genu to reach the medial wall of the frontal lobe.

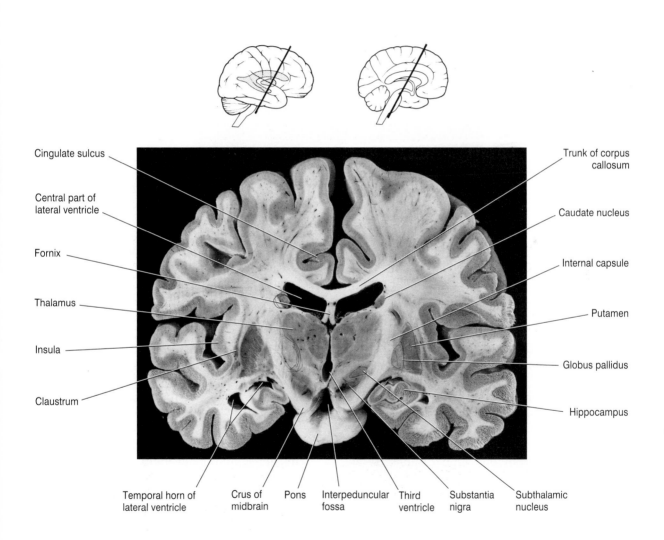

Figure 2.15 Coronal section of fixed brain at the level indicated at top. (Photograph reproduced from Gluhbegovic and Williams (1980) with kind permission of the authors and of J.B. Lippincott, Inc.)

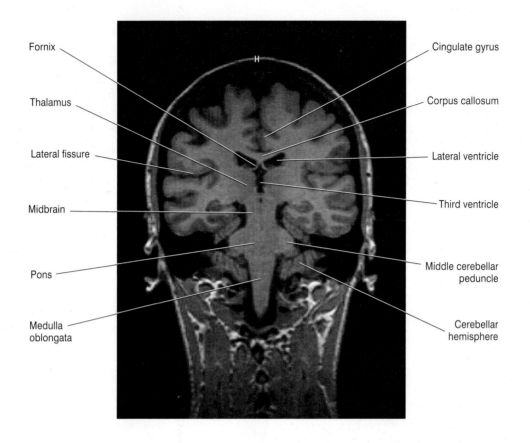

Fornix

Thalamus

Lateral fissure

Midbrain

Pons

Medulla
oblongata

Cingulate gyrus

Corpus callosum

Lateral ventricle

Third ventricle

Middle cerebellar
peduncle

Cerebellar
hemisphere

Figure 2.16 Coronal MRI 'slice' at the level indicated at top. (From a series kindly provided by Dr. J. Paul Finn, Director, MR Research and Development, Siemens Medical Systems Inc., Iselin, New Jersey.)

Minor Commissures

The **anterior commissure** interconnects the anterior parts of the temporal lobes, as well as the two olfactory tracts (*Figure 2.20*).

The **posterior commissure** and the **habenular commissure** lie directly in front of the pineal gland.

The **commissure of the fornix** contains some fibers traveling from one hippocampus to the other by way of the two crura.

LATERAL AND THIRD VENTRICLES

The **lateral ventricle** consists of a **central part** (**body**) within the parietal lobe, and **frontal (anterior)**, **occipital (posterior)** and **temporal (inferior)** horns (*Figure 2.21*). The anterior limit of the central part is the **interventricular foramen**, located between thalamus and anterior pillar of the fornix, through which it communicates with the third ventricle (*Figure 2.20*). The central part joins the occipital and temporal horns at the **trigone** (*Figure 2.22*).

The relationships of the lateral ventricle are listed below.

Frontal horn: lies between head of caudate nucleus and septum pellucidum. Its other boundaries are formed by the corpus callosum: trunk above, genu in front, rostrum below.

Central part: lies below the trunk of the corpus callosum and above the thalamus and anterior part of the body of the fornix. Medially is the septum pellucidum, which tapers away posteriorly where the fornix rises to meet the corpus callosum. The **septum pellucidum** is formed of the thinned out walls of the two cerebral hemispheres. Its bilateral origin may be indicated by a central cavity (**cavum**).

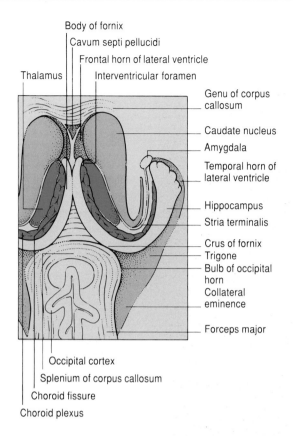

Body of fornix
Cavum septi pellucidi
Frontal horn of lateral ventricle
Thalamus
Interventricular foramen
Genu of corpus callosum
Caudate nucleus
Amygdala
Temporal horn of lateral ventricle
Hippocampus
Stria terminalis
Crus of fornix
Trigone
Bulb of occipital horn
Collateral eminence
Forceps major
Occipital cortex
Splenium of corpus callosum
Choroid fissure
Choroid plexus

Figure 2.17 Continuity of structures in central part and temporal horn of lateral ventricle. Note: Amygdala, stria terminalis, and tail of caudate nucleus occupy the roof of the temporal horn.

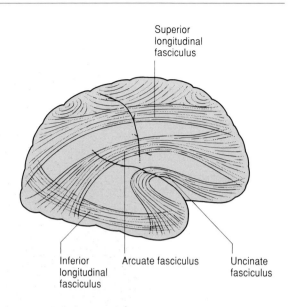

Superior longitudinal fasciculus
Inferior longitudinal fasciculus
Arcuate fasciculus
Uncinate fasciculus

Figure 2.18 Lateral view of right cerebral hemisphere showing position of long association fiber bundles.

Occipital horn: lies below the splenium and medial to the tapetum of the corpus callosum. On the medial side, the forceps major forms the **bulb** of the posterior horn (*Figure 2.17*).

Temporal horn: lies below the tail of the caudate nucleus and, at the anterior end, the **amygdala** (*Figure 2.17*), a nucleus belonging to the limbic system. The hippocampus and its associated structures occupy the full length of the floor. Outside these is the **collateral eminence**, created by the collateral sulcus.

The **third ventricle** is the cavity of the diencephalon. Its boundaries are shown in *Figure 2.20*. A **choroid plexus** hangs from its roof, which is formed of a double layer of pia mater called the **tela choroidea**. Above this are the fornix and corpus callosum. In each side wall are the thalamus and hypothalamus. The anterior wall is formed by the anterior commissure, the **lamina terminalis**, and the **optic chiasm**. In the floor are the **infundibulum**, the **tuber cinereum**,

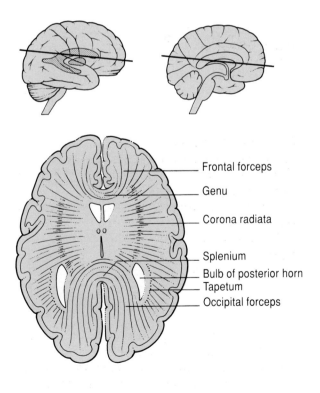

Frontal forceps
Genu
Corona radiata
Splenium
Bulb of posterior horn
Tapetum
Occipital forceps

Figure 2.19 Horizontal section through genu and splenium of corpus callosum. Fibers passing laterally from the trunk intersect the corona radiata.

21

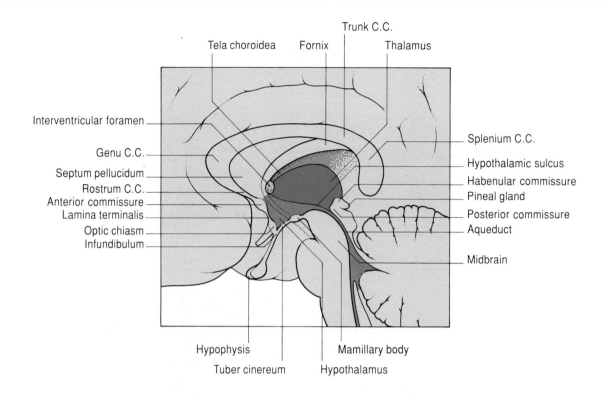

Figure 2.20 Sagittal section of diencephalon and surroundings. C.C., corpus callosum.

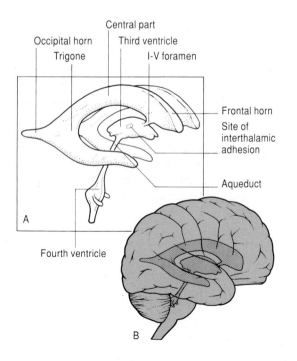

Figure 2.21 Ventricular system. **(A)** isolated cast; **(B)** ventricular system in situ.

the **mamillary bodies** (also spelt 'mammillary'), and the upper end of the midbrain. The **pineal gland** and related commissures form the posterior wall. The pineal is often calcified, and the **habenular commissure** is sometimes calcified, as early as the second decade of life, thereby becoming detectable even on plain radiographs of the skull. The pineal is sometimes displaced to one side by a tumor, hematoma or other space-occupying lesion within the cranial cavity.

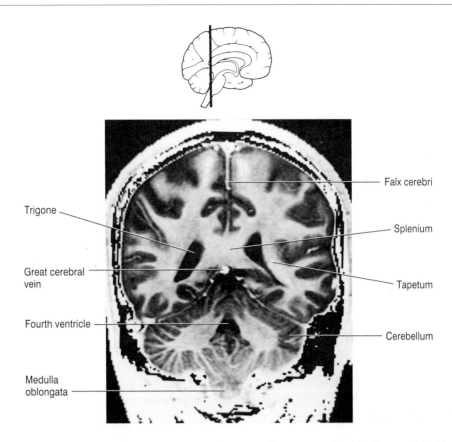

Trigone

Great cerebral vein

Fourth ventricle

Medulla oblongata

Falx cerebri

Splenium

Tapetum

Cerebellum

Figure 2.22 Coronal MRI 'slice' at the level indicated at top. (From a series kindly provided by Dr. J. Paul Finn, Director, MR Research and Development, Siemens Medical Systems Inc., Iselin, New Jersey.)

CORE INFORMATION

On the lateral surface of the cerebrum, four lobes are defined by the lateral and central sulci and an imaginary T-shaped line. The frontal lobe has six named gyri, the parietal lobe has seven, the occipital lobe five, the temporal lobe four. The insula is in the floor of the lateral sulcus.

On the medial surface, the corpus callosum comprises splenium, trunk, genu and rostrum; the rostrum is attached to the anterior commissure. The septum pellucidum stretches from the corpus callosum to the trunk of the fornix. Separating fornix from thalamus is the choroidal fissure through which the choroid plexus invaginates into the lateral ventricle. The third ventricle has the fornix in its roof; thalamus and hypothalamus in its side wall; infundibulum, tuber cinereum and mamillary bodies in its floor. Behind it is the pineal gland, often calcified.

The basal ganglia comprise the corpus stria-tum (caudate and lentiform nuclei), subthalamic nucleus and substantia nigra. The lentiform nucleus comprises putamen and globus pallidus. The striatum is made up of caudate and putamen, the pallidum of globus pallidus alone.

The internal capsule is the white matter separating the lentiform nucleus from the thalamus and head of caudate nucleus. The corticospinal tract descends through the corona radiata, internal capsule and crus of midbrain.

Association fibers (e.g. longitudinal, arcuate, uncinate fasciculi) link different areas within a hemisphere; commissural fibers (e.g. corpus callosum, anterior and posterior commisssures) link matching areas across the midline; projection fibers (e.g. corticothalamic, corticobulbar, corticospinal) pass to thalamus and brainstem. The lateral ventricles have a central part and three horns. Structures determining ventricular shape include corpus callosum, caudate nucleus, thalamus, amygdala and hippocampus.

SELF TEST

Answer A if 1, 2, and 3 only are correct
B if 1 and 3 only are correct
C if 2 and 4 only are correct
D if 4 only is correct
E if all four are correct

1 **The following structures are found in the floor of third ventricle:**

1 Lamina terminalis
2 Infundibulum
3 Anterior commissure
4 Mamillary bodies

2 **The following structures belong to the diencephalon:**

1 Hypothalamus
2 Inferior colliculi
3 Thalamus
4 Superior colliculi

3 **The following belong(s) to the basal ganglia:**

1 Caudate nucleus
2 Lentiform nucleus
3 Subthalamic nucleus
4 Substantia nigra

4 **The following belong(s) to the temporal lobe of the brain:**

1 Parahippocampal gyrus
2 Uncus
3 Hippocampus
4 Cuneus

5 **Nerve pathways running from the cerebral cortex through the brainstem pass through the:**

1 Corona radiata
2 Internal capsule
3 Crus cerebri
4 Corpus callosum

6 **The following is/are composed of association fibers:**

1 Anterior commissure
2 Frontal forceps
3 Tapetum
4 Arcuate fasciculus

REFERENCES

DeArmond, S.J., Fusco, M.M. and Dewey, M.M. (1976) *Structure of the Human Brain: a Photographic Atlas,* 2nd edn. Oxford: Oxford University Press.

Gluhbegovic, N. and Williams, T.H. (1980) *The Human Brain: a Photographic Guide.* New York: Harper & Row.

Kretschmann, H-J. and Weinrich, W. (1992) *Clinical Neuroanatomy and Neuroimaging.* Stuttgart: Georg Thieme.

Ludwig, E. and Klingler, J. (1956) *Atlas Cerebri Humani.* Boston: Little Brown & Co.

Niewenhuys, R., Voogd, J. and van Huijzen, C. (1988) *The Human Central Nervous System: a Synopsis and Atlas,* 3rd edn. New York: Springer-Verlag.

Roberts, M., Hanaway, J. and Morest, D.K. (1987) *Atlas of the Human Brain in Section,* 2nd edn. Philadelphia: Lea & Febiger.

Wicke, L. (1994) *Atlas of Radiologic Anatomy.* Philadelphia: Lea & Febiger.

3

MIDBRAIN, HINDBRAIN, SPINAL CORD

Chapter Summary	Study Guidelines
Brainstem Ventral view Dorsal view Sectional views **Cerebellum** **Spinal cord** General features Internal anatomy	1 Become familiar with the locations of the corticospinal tract and of ascending sensory pathways at the eight levels shown. 2 Get to grips with the nomenclature used for sections of the midbrain. 3 Relate the three cerebellar peduncles to the fourth ventricle as seen in cross sections. 4 Be able to divide the 31 spinal nerves into five groups.

The midbrain connects the diencephalon to the hindbrain. As explained in Chapter 1, the hindbrain is made up of the pons, medulla oblongata, and cerebellum. The medulla oblongata joins the spinal cord within the foramen magnum of the skull.

trigeminal nerve (V). The **middle cerebellar peduncle** plunges into the hemisphere of the cerebellum.

At the lower border of the pons are the attachments of the **abducens** (VI), **facial** (VII), and **vestibulocochlear** (VIII) nerves.

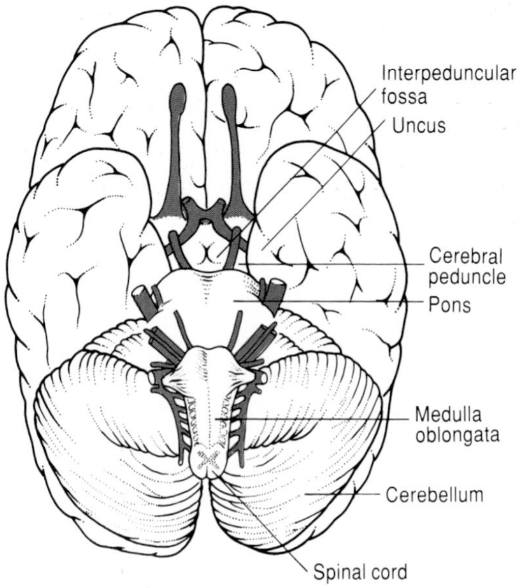

BRAINSTEM

VENTRAL VIEW (FIGURES 3.1, 3.2)

Midbrain

The ventral surface of the midbrain shows two massive **cerebral peduncles** bordering the **interpeduncular fossa**. The **optic tracts** wind around the midbrain at its junction with the diencephalon. Lateral to the midbrain is the **uncus** of the temporal lobe. The **oculomotor nerve** (III) emerges from the medial surface of the cerebral peduncle. The **trochlear nerve** (IV) can be seen between the peduncle and the uncus.

Pons

The bulk of the pons is composed of **transverse fibers** which raise numerous surface ridges. On each side, the pons is marked off from the middle cerebellar peduncle by the attachment of the

Figure 3.1 Ventral view of the brainstem, in situ.

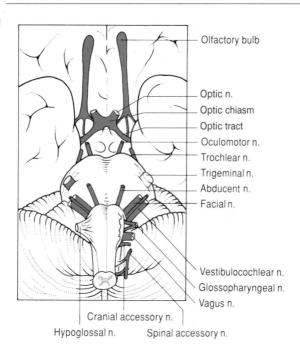

Figure 3.2 Cranial nerves. The olfactory bulb receives the olfactory nerve from the nose.

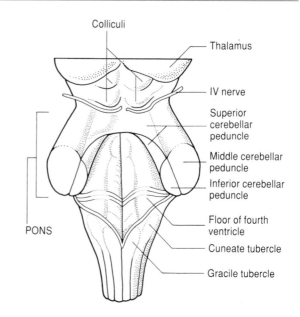

Figure 3.3 Dorsal view of brainstem, following removal of the cerebellum.

Medulla oblongata

The **pyramids** are alongside the anterior median fissure. Just above the spinomedullary junction, the fissure is invaded by the **decussation of the pyramids,** where fibers of the two pyramids intersect while crossing the midline. Lateral to the pyramid is the **olive,** and behind the olive is the **inferior cerebellar peduncle.** Attached between pyramid and olive is the **hypoglossal nerve** (XII). Attached between olive and inferior cerebellar peduncle are the **glossopharyngeal** (IX), **vagus** (X) and **cranial accessory** (XIc) nerves. The **spinal accessory nerve** (XIs) arises from the spinal cord and runs up through the foramen magnum to join the cranial accessory.

DORSAL VIEW *(FIGURE 3.3)*

The roof or **tectum** of the midbrain is composed of four colliculi. The **superior colliculi** belong to the visual system and the **inferior colliculi** belong to the auditory system. The **trochlear nerve** (IV) emerges below the inferior colliculus on each side.

The diamond-shaped **fourth ventricle** lies behind the pons and upper medulla oblongata, under cover of the cerebellum. The upper half of the diamond is bounded by the **superior cerebel-**

lar peduncles which are attached to the midbrain. The lower half is bounded by the **inferior cerebellar peduncles,** which are attached to the medulla oblongata. The **middle cerebellar peduncles** enter from the pons and overlap the other two.

Below the fourth ventricle, the medulla oblongata shows a pair of **gracile tubercles** flanked by a pair of **cuneate tubercles.**

SECTIONAL VIEWS

Sagittal section *(Figure 3.4A)*

In the midbrain, the central canal of the embryonic neural tube is represented by the **aqueduct.** Behind the pons and upper medulla oblongata, it is represented by the fourth ventricle, which is tent shaped in this view. The central canal resumes at mid-medullary level; it is continuous with the central canal of the spinal cord, although movement of cerebrospinal fluid into the cord canal is negligible.

The intermediate region of the brainstem is called the **tegmentum.** Ventral to this in the pons is the **basilar region.** Ventral to it in the medulla oblongata are the **pyramids.**

Transverse sections

The tegmentum of the entire brainstem is perme-

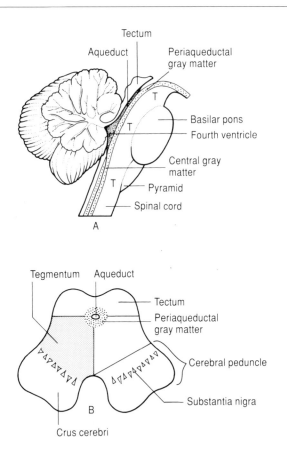

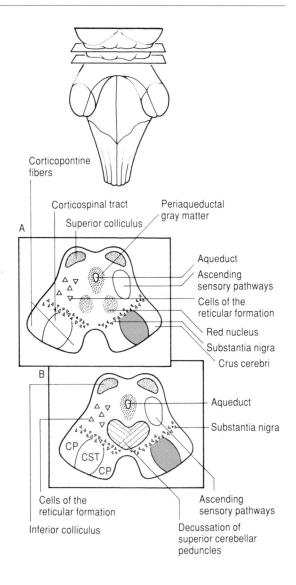

Figure 3.4 **(A)** Named parts of the brainstem in sagittal section; **(B)** named parts of the midbrain.

ated by an important network of neurons, the **reticular formation**. The tegmentum also contains *ascending sensory pathways* carrying general sensory information from the trunk and limbs. *Motor pathways* to cell groups in the brainstem and spinal cord are placed more ventrally: they occupy the crura of the midbrain, the basilar pons, and the pyramids of the medulla oblongata. The largest motor pathways are corticopontine, to the pons, and corticospinal, to the spinal cord.

Note: In this introductory account the positions of the cranial nerve nuclei are not included. (For these, see Chapter 14.) In the tegmentum, the reticular formation is shown on one side and ascending sensory pathways on the other side. In life, both exist bilaterally.

Midbrain

The midbrain comprises the tectum, the tegmentum, and the crus cerebri (*Figure 3.4B*). The central gray matter surrounds the aqueduct; it is called the **periaqueductal gray matter**.

Figure 3.5 Transverse sections of midbrain. **(A)** Level of superior colliculi; **(B)** Level of inferior colliculi.

The most ventral structure in the tegmentum is the **substantia nigra**. The crus cerebri contains motor pathways descending from the cerebral cortex to the brainstem and spinal cord. The lateral part of the tegmentum contains sensory pathways ascending to the thalamus. The cerebral peduncle of gross anatomy includes the ventral part of the tegmentum.

The **red nucleus** occupies the tegmentum on each side at the level of the superior colliculi (*Figure 3.5A*). The **decussation of the superior cerebellar peduncles** straddles the midline at the level of the inferior colliculi (*Figure 3.5B*).

Pons

The cavity of the fourth ventricle is bordered laterally by the superior cerebellar peduncles above and by the inferior cerebellar peduncles below (*Figure 3.6*). Ventral to it is the central gray matter. The tegmentum contains ascending sensory pathways as well as elements of the reticular formation. The basilar region contains descending motor pathways, as well as millions of transverse fibers which enter the middle cerebellar peduncle.

Medulla Oblongata

The medulla oblongata shows distinctive features at three different levels. The upper third shows the wrinkled **inferior olivary nucleus**, which creates the olive of gross anatomy (*Figure 3.7A*).

The middle third shows the **gracile and cuneate nuclei,** which create the gracile and cuneate tubercles (*Figure 3.7B*). (The gracile and cuneate nuclei are also called the *posterior column nuclei* because they receive massive inputs from the posterior white columns of the spinal cord.) The lower third of the medulla shows the decussation of the pyramids (*Figure 3.7C*).

The tegmentum contains ascending sensory pathways and elements of the reticular formation.

CEREBELLUM

The cerebellum is made up of two hemispheres

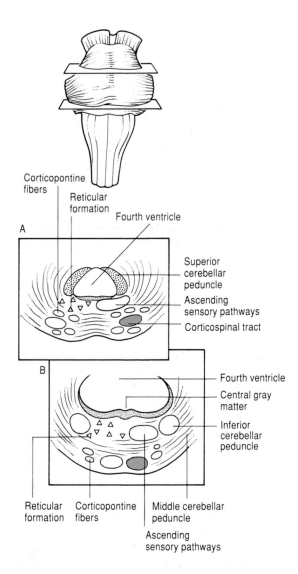

Figure 3.6 Transverse sections of pons. **(A)** Upper; **(B)** lower.

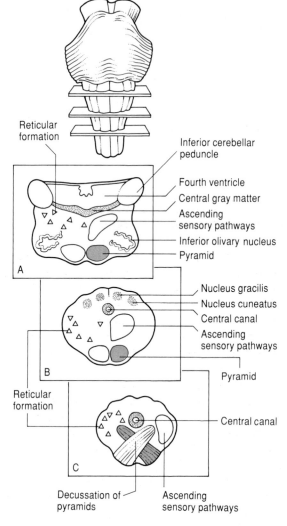

Figure 3.7 Transverse sections of medulla oblongata. **(A)** Upper third; **(B)** middle third; **(C)** lower third.

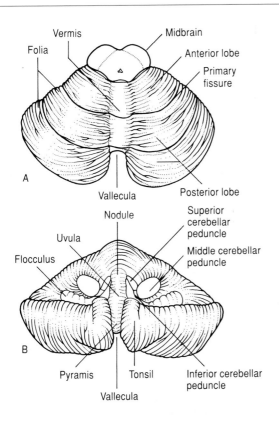

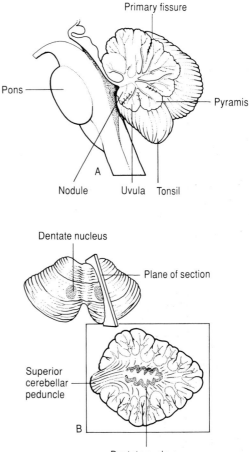

Figure 3.8 Cerebellum. **(A)** Viewed from above; **(B)** viewed from the position of the pons.

Figure 3.9 **(A)** Sagittal section of hindbrain; **(B)** Oblique section of cerebellum.

connected by the **vermis** in the midline (*Figure 3.8*). The vermis is distinct only on the under surface, where it occupies the floor of a deep groove, the **vallecula**. The hemispheres show numerous deep **fissures**, with **folia** between (*Figure 3.9A*). About 80% of the cortex (surface gray matter) is hidden from view on the surfaces of the folia.

The oldest part of the cerebellum (present even in fishes) is the flocculonodular lobe consisting of the **nodule** of the vermis and the **flocculus** in the hemisphere on each side. More recent is the **anterior lobe** which is bounded posteriorly by the **fissura prima** and contains the **pyramis** and the **uvula**. Most recent is the **posterior lobe**. A prominent feature of the posterior lobe is the **tonsil**. This tonsil lies directly above the foramen magnum of the skull; if the intracranial pressure is raised (for example by a brain tumor), one or both tonsils may descend into the foramen and pose a threat to life by compressing the medulla oblongata.

The white matter contains several **deep nuclei**. The largest of these is the **dentate nucleus** (*Figure 3.9B*).

SPINAL CORD

GENERAL FEATURES

The spinal cord occupies the upper half of the vertebral canal. Thirty-one pairs of spinal nerves are attached to it, by means of **anterior** and **posterior nerve roots** (*Figure 3.10A*). The cord shows **cervical** and **lumbar enlargements** which accommodate nerve cells supplying the upper and lower limbs.

INTERNAL ANATOMY

■ In transverse sections, the cord shows butterfly-shaped gray matter surrounded by three columns or **funiculi** of white matter:

■ an anterior funiculus in the interval between the anterior median fissure and the emerging anterior nerve roots;

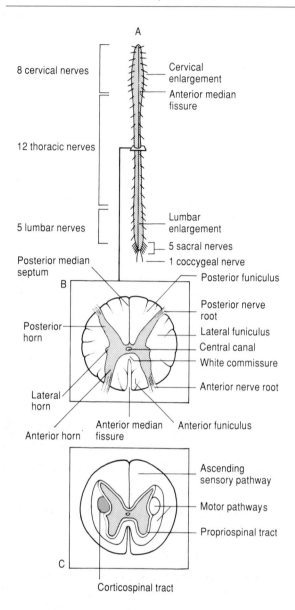

Figure 3.10 Spinal cord. **(A)** Anterior view, with nerve attachments; **(B)** transverse section at thoracic level; **(C)** general arrangement of pathways in the white matter.

- a lateral funiculus between the anterior and posterior nerve roots; and
- a posterior funiculus between the posterior roots and the **posterior median septum** (*Figure 3.10B*).

The gray matter consists of **central gray matter** surrounding a minute central canal, and **anterior** and **posterior gray horns**. At the levels of attachment of the twelve thoracic and upper two or three lumbar nerve roots a **lateral gray horn** is present as well.

Axons pass from one side of the spinal cord to the other in the **gray commissures,** and in the **white commissure** deep to the anterior median fissure.

Location of pathways *(Figure 3.10C)*

Adjacent to the central gray matter is the **propriospinal tract,** containing fibers linking one level of the cord with another. Outside this are motor pathways descending from the brain. Outermost are sensory pathways ascending to the brainstem and thalamus.

REFERENCES

See list for Chapter 2.

CORE INFORMATION

Brainstem

Descending motor pathways occupy the crus of midbrain, the basilar pons and the pyramid of medulla oblongata. The brain stem tegmentum contains reticular formation and ascending sensory pathways. The central canal forms the aqueduct in the midbrain and the fourth ventricle at the back of pons and upper medulla. Two cranial nerves are attached to the midbrain, four to the pons and four to the medulla. The inferior cerebellar peduncles enter the cerebellum from the side of the medulla and the middle peduncles enter from the side of the pons; the superior peduncles leave the cerebellum and decussate in the isthmus (lowest part of midbrain).

Cerebellum

The hemispheres are deeply fissured and are linked by the vermis. The oldest part is the flocculonodular lobe. More recent is the anterior lobe. Most recent is the posterior lobe, which includes the tonsils. The white matter contains several nuclei including the dentate nucleus.

Spinal cord

The spinal cord occupies only the upper half of the vertebral canal, the sacral nerve roots being attached to it at the level of the first lumbar vertebra. In all, 31 pairs of roots are attached. The gray matter is most abundant at the levels of attachment of the brachial and lumbosacral plexuses. Anterior and posterior horns are present at all levels, and lateral horns at the level of thoracic and upper lumbar root attachments. The white matter comprises anterior, lateral and posterior funiculi. Axons cross the midline in the gray commissures and in the white commisure. In general, propriospinal pathways are innermost, motor pathways are intermediate and sensory pathways are outermost.

SELF TEST

Select the false statement:

1 In the midbrain:

  A The most ventral structure in the tegmentum is the substantia nigra
  B The tegmentum contains the red nucleus
  C The central canal is represented by the aqueduct
  D The oculomotor nerve is attached
  E 'Cerebral peduncle' is synonymous with 'crus cerebri'

2 In the pons:

  A The basilar region contains the corticospinal tract
  B The tegmentum contains sensory pathways
  C Transverse fibers enter the middle cerebellar peduncle
  D The trigeminal nerve is attached
  E The hypoglossal nerve is attached

3 In the medulla oblongata:

  A The upper third contains part of the fourth ventricle
  B The middle third contains the posterior column nuclei
  C The lower third contains the decussation of the pyramids
  D The abducens nerve is attached
  E The spinomedullary junction occupies the foramen magnum

4 In the cerebellum:

  A The flocculonodular lobe is the most recent phylogenetically
  B The tonsils are close to the foramen magnum
  C The superior cerebellar peduncle passes to the midbrain
  D Most of the cortex occupies the walls of fissures
  E The vermis occupies the roof of the vallecula

5 In the spinal cord:

  A Eight pairs of cervical nerves are attached
  B The anterior median fissure is bounded by anterior funiculi
  C The corticospinal tracts occupy the lateral funiculi
  D Motor pathways lie internal to sensory pathways
  E The propriospinal pathway is outermost

4

MENINGES

Chapter Summary	Study Guidelines
Cranial meninges Dura mater Meningeal arteries Arachnoid mater Pia mater Subarachnoid cisterns Sheath of the optic nerve **Spinal meninges** **Circulation of cerebrospinal fluid** CLINICAL PANELS Extradural/subdural hematomas Hydrocephalus	1 Be able to compare the structure of the dura mater with that of the pia-arachnoid. 2 Be able to follow a drop of blood from the superior sagittal sinus to the internal jugular vein; and from an ophthalmic vein to the sigmoid sinus. 3 Name the nerves supplying: (a) the supratentorial dura; (b) the infratentorial dura. 4 Identify the different vessels responsible for extradural, subdural and subarachnoid bleeding. 5 Appreciate the mechanism of papilledema, and why lumbar puncture should not be undertaken in its presence. 6 Trace a drop of CSF from a lateral ventricle to: (a) its point of entry into the bloodstream; (b) a lumbar puncture needle. 7 Know about a major cause of hydrocephalus: (a) in infancy; (b) in adults; and why both are examples of 'outlet obstruction.'

The meninges surround the central nervous system and suspend it in the protective jacket provided by the cerebrospinal fluid. The meninges comprise the tough **dura mater** or **pachymeninx** (Greek, thick membrane), and the **leptomeninges** (Greek, slender membranes) consisting of the **arachnoid mater** and **pia mater**. Between the arachnoid and the pia is the **subarachnoid space** filled with cerebrospinal fluid.

CRANIAL MENINGES

DURA MATER

The terminology used to describe the cranial dura mater varies among different authors. It seems best to regard it as a single, tough layer of fibrous tissue which is fused with the inner periosteum of the skull except where it is reflected into the interior of the vault or is stretched across the skull base. Wherever it separates from the periosteum, the intervening space contains venous sinuses (*Figure 4.1*).

Two great dural folds extend into the cranial cavity and help to stabilize the brain. These are the **falx cerebri** and the **tentorium cerebelli**.

The falx cerebri occupies the longitudinal fissure between the cerebral hemispheres. Its attached border extends from the crista galli of the ethmoid bone to the upper surface of the tentorium cerebelli. Along the vault of the skull it encloses the **superior sagittal sinus**. Its free border contains the **inferior sagittal sinus** which unites with the **great cerebral vein** to form the **straight sinus** (*Figure 4.2*). The straight sinus travels along the line of attachment of falx to tentorium and meets the superior sagittal sinus at the **confluence of the sinuses**.

The tentorium cerebelli arches like a tent above the posterior cranial fossa, being lifted up by the falx cerebri in the midline. The attached margin of the tentorium encloses the **transverse sinuses** on the inner surface of the occipital bone and the **superior petrosal sinuses** along the upper border of the petrous temporal bone. The attached margin reaches to the posterior clinoid processes of the sphenoid bone. Most of the

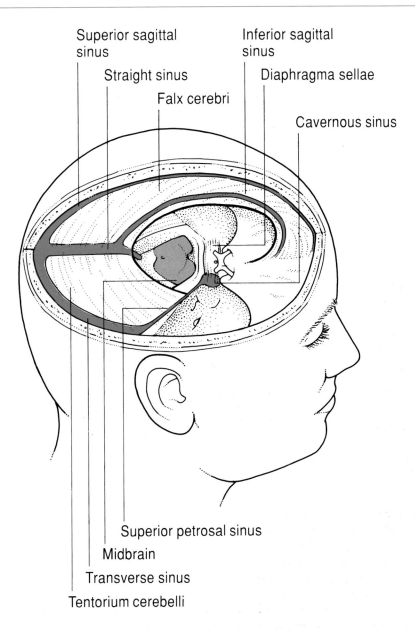

Superior sagittal sinus

Inferior sagittal sinus

Straight sinus

Diaphragma sellae

Falx cerebri

Cavernous sinus

Superior petrosal sinus

Midbrain

Transverse sinus

Tentorium cerebelli

Figure 4.1 Dural reflections and venous sinuses. The midbrain occupies the tentorial notch.

blood from the superior sagittal sinus enters the right transverse sinus (*Figure 4.3*).

The free margin of the tentorium is U-shaped. The tips of the U are attached to the anterior clinoid processes. Just behind this, the two limbs of the U are linked by a sheet of dura, the **diaphragma sellae,** which is pierced by the pituitary stalk. Laterally, the dura falls away into the middle cranial fossae from the limbs of the U, creating the **cavernous sinus** on each side. Behind the sphenoid bone, the concavity of the U encloses the midbrain.

The cavernous sinus receives blood from the orbit via the **ophthalmic veins** (*Figure 4.2*). The superior petrosal sinus joins the transverse sinus at its junction with the **sigmoid sinus.** The sigmoid sinus descends along the occipital bone and discharges into the bulb of the internal jugular vein. The bulb receives the **inferior petrosal sinus** which descends along the edge of the occipital bone.

The tentorium cerebelli divides the cranial cavity into a **supratentorial compartment** containing the forebrain and an **infratentorial compartment** containing the hindbrain.

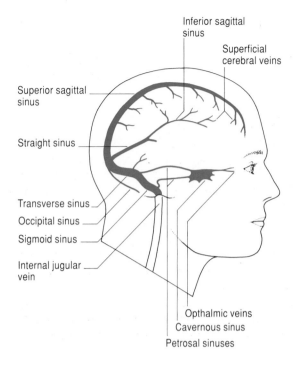

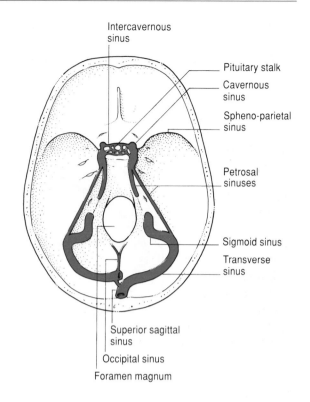

Figure 4.2 Side view of intracranial venous sinuses and their tributaries.

Figure 4.3 Venous sinuses on the base of the skull.

Innervation of the cranial dura mater

The dura mater lining the supratentorial compartment of the cranial cavity receives sensory innervation from the trigeminal nerve. Stretching or inflammation of the supratentorial dura gives rise to frontal or parietal headache.

The dura mater lining the infratentorial compartment is supplied by branches of the upper cervical spinal nerves. Occipital and posterior neck pains accompany disturbance of the infratentorial dura. Acute meningitis involving the posterior cranial fossa is associated with *neck rigidity* and often with *head retraction* brought about by reflex contraction of the posterior nuchal muscles, which are supplied by cervical nerves.

MENINGEAL ARTERIES

Embedded in the inner periosteum of the skull are several **meningeal arteries** whose main function is to supply the diploe (bone marrow). Much the largest is the **middle meningeal artery**, which ramifies over the inner surface of the temporal and parietal bones. Tearing of this artery, with its accompanying vein, is the usual source of an *extradural hematoma (Panel 4.1)*.

ARACHNOID MATER

The arachnoid (Greek, spidery) is a thin, fibrocellular layer in direct contact with the dura mater (*Figure 4.4*). The outermost cells of the arachnoid are bonded to one another by tight junctions which seal the subarachnoid space. Innumerable **arachnoid trabeculae** cross the space to reach the pia mater.

PIA MATER

The pia mater invests the brain closely, following its contours and lining the various sulci (*Figure 4.4*). Like the arachnoid, it is fibrocellular. The cellular component of the pia is external and is permeable to cerebrospinal fluid. The fibrous component occupies a narrow **subpial space** which is continuous with **perivascular spaces** around cerebral blood vessels penetrating the brain surface.

Note: Although the subarachnoid and subpial spaces are proven, there is no sign of any 'subdural space' in properly fixed material. Such a space can be created, however, by leakage of blood into

EXTRADURAL/SUBDURAL HEMATOMAS

An *extradural (epidural) hematoma* is typically caused by a blow to the side of the head severe enough to cause a fracture with associated tearing of the anterior or posterior branch of the middle meningeal artery. Following the initial *concussion* of the brain, with loss of consciousness, there may be a *lucid interval* of several hours. Onset of increasing headache and drowsiness signals *cerebral compression* produced by expansion of the hematoma. Coma and death will supervene unless the hematoma is drained though a burr-hole drilled close to the fracture line.

Subdural hematomas are caused by rupture of superficial cerebral veins in transit from the brain to an intracranial venous sinus.

An *acute subdural hematoma* most often follows severe head injury in children. It must always be suspected where a child remains unconscious after a head injury. Child battering is a possible explanation where this situation arises in the home.

A *subacute subdural hematoma* may follow head injury at any age. Symptoms and signs of raised intracranial pressure (described in Chapter 6) develop up to 3 weeks after the injury.

Chronic subdural hematomas occur in older people, where the transit veins have become brittle and made taut by shrinkage of the aging brain. Head injury may be mild or even absent. A significant number of these patients are alcoholics with reduced blood clotting. Presenting symptoms are variable and include personality changes, headaches and epileptic seizures.

the cellular layer of the dura mater following a tear of a cerebral vein at its point of anchorage to the fibrous layer. (See subdural hematoma in Panel 4.1.)

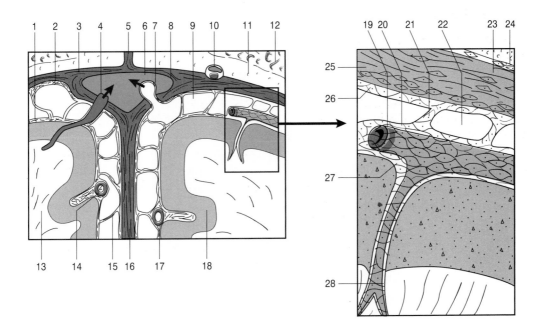

Figure 4.4 Coronal section of the superior sagittal sinus and related structures. **1,** pia mater; **2,** arachnoid mater; **3,** dura mater; **4,** superficial cerebral vein; **5,** sagittal suture; **6,** superior sagittal sinus; **7,** arachnoid granulation; **8,** arachnoid mater; **9,** subarachnoid space; **10,** meningeal vessels; **11,** inner table of skull; **12,** diploë; **13,** white matter;**14,** cerebral artery; **15,** arachnoid trabecula; **16,** falx cerebri; **17,** pia mater; **18,** cerebral cortex; **19,** cerebral artery; **20,** pia mater; **21,** arachnoid trabecula; **22,** subarachnoid space; **23,** fibrous layer of dura mater; **24,** periosteum; **25,** cellular layer of dura mater; **26,** arachnoid mater; **27,** subpial space; **28,** perivascular space.

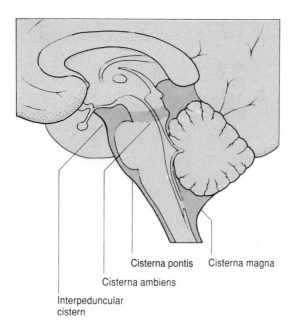

Cisterna pontis   Cisterna magna

Cisterna ambiens

Interpeduncular
cistern

Figure 4.5   Subarachnoid cisterns.

SUBARACHNOID CISTERNS

Along the base of the brain and the sides of the brainstem, pools of cerebrospinal fluid occupy subarachnoid cisterns (*Figure 4.5*). The largest of these is the **cisterna magna,** in the interval between the cerebellum and the medulla oblongata. More rostrally are the **cisterna pontis** ventral to the pons, the **interpeduncular cistern** between the cerebral peduncles, and the **cisterna ambiens** at the side of the midbrain (*Figure 4.6*).

SHEATH OF THE OPTIC NERVE

The optic nerve is composed of CNS white matter, and it has a complete meningeal investment. The central vessels of the retina pierce the meninges to enter it (*Figure 4.7*). Any sustained elevation of intracranial pressure will be transmitted to the subarachnoid space surrounding the nerve. The **central vein** will be compressed, resulting in swelling of the retinal tributaries of

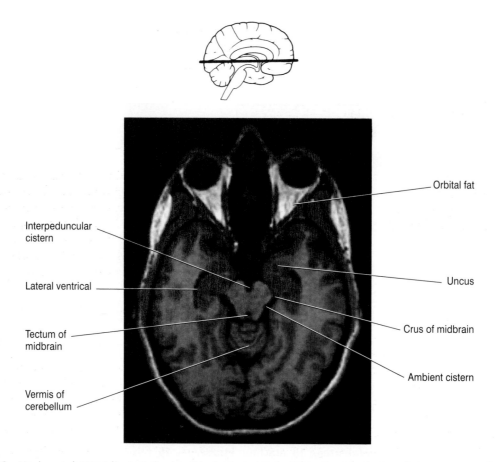

Interpeduncular
cistern

Lateral ventrical

Tectum of
midbrain

Vermis of
cerebellum

Orbital fat

Uncus

Crus of midbrain

Ambient cistern

Figure 4.6   Horizontal MRI 'slice' at the level indcated at top. Note the proximity of the uncus to the crus of the midbrain (cf. uncal herniation in Chapter 6). (From a series kindly provided by Dr. J. Paul Finn, Director, MR Research and Development, Siemens Medical Systems Inc., Iselin, New Jersey)

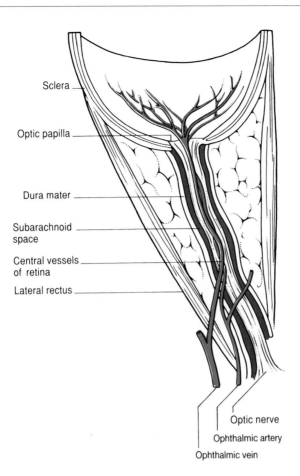

Sclera

Optic papilla

Dura mater

Subarachnoid space

Central vessels of retina

Lateral rectus

Optic nerve
Ophthalmic artery
Ophthalmic vein

Figure 4.7 Horizontal section of the left orbit.

the vein and edema of the optic papilla, where the optic nerve begins. The condition is known as *papilledema* (*Figure 4.8*). It can be recognized on inspection of the retina with an ophthalmoscope.

SPINAL MENINGES *(Figure 4.9)*

The spinal dural sac is like a test tube, attached to the rim of the foramen magnum and reaching down to the level of the second sacral vertebra. The outer surface of the tube is adherent to the posterior longitudinal ligament of the vertebrae in the midline; elsewhere it is surrounded by fat containing an epidural (internal vertebral) plexus of veins (Chapter 11).

The internal surface of the dura is lined with arachnoid mater. The pia mater lines the surface of the spinal cord and is attached to the dura mater at regular intervals by the serrated **ligamentum denticulatum.**

Because the spinal cord reaches only to first or second lumbar vertebral level, a large **lumbar cistern** is created, containing the free-floating roots of the sacral and lower lumbar spinal nerves (Chapter 11). The lumbar cistern may be tapped to procure samples of cerebrospinal fluid for analysis ('lumbar puncture' or 'spinal tap').

CIRCULATION OF CEREBROSPINAL FLUID

The principal source of the cerebrospinal fluid is the secretion of the choroid plexuses into the ventricles of the brain. From the lateral ventricles the CSF enters the third through the interventricular foramen. It descends to the fourth through the aqueduct, and gains the subarachnoid space through the median and lateral apertures. (Flow within the central canal of the spinal cord is negligible.)

37

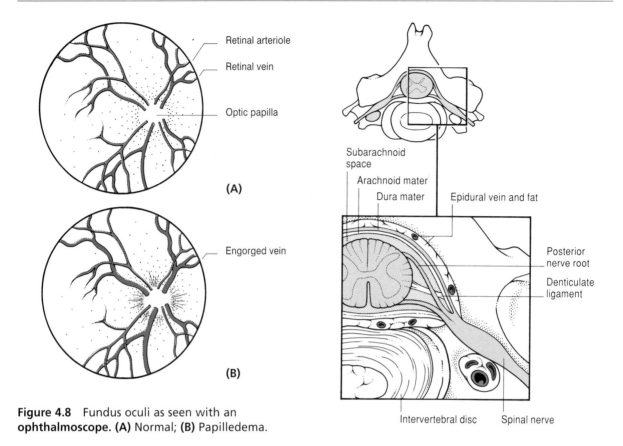

Figure 4.8 Fundus oculi as seen with an **ophthalmoscope. (A)** Normal; **(B)** Papilledema.

Figure 4.9 Contents of cervical vertebral canal.

CLINICAL PANEL 4.2

HYDROCEPHALUS

Hydrocephalus (Greek, *water in the head*) denotes accumulation of cerebrospinal fluid (CSF) in the ventricular system. With the exception of overproduction of CSF by a rare papilloma of the choroid plexus, hydrocephalus results from obstruction of the normal CSF circulation, with consequent dilatation of the ventricles. The term is not used to describe the accumulation of fluid in the ventricles and subarachnoid space in association with senile atrophy of the brain.

In the great majority of cases, hydrocephalus is caused by obstruction of the outlets from the fourth ventricle into the subarachnoid space. A major cause of outlet obstruction in *infancy* is the *Arnold-Chiari malformation*, in which the cerebellum is partly extruded into the vertebral canal during fetal life because the posteri-or cranial fossa is underdeveloped. In untreated cases the child's head may become as large as a football and the cerebral hemispheres paper thin. The condition is nearly always associated with spina bifida (Chapter 11). Early treatment is essential to prevent severe brain damage. The obstruction can be bypassed by means of a catheter having one end inserted into a lateral ventricle and the other inserted into the internal jugular vein.

A major cause of outlet obstruction in *adults* is displacement of the cerebellum into the foramen magnum by a space-occupying lesion such as a tumor or hematoma (see Chapter 6).

Meningitis can cause hydrocephalus at any age. The development of leptomeningeal adhesions may compromise CSF circulation at the level of the ventricular outlets, the tentorial notch, and/or the arachnoid granulations.

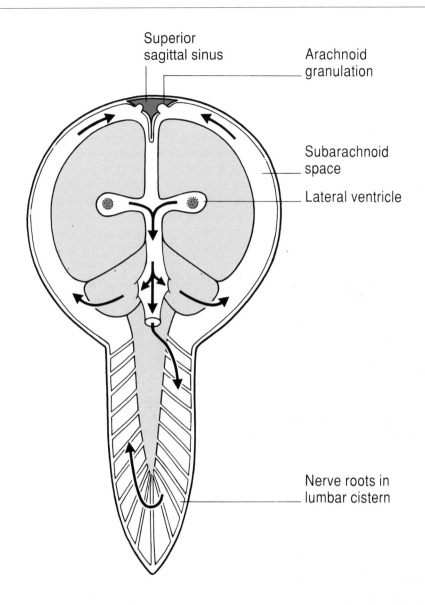

Figure 4.10 Circulation of cerebrospinal fluid.

Within the subarachnoid space, some of the CSF descends through the foramen magnum, reaching the lumbar cistern in about 12 hours. A small amount is absorbed into spinal segmental veins; the rest returns to the cranial subarachnoid space. From the subarachnoid space at the base of the brain, the CSF ascends through the tentorial notch and bathes the surface of the cerebral hemispheres before being returned to the blood through the **arachnoid granulations** (*Figure 4.4*). The arachnoid granulations are pinhead pouches of arachnoid mater projecting through the dural wall of the major venous sinuses—especially the superior sagittal sinus and the small venous **lacunae** that open into it. CSF is transported across the arachnoid epithelium in giant vacuoles.

About 300 ml of CSF are secreted by the choroid plexuses every 24 hours. Another 200 ml are produced from other sources, as described in Chapter 5. Blockage of flow through the ventricular system or cranial subarachnoid space will cause back-up within the ventricular system: a state of *hydrocephalus* (*Panel 4.2*).

CORE INFORMATION

Meninges

The meninges comprise dura, arachnoid and pia mater. The subarachnoid space contains cerebrospinal fluid.

The cranial dura mater shows two large folds: the falx cerebri encloses the superior sagittal sinus, which usually enters the right of the two transverse sinuses enclosed by the tentorium cerebelli. The inferior sagittal sinus joins the great cerebral vein, forming the straight sinus which joins the confluence of the sagittal and transverse sinuses. The transverse sinus enters the sigmoid sinus which empties into the internal jugular vein. The midbrain is partly enclosed by the free edge of the tentorium, which is attached to the anterior clinoid processes of the sphenoid bone; dura drapes from the free edge into the middle cranial fossa, creating the cavernous sinus on each side. The supratentorial dura mater is innervated by the trigeminal nerve, the infratentorial dura by upper cervical nerves. The meningeal vessels run extradurally to supply the diploë; if torn by skull fracture, they may form an extradural hematoma compressing the brain.

Cerebrospinal fluid

Pools of CSF at the base of the brain include the cisterna magna, the c. pontis, the interpeduncular c., and the c. ambiens. CSF also extends along the meningeal sheath of the optic nerve, and raised intracranial pressure may compress the central vein of the retina, causing papilledema.

The spinal dural sac extends down to S2 vertebral level. The lumbar cistern contains spinal nerve roots and is accessible for lumbar puncture (spinal tap). CSF secreted by the choroid plexuses escapes into the subarachnoid space through the three fourth-ventricular apertures. Some descends to the lumbar cistern. The CSF ascends through the tentorial notch and the cerebral subarachnoid space to reach the superior sagittal sinus and its lacunae via the arachnoid granulations. Blockage of CSF flow anywhere along its course leads to hydrocephalus.

SELF TEST

Select the best response:

1 **The superior sagittal sinus receives:**

   A Superficial cerebral veins
   B Cerebrospinal fluid
   C Deep cerebral veins
   D All of the above
   E A and B only

2 **Which of the following travel across the subarachnoid space?**

   A Cerebral arteries
   B Superficial cerebral veins
   C Diploic veins
   D All of the above
   E A and B only

3 **The tentorial notch is occupied by the:**

   A Medulla oblongata
   B Pons
   C Cerebellum
   D Midbrain
   E Diencephalon

4 **Meningitis in the posterior cranial fossa may give rise to pain referred to the:**

   A Forehead
   B Face
   C Front of neck
   D Back of neck
   E Jaw

5 **Extradural hematomas arise from rupture of the following vessels:**

   A Diploic
   B Meningeal
   C Cerebral
   D All of the above
   E A and B only

6 **Which of the following are possible sites of obstruction to CSF circulation:**

   A Aqueduct
   B Ventricular exit foramina
   C Tentorial notch
   D Arachnoid granulations
   E All of the above

REFERENCES

Alskne, J.F. and Lovings, E.T. (1972) Functional ultrastructure of the arachnoid villus. *Arch. Neurol.* **27**: 371—377.

Hutchings, M. and Weller, R.O. (1986) Anatomical relationships of the pia mater to cerebral blood vessels in man. *J. Neurosurg.* **65**: 316—325.

Nicholas, D.S. and Weller, R.O. (1988) The fine anatomy of the human spinal meninges. *J. Neurosurg.* **69**: 276—282.

Prockop, L.D. and Shah, C.P. (1989) Hydrocephalus. In *Merritt's Textbook of Neurology*, 8th edn (Rowland, L.P., ed.). Philadelphia: Lea & Febiger.

5

BLOOD SUPPLY OF THE BRAIN

Chapter Summary

Arterial supply of the forebrain
Anterior cerebral artery
Middle cerebral artery
Posterior cerebral artery

Blood supply of the brainstem
Vertebral branches
Basilar branches

Venous drainage of the brain
Superficial veins
Deep veins

Regulation of blood flow

The blood–brain barrier
Blood–CSF barrier
Blood–ECF barrier
Functions of the blood–brain barrier

CLINICAL PANEL
Blood–brain barrier pathology

Study Guidelines

Because interpretation of the symptoms produced by cerebrovascular accidents requires prior knowledge of brain function, Clinical Panels on this subject are placed in the final chapter. On the other hand, a Clinical Panel on blood–brain barrier pathology is placed in the present chapter because the symptoms are of a general nature.

1 On simple outline drawings of a hemisphere, shade in the territories of the three cerebral arteries.
2 Identify the several sources of arterial supply to the internal capsule.
3 Become familiar with carotid and vertebral angiograms.
4 Be able to list the areas supplied by the vertebral and basilar arteries.
5 Identify the two blood–brain barriers. Be able to understand why, for example, shallow breathing after abdominal surgery can tip a patient into coma.

The brain is absolutely dependent upon a continuous supply of oxygenated blood. The brain controls the delivery of its blood by sensing the momentary pressure changes in its main artery of supply. It controls its arterial oxygen tension by monitoring respiratory gas levels in the the internal carotid artery and in the cerebrospinal fluid beside the medulla oblongata (Chapter 19). The control systems used by the brain are exquisitely sophisticated, but they can be brought to nothing if a distributing artery ruptures spontaneously or is rammed shut by an embolus.

ARTERIAL SUPPLY OF THE FOREBRAIN

The blood supply to the forebrain is derived from the two **internal carotid arteries** and from the **basilar artery** (*Figure 5.1*).

Each internal carotid artery enters the subarachnoid space by piercing the roof of the cavernous sinus. In the subarachnoid space it gives off **ophthalmic, posterior communicating** and **anterior choroidal arteries** before dividing into the **anterior** and **middle cerebral arteries**.

The basilar artery divides at the upper border of the pons into the two **posterior cerebral arteries**. The **arterial circle of Willis** is completed by a linkage of the posterior communicating artery with the posterior cerebral on each side, and by linkage of the two anterior cerebrals by the **anterior communicating artery**.

The choroid plexus of the lateral ventricle is supplied from the **anterior choroidal** branch of

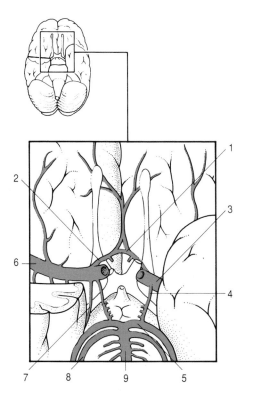

Figure 5.1   Arteries at the base of the brain. Arteries forming the circle of Willis: **1,** anterior communicating; **2,** anterior cerebral; **3,** internal carotid; **4,** posterior communicating; **5,** posterior cerebral. Other arteries: **6,** middle cerebral; **7,** anterior choroidal; **8,** superior cerebellar; **9,** basilar.

Table 5.1   Named cortical* branches of the anterior cerebral artery

Branch	Territory
Orbital	Orbital surface of frontal lobe
Frontopolar	Frontal pole
Callosomarginal	Cingulate and superior frontal gyri; paracentral lobule
Pericallosal	Corpus callosum

*The term 'cortical' is conventional. The official term 'terminal' is better because these arteries supply the subjacent white matter as well.

ANTERIOR CEREBRAL ARTERY (*FIGURE 5.2*)

The anterior cerebral artery passes above the optic chiasm to gain the medial surface of the cerebral hemisphere. It forms an arch around the genu of the corpus callosum, making it easy to identify in a carotid angiogram (*Figure 5.4*). Close to the anterior communicating artery it gives off a final central branch, the **recurrent artery of Heubner** (pron. 'Hoibner') which supplies the anterior limb and genu of the internal capsule. Cortical branches of the anterior cerebral supply the medial surface of the hemisphere as far back as the parieto-occipital sulcus (*Table 5.1*). The branches overlap onto the orbital and lateral surfaces of the hemisphere.

MIDDLE CEREBRAL ARTERY (*FIGURE 5.3*)

The middle cerebral artery is the main continuation of the internal carotid, receiving 80% of the carotid blood flow. It immediately gives off important central branches, then passes along the depth of the lateral fissure to reach the surface of the insula (*Figure 5.4*). There it usually breaks into upper and lower divisions. The upper division supplies the frontal and anterior parietal lobes; the lower division supplies the posterior parietal lobe, the temporal lobe, and the midregion of the optic radiation. Named cortical branches are listed in *Table 5.2* and shown in *Figure 5.3*. Overall, the middle cerebral supplies two-thirds of the lateral surface of the hemisphere.

The **central branches** of the middle cerebral are **medial** and **lateral striate** arteries (*Figure 5.5*). These arteries supply the corpus striatum, internal capsule, and thalamus. Occlusion of one of the lateral striate arteries is the chief cause of classical *stroke*, where damage to the pyramidal

the anterior cerebral artery and by a **posterior choroidal** branch from the posterior cerebral artery.

Dozens of fine **central (perforating) branches** are given off by the constituent arteries of the circle of Willis. They enter the brain through the **anterior perforated substance** beside the optic chiasm, and through the **posterior perforated substance** behind the mamillary bodies. They have been classified in various ways but can be conveniently grouped into short and long branches. **Short central branches** arise from all of the constituent arteries and from the two choroidal arteries. They supply the optic nerve, chiasm and tract, and the hypothalamus. **Long central branches** arise from the three cerebral arteries. They supply the thalamus, corpus striatum, and internal capsule. They include the **striate branches** of the anterior and middle cerebral arteries.

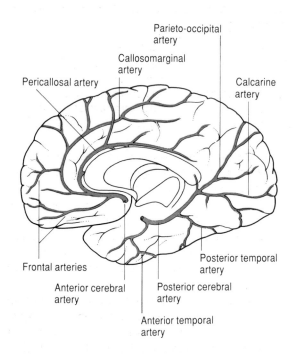

Figure 5.2 Cortical branches of the anterior and posterior cerebral arteries.

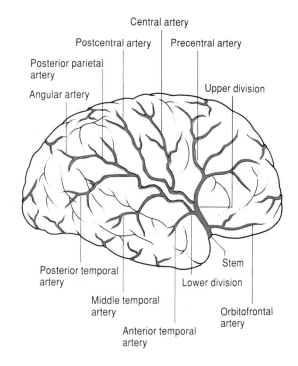

Figure 5.3 Cortical branches of the middle cerebral artery.

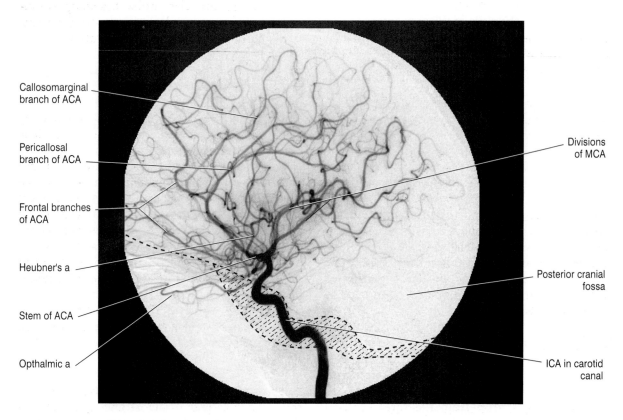

Figure 5.4 Arterial phase of a carotid angiogram. Contrast medium injected into the left internal carotid artery is passing through the anterior and middle cerebral arteries (ACA, MCA). The base of the skull is shown in hatched outline. ICA, internal carotid artery. (From an original series kindly provided by Dr. Michael Modic, Department of Radiology, The Cleveland Clinic Foundation)

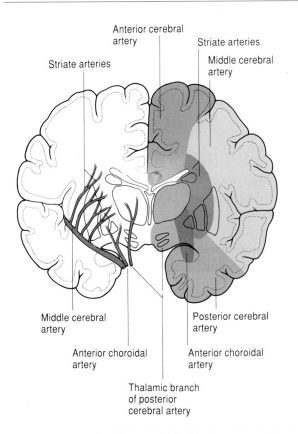

Figure 5.5 Distribution of perforating branches of the middle cerebral, anterior choroidal, and posterior cerebral arteries (schematic).

tract in the posterior limb of the internal capsule causes *hemiplegia,* a term denoting paralysis of the contralateral arm, leg and lower part of face. (For varieties of stroke, see Chapter 27).

POSTERIOR CEREBRAL ARTERY *(FIGURE 5.2)*

The two posterior cerebral arteries are the terminal branches of the basilar. However, in embryonic life they originated from the internal carotid, and in about 25% of individuals the

Table 5.2 Cortical branches of the middle cerebral artery and their territories

Branch	Territory
Orbitofrontal	Orbitofrontal cortex
Precentral	Motor/premotor/Broca areas
Postcentral	Primary sensory cortex
Posterior parietal	Posterior parietal cortex
Angular	Angular gyrus
Anterior temporal	Temporal polar area
Middle temporal	Auditory/Wernicke areas
Posterior temporal	Posterior temporal cortex

Table 5.3 Named cortical branches of the posterior cerebral artery

Branch	Territory
Anterior temporal	Parahippocampal gyrus, hippocampal formation
Posterior temporal	Occipitotemporal gyri
Calcarine	Walls of calcarine sulcus
Parieto-occipital	Cuneus, precuneus

internal carotid persists as the primary source of blood on one or both sides, by way of a large posterior communicating artery.

Close to its origin, each posterior cerebral gives branches to the midbrain and a **posterior choroidal artery** to the choroid plexus of the lateral ventricle. Additional, **central branches** are sent into the posterior perforated substance (*Figure 5.1*).

The main artery winds around the midbrain in company with the optic tract. It supplies the splenium of the corpus callosum and the cortex of the occipital and temporal lobes. Named cortical branches and their territories are given in *Table 5.3.*

The central branches, called **thalamoperforating** and **thalamogeniculate,** supply the thalamus, subthalamic nucleus, and optic radiation.

BLOOD SUPPLY OF THE BRAINSTEM

The brainstem and cerebellum are supplied by the vertebral and basilar arteries and their branches (*Figure 5.6*).

The two **vertebral** arteries arise from the subclavian arteries and ascend the neck in the foramina transversaria of the upper six cervical vertebrae. They enter the skull through the foramen magnum and unite at the lower border of the pons to form the **basilar artery.** The basilar artery ascends to the upper border of the pons and divides into two posterior cerebral arteries (*Figure 5.7*).

All of the primary branches of the vertebral and basilar arteries give branches to the brainstem.

VERTEBRAL BRANCHES

The **posterior inferior cerebellar artery** supplies the side of the medulla before giving branches to the cerebellum. **Anterior** and **posterior spinal arteries** supply the ventral and dorsal medulla, respectively, before descending through the foramen magnum.

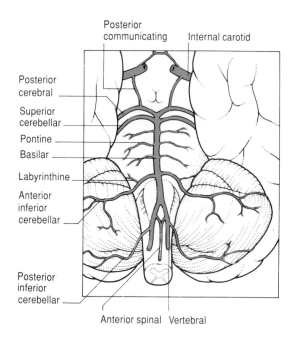

Figure 5.6 Arterial supply of brainstem.

BASILAR BRANCHES

The **anterior inferior cerebellar** and **superior cereb-ellar arteries** supply the side of the pons before giving branches to the cerebellum. The anterior inferior cerebellar usually gives off the **labyrinthine artery** to the inner ear.

About a dozen **pontine arteries** supply the full thickness of the medial part of the pons.

The midbrain is supplied by the **posterior cerebral artery,** and by the **posterior communicating artery** linking the posterior cerebral to the internal carotid.

VENOUS DRAINAGE OF THE BRAIN

The venous drainage of the brain is of great importance in relation to neurosurgical procedures. It is also important to the professional neurologist because a variety of clinical syndromes can be produced by venous obstruction,

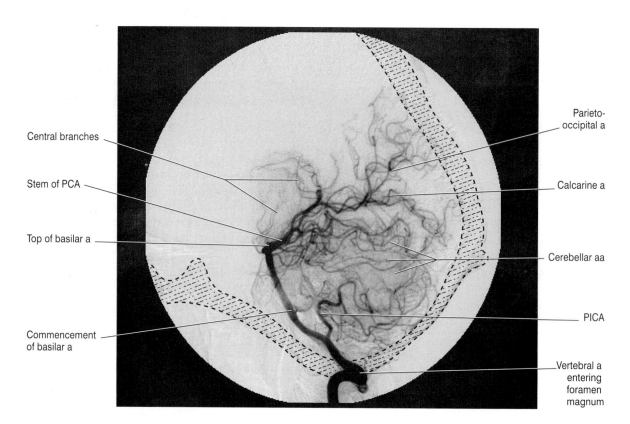

Figure 5.7 Vertebrobasilar angiogram. Contrast medium was injected into the left vertebral artery. PCA, posterior cerebral artery; PICA, posterior inferior cerebellar artery. Basilar supply to the upper half of the cerebellum are somewhat obscured by overlying posterior parietal branches of the PCA. (From an original series kindly provided by Dr Michael Modic, Department of Radiology, The Cleveland Clinic Foundation.)

venous thrombosis, and congenital arteriovenous communications. In general medical practice, however, problems caused by cerebral veins are rare in comparison with arterial disease.

The cerebral hemispheres are drained by superficial and deep cerebral veins. Like the intracranial venous sinuses, they are devoid of valves.

SUPERFICIAL VEINS

The **superficial cerebral veins** lie in the subarachnoid space overlying the hemispheres. They drain the cerebral cortex and underlying white matter and empty into intracranial venous sinuses (*Figures 5.8A and 5.9*).

The upper part of each hemisphere drains into the superior sagittal sinus. The middle part drains into the cavernous sinus (as a rule) by way of the **superficial middle cerebral vein**. The lower part drains into the transverse sinus.

DEEP VEINS (*FIGURE 5.8B*)

The deep cerebral veins drain the corpus striatum, thalamus, and choroid plexuses.

A **thalamostriate vein** drains the thalamus and caudate nucleus. Together with a **choroidal vein** it forms the **internal cerebral vein**. The two internal cerebral veins unite beneath the corpus callosum to form the **great cerebral vein** (of Galen).

A **basal vein** is formed beneath the anterior perforated substance by the union of **anterior** and **deep middle cerebral veins**. The basal vein runs around the crus cerebri and empties into the great cerebral vein.

Finally, the great cerebral vein enters the midpoint of the tentorium cerebelli. As it does so, it

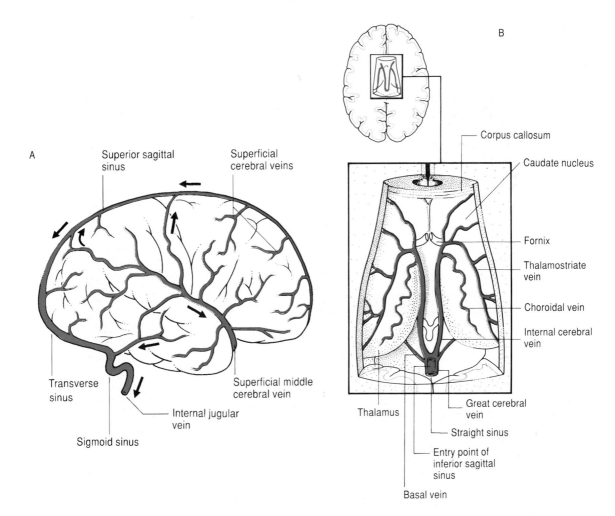

Figure 5.8 Cerebral veins. **(A)** Superficial veins viewed from the right side; arrows indicate direction of blood flow. **(B)** Deep veins viewed from above.

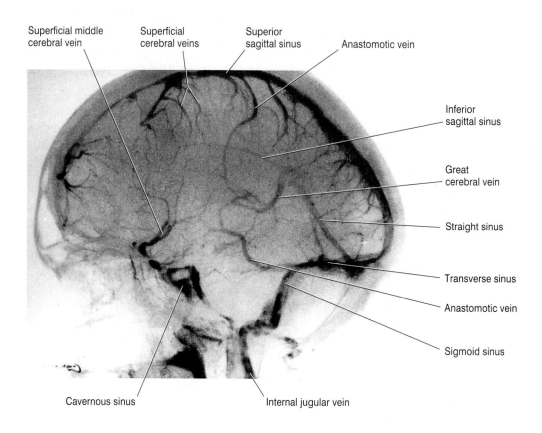

Figure 5.9 Internal carotid angiogram, venous phase. The dye is draining into the dural venous sinuses. (Photograph kindly provided by Dr James Toland, Department of Radiology, Beaumont Hospital, Dublin.)

unites with the **inferior sagittal sinus** to form the **straight sinus**. The straight sinus empties in turn into the **left transverse sinus**.

REGULATION OF BLOOD FLOW

Blood flow in the cerebral vessels is primarily controlled by *autoregulation,* which is defined as the capacity of a tissue to regulate its own blood supply.

The most powerful source of autoregulation in the CNS is the *H+ ion concentration* in the extracellular fluid surrounding the arterioles within the brain parenchyma. Generalized relaxation of arteriolar smooth muscle tone is produced by hypercapnia (excess plasma PCO_2) On the other hand, hypocapnia causes arteriolar vasoconstriction.

A second powerful source of autoregulation is the *intraluminal pressure* within the arterioles. Any increase in pressure elicits a direct, myogenic response. When other factors are controlled (in animal experiments), the myogenic response is sufficient to maintain steady-state perfusion of the brain within a systemic blood pressure range of 80–180 mmHg (11-24 kPa).

Focal blood flow increases within cortical foci and deep nuclei involved in particular motor, sensory or cognitive tasks. The local arteriolar relaxation can be accounted for by a rise in K+ levels caused by propagation of action potentials, and by a rise in H+ caused by increased cell metabolism. At precapillary level neuronal peptides and amines may be significant, the most promising candidate being VIP (vasoactive intestinal polypeptide).

A large number of vasoactive substances have been identified in neural networks surrounding the cerebral conducting arteries and the arterioles. A specific role is difficult to assign to any of them, within the physiological range of blood flow.

THE BLOOD–BRAIN BARRIER

The nervous system is isolated from the blood by a barrier system that provides a stable and chemically optimal environment for neuronal function. The neurons and neuroglia are bathed in brain *extracellular fluid* (ECF) which accounts for 15% of total brain volume.

The extracellular compartments of the CNS are shown diagrammatically in *Figure 5.10*. As previously described (Chapter 4), cerebrospinal fluid (CSF) secreted by the choroid plexuses circulates through the ventricular system and the subarachnoid space before passing through the arachnoid villi into the dural venous sinuses. In addition, CSF diffuses passively through the ependyma–glial membrane lining the ventricles and enters the brain extracellular spaces. It adds to the ECF produced by the capillary bed and by cell metabolism, and it diffuses through the pia–glial membrane into the subarachnoid space. This 'sink' movement of fluid compensates for the absence of lymphatics from the CNS.

Metabolic water is the only component of the CSF which does not pass through the blood–brain barrier. It carries with it any neurotransmitter substances that have not been recaptured following liberation by neurons, and it accounts for the presence in the subarachnoid space of transmitters and transmitter metabolites that could not penetrate the blood–brain barrier.

Relative contributions to the CSF obtained from a spinal tap are approximately as follows:

Choroid plexuses	60%
Capillary bed	30%
Metabolic water	10%

The blood–brain barrier has two components. One is at the level of the choroid plexus, the other resides in the CNS capillary bed.

Blood–CSF barrier

The blood–CSF barrier occupies in the specialized ependymal lining of the choroid plexuses. This **choroidal epithelium** differs from the general ependymal epithelium in three ways:

1 Cilia are almost completely replaced by microvilli.
2 The cells are bonded by tight junctions. These pericellular belts of membrane fusion are the actual site of the blood–CSF barrier.

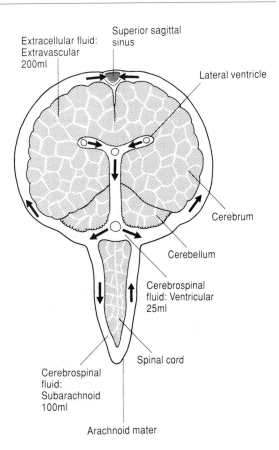

Figure 5.10 Extracellular compartments of the brain. Arrows indicate circulation of cerebrospinal fluid.

3 The epithelium contains numerous enzymes specifically involved in transport of ions and metabolites.

Blood–ECF barrier

The blood–ECF barrier resides in the CNS capillary bed, which differs from that of other tissues in three ways:

1 The endothelial cells are bonded by tight junctions.
2 Pinocytotic vesicles are rare, and fenestrations are absent.
3 The cells contain the same transport systems as those of the choroidal epithelium.

The surface area of the brain capillary bed is about the size of a tennis court. This huge area accounts for the brain's consumption of 20% of basal oxygen intake by the lungs.

FUNCTIONS OF THE BLOOD–BRAIN BARRIER

■ Modulation of the entry of metabolic substrates. Glucose, in particular, is a fundamental source of energy for neurons. The level of glucose in the brain ECF is more stable than that of the blood because the specific carrier becomes saturated when blood glucose rises and becomes hyperactive when it falls.

■ Control of ion movements. Na^+–K^+ ATPase in the barrier cells pumps sodium into the CSF and pumps potassium out of the CSF into the blood.

■ Prevention of access to the CNS by toxins and by peripheral neurotransmitters escaping into the blood stream from autonomic nerve endings.

For some clinical notes concerning the blood-brain barrier, see *Panel 5.1*.

CLINICAL PANEL 5.1

BLOOD–BRAIN BARRIER PATHOLOGY

The following five conditions are associated with breakdown of the blood-brain barrier:

1 Patients suffering from hypertension are liable to attacks of hypertensive encephalopathy should the blood pressure exceed the power of the arterioles to control it. The pressure may then open the tight junctions of the brain capillary endothelium. Rapid exudation of plasma causes cerebral edema with severe headache and vomiting, sometimes progressing to convulsions and coma.

2 In patients with severe hypercapnia brought about by reduced ventilation of the lungs (as in pulmonary or heart disease, or after surgery), relaxation of arteriolar muscle may be sufficient to induce cerebral edema even if the blood pressure is normal. In this case the edema may be expressed by mental confusion and drowsiness progressing to coma.

3 Brain injury, whether from trauma or spontaneous hemorrhage, leads to edema due to the osmotic effects of tissue damage (and other factors).

4 Infections of the brain or meninges are accompanied by breakdown of the blood-brain barrier, perhaps because of the large-scale emigration of leukocytes through the brain capillary bed. The breakdown can be exploited because the porous capillary walls will permit the passage of non-lipid-soluble antibiotics.

5 The capillary bed of brain tumors is fenestrated. As a result, radioactive tracers too large to penetrate healthy brain capillaries can be detected within tumors.

CORE INFORMATION

Arteries

The circle of Willis comprises the anterior communicating artery and two anterior cerebral arteries, the internal carotids, two posterior communicating arteries, and the two posterior cerebral arteries.

The anterior cerebral gives off Heubner's artery to the anteroinferior internal capsule, then arches around the corpus callosum and supplies the medial surface of hemisphere as far back as the parieto–occipital sulcus, with overlap on to the lateral surface.

The middle cerebral artery enters the lateral sulcus and supplies two-thirds of the lateral surface of the hemisphere. Its central branches include the leak-prone lateral striate supplying the upper part of the internal capsule.

The posterior cerebral artery arises from the basilar; it supplies the splenium of corpus callosum and the occipital and temporal cortex.

The vertebral arteries enter the foramen magnum. They supply spinal cord, posterior-inferior cerebellum and medulla oblongata before uniting to form the basilar.

The basilar artery supplies the anterior–inferior and superior cerebellum, the pons and inner ear, before dividing into posterior cerebral arteries.

Veins

Superficial cerebral veins drain the cerebral cortex and empty into dural venous sinuses. The internal cerebral veins drain the thalami and unite as the great cerebral vein. The great veins drain the corpus striatum via the basal vein before entering the straight sinus.

Autoregulation

Hypercapnia causes arteriolar dilatation; hypocapnia causes constriction. A rise of intraluminal pressure produces a direct, myogenic response by arteriolar walls.

Blood–brain barrier

A blood–CSF barrier resides in the choroidal epithelium (modified ependyma) of the ventricles. A blood–ECF barrier resides in the endothelium of the brain capillary bed.

SELF TEST

Select the best response:

1 Which of the following is/are in the territory of the anterior cerebral artery:

A Precentral gyrus
B Postcentral gyrus
C Frontal pole
D All of the above
E A and B only

2 Which of the following is/are in the territory of the middle cerebral artery:

A Precentral gyrus
B Postcentral gyrus
C Temporal pole
D All of the above
E A and B only

3 Which of the following is/are in the territory of the posterior cerebral artery:

A Precentral gyrus
B Postcentral gyrus
C Occipital pole
D All of the above
E A and B only

4 The superficial middle cerebral vein empties into:

A Superior sagittal sinus
B Inferior sagittal sinus
C Transverse sinus
D Straight sinus
E None of the above

5 Sites of the blood brain barrier include:

A Choroidal epithelium
B Brain capillary endothelium
C Astrocyte network
D All of the above
E A and B only

6 Ultrastructural features of the blood brain barrier include:

A Desmosomes
B Tight junctions
C Pinocytotic vesicles
D All of the above
E A and B only

REFERENCES

Duvernoy, H.M. (1978) *Human Brainstem Vessels*. New York: Springer-Verlag.

Gloger, S., Gloger, A., Vogt., H. and Kretschmann, H.-J. (1994) Computer-assisted 3D reconstruction of the terminal branches of the cerebral arteries. *Neuroradiol.* **36:** 173-180; 181-187; 251-257.

Kapp, J.P. (1984) *The Cerebral Venous System and its Disorders*. Orlando: Grune & Stratton.

Sage, M.R. and Wilson, A.J. (1994) The blood-brain barrier: an important concept in neuroimaging. *Am. J. Neuroradiol.* **94:** 601-622.

Wahl, M. and Schilling, L. (1993) Regulation of cerebral blood flow - a brief review. *Acta Neurochir.* **59:** 3-10.

6
NEURONS AND NEUROGLIA

Chapter Summary

Neurons
Internal structure of neurons

Synapses
Electrical synapses
Chemical synapses

Neuroglial cells of the CNS
Astrocytes
Oligodendrocytes
Microglia
Ependyma

CLINICAL PANELS
Clinical relevance of neuronal
   transport
Gliomas
Multiple sclerosis

Study Guidelines

1 Appreciate the challenge faced by many neurons in having to deliver/retrieve materials over enormous distances, and the economy of recycling at nerve endings.
2 Appreciate how a healthy transport system can spread disease in the nervous system.
3 Visualize the three methods of production and loading of synaptic vesicles.
4 Visualize the 'lock and key' analogy used in pharmacology.
5 Draw an axodendritic synapse; then add another axon exerting both pre- and postsynaptic inhibition.
6 Understand why demyelinating disorders compromise conduction.
7 Draw up a structure/function list for neuroglial cells.
8 Gliomas will obviously interfere with brain function in the region they grow. Try to understand how they exert distance effects.

Nerve cells, or **neurons,** are the structural and functional units of the nervous system. They generate and conduct electrical changes in the form of nerve impulses. They communicate chemically with other neurons at points of contact called **synapses. Neuroglia** (literally, 'nerve glue') is the connective tissue of the nervous system.

Neuroglial cells outnumber neurons by about ten to one. They have important nutritive and supportive functions.

NEURONS

Billions of neurons form a shell, or **cortex,** on the surface of the cerebral and cerebellar hemispheres. **Nuclei** are aggregates of neurons buried within the white matter.

In the central nervous system, almost all neurons are multipolar, their cell bodies or **somas** having multiple poles or angles. At every pole but

one, a **dendrite** emerges and divides repeatedly (*Figure 6.1*). On some neurons the shafts of the dendrites are smooth. On others the shafts show numerous short **spines**. The dendrites receive synaptic contacts from other neurons, both on the spines and on the shaft surface.

The remaining pole of the soma gives rise to the **axon,** which conducts nerve impulses. Most axons give off **collateral branches** (*Figure 6.2*). **Terminal** *branches* synapse upon target neurons.

Most synaptic contacts between neurons are either **axodendritic** or **axosomatic.** Axodendritic synapses are usually excitatory in their effect upon target neurons, whereas most axosomatic synapses have an inhibitory effect.

INTERNAL STRUCTURE OF NEURONS

All parts of neurons are permeated by **microtubules** and **neurofilaments** (*Figure 6.3*). The soma contains the nucleus and the cytoplasm or

53

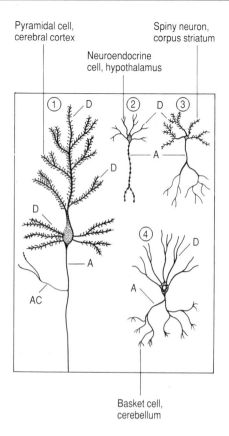

Pyramidal cell, cerebral cortex

Neuroendocrine cell, hypothalamus

Spiny neuron, corpus striatum

Basket cell, cerebellum

Figure 6.1 Profiles of neurons from the brain. **1**, pyramidal cell, cerebral cortex; **2**, neuroendocrine cell, hypothalamus; **3**, spiny neuron, corpus striatum; **4**, basket cell, cerebellum. Neurons **1** and **3** show dendritic spines. A, axon; AC, axon collateral; D, dendrite.

perikaryon (Greek, around the nucleus). The perikaryon contains clumps of granular endoplasmic reticulum known as *Nissl bodies*; also Golgi complexes, free ribosomes, mitochondria, and smooth endoplasmic reticulum (SER).

Intracellular transport

Turnover of membranous and skeletal material takes place in all cells. In neurons, fresh components are continuously synthesized in the soma and moved into the axon and dendrites by a process of *anterograde transport*. At the same time, worn out materials are returned to the soma by *retrograde transport*, for degradation in lysosomes (see also *target recognition*, later).

Anterograde transport is of two kinds, rapid and slow. Included in *rapid* transport (at a speed of 300–400 mm per day) are free elements such as synaptic vesicles, transmitter substances (or their precursor molecules), and mitochondria. Also included are lipid and protein molecules (including receptor proteins) for insertion into the plasma membrane. Included in *slow* transport (at 5–10 mm per day) are the skeletal elements, and soluble proteins including those involved in transmitter release at nerve endings. Microtubules seem to be largely constructed within the axon. They are exported from the soma in preassembled short sheaves which propel one another along the initial segment of the axon; further progress is mainly by a process of elongation (up to 1 mm apiece) performed by the addition of tubulin polymers at their distal ends, with some disassembly at their proximal ends. The bulk movement of neurofilaments slows down to almost zero distally; there, the filaments are refreshed by insertion of filament polymers moving from the soma by slow transport.

Retrograde transport of worn out mitochondria, SER and plasma membrane (including receptors therein) is fairly rapid (150–200 mm per day). In addition to its function in waste disposal, retrograde transport is involved in *target cell recognition*. At synaptic contacts, axons constantly 'nibble' the plasma membrane of target neurons by means of endocytotic vesicular uptake, the vesicles being brought to the soma and incorporated into Golgi complexes there. Uptake of target cell 'marker' molecules is important for cell recognition during development. It may also be necessary for viability later on because adult neurons shrink and may even die if their axons are severed proximal to their first branches.

Transport Mechanisms

Microtubules are the supporting structures for neuronal transport. Microtubule-associated proteins, in the form of ATPases, propel organelles and molecules along the outer surface of the microtubules. Distinct ATPases are used for anterograde and retrograde work.

Neurofilaments do not seem to be involved in the transport mechanism. They are rather evenly spaced, having side-arms that keep them apart and provide skeletal stability by attachment to proteins beneath the axolemmal membrane. Neurofilament numbers are in direct proportion to axonal diameter and the filaments may in truth *determine* axonal diameter.

Some points of clinical relevance are highlighted in Panel 6.1.

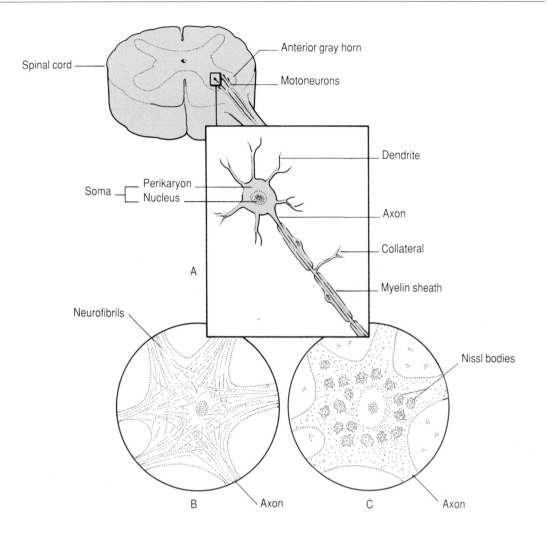

Figure 6.2 Motoneuron from the anterior gray horn of the spinal cord. **(A)** General features; **(B)** neurofibrils (matted neurofilaments) seen after staining with silver salts; **(C)** Nissl bodies (clumps of granular endoplasmic reticulum) seen after staining with a cationic dye such as thionin.

SYNAPSES

CHEMICAL SYNAPSES

Synapses are the points of contact between neurons. Conventional synapses are *chemical*, depending for their effect on the release of a **transmitter substance**. The typical chemical synapse comprises a **presynaptic membrane**, a **synaptic cleft**, and a **postsynaptic membrane** (*Figure 6.4*). The presynaptic membrane belongs to the terminal bouton, the **postsynaptic** membrane to the target neuron. Transmitter substance is released from the bouton by exocytosis, traverses the narrow synaptic cleft and activates receptors in the postsynaptic membrane.

Underlying the postsynaptic membrane is a **subsynaptic web**, in which numerous biochemical changes are initiated by receptor activation.

The bouton contains **synaptic vesicles** loaded with transmitter substance, together with numerous mitochondria and sacs of SER. Following conventional methods of fixation presynaptic dense projections are visible, and microtubules seem to guide the synaptic vesicles to active zones in the intervals between the projections.

Transmitter-loaded synaptic vesicles have three possible sources, as shown in *Figure 6.5*:

1 Some vesicles are formed and loaded in the Golgi apparatus and shipped to the synaptic boutons by rapid transport.

2 Some transmitter precursors and requisite enzymes are shipped to the boutons individually, before being taken into vesicles budded from terminal sacs of SER.

3 Some transmitter molecules are retrieved from the synaptic cleft by endocytosis and returned to the synaptic vesicular pool.

RECEPTOR ACTIVATION

Transmitter molecules cross the synaptic cleft and activate receptor proteins which straddle the postsynaptic membrane (*Figure 6.5*). The activated receptors initiate ionic events that either raise or lower the postsynaptic membrane potential (depending upon the receptor type). The voltage change passes over the soma in a decremental wave called *electrotonus*, and alters the resting potential of the first part or **initial segment** of the axon. (See physiology texts for details of the ionic events.) If excitatory postsynaptic potentials are dominant, the initial segment will be depolarized to threshold and generate a burst of action potentials.

In the CNS, the commonest excitatory transmitter is glutamate; the commonest inhibitory one is γ-aminobutyric acid (GABA). In the PNS, the transmitter for motoneurons supplying muscle is *acetylcholine*; the main transmitter for sensory neurons is *glutamate*.

Many sensory neurons liberate one or more peptides as well as glutamate; the peptides may be shed from any part of the neuron, but their

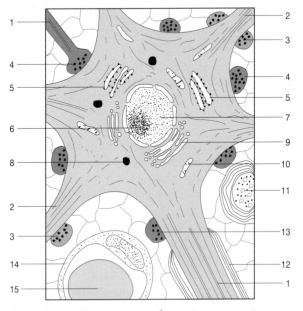

Figure 6.3   Ultrastructure of a motoneuron. **1,** axon; **2,** dendrite; **3,** axodendritic synapse; **4,** axosomatic synapse; **5,** Nissl body; **6,** nucleolus; **7,** nucleus; **8,** lysosome; **9,** Golgi complex; **10,** mitochondrion; **11,** neighboring axon; **12,** myelin; **13,** axo-axonic synapse; **14,** capillary; **15,** erythrocyte.

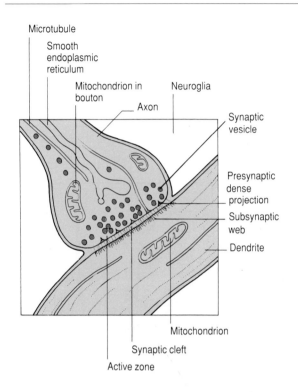

Figure 6.4 Ultrastructure of an axodendritic synapse following conventional tissue fixation.

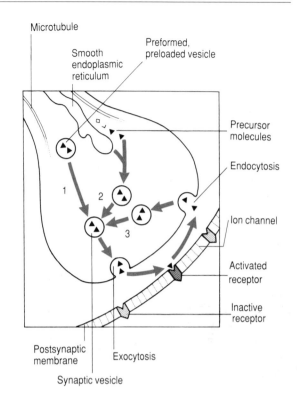

Figure 6.5 Diagram to show origin and fate of synaptic vesicles, and transmitter-receptor binding. For numbers, see text.

usual role is to modulate (raise or lower) the effectiveness of the transmitter.

Lock and key analogy for drug therapy

The receptor may be likened to a lock, the transmitter being the key that operates it. The transmitter output of certain neurons may falter as a consequence of age or disease, and a duplicate key can often be provided in the form of a drug which mimics the action of the transmitter. Such a drug is called an *agonist*. On the other hand, excessive production of a transmitter may be countered by a *receptor blocker*—the equivalent of a dummy key which will occupy the lock without activating it.

Less common chemical synapses

Two varieties of **axo-axonic** synapses are recognized. In both cases the boutons belong to inhibitory neurons. One variety occurs on the initial segment of the axon, where it exercises a powerful veto on impulse generation (*Figure 6.6*). In the second kind, the boutons are applied

to excitatory boutons of other neurons, and they inhibit transmitter release. The effect is called *presynaptic inhibition,* any conventional contact being *postsynaptic* in this context (Figure 6.7).

Dendrodendritic (D-D) synapses occur between dendritic spines of contiguous spiny neurons and alter the electrotonus of the target neuron rather than generating nerve impulses. In *one-way* D-D synapses, one of the two spines contains synaptic vesicles. In *reciprocal* synapses, both do. Excitatory D-D synapses are shown in *Figure 6.8*. Inhibitory D-D synapses are numerous in relay nuclei of the thalamus (Chapter 22).

Somatodendritic and **somatosomatic** synapses have also been identified, but they are scarce.

ELECTRICAL SYNAPSES

Electrical synapses consist of gap junctions (nexuses) between dendrites or somas of contiguous neurons. They permit electrotonic changes to pass from one neuron to another. Their function seems to be to ensure synchronous activity of neurons having a common action. An example is the inspiratory center in the medulla oblongata,

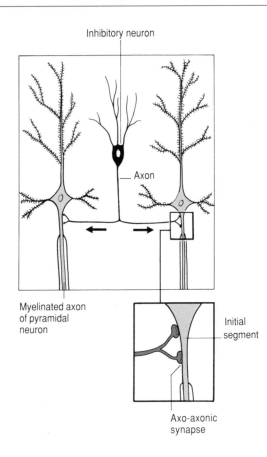

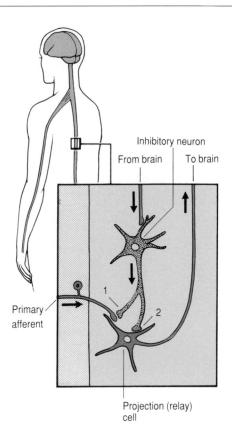

Figure 6.6 Axo-axonic synapses in the cerebral cortex. Arrows indicate direction of impulse conduction.

Figure 6.7 1, Presynaptic and 2, postsynaptic inhibition of a spinal neuron projecting to the brain. Arrows indicate directions of impulse conduction (relay cell may be silenced by inhibitory cell activity).

where all of the cells exhibit synchronous discharge during inspiration.

NEUROGLIAL CELLS OF THE CNS

Four different types of neuroglial cell are found in the CNS: astrocytes, oligodendrocytes, microglia, and ependymal cells.

ASTROCYTES

Astrocytes are bushy cells with dozens of fine radiating processes (*Figure 6.9*). The cytoplasm contains abundant intermediate filaments. This confers a degree of rigidity on these cells which helps to support the brain as a whole. Glycogen granules, which are also abundant, provide an immediate source of glucose for the neurons.

Some astrocyte processes form **glial limiting membranes** on the inner (ventricular) and outer (pial) surfaces of the brain. Other astrocyte pro-

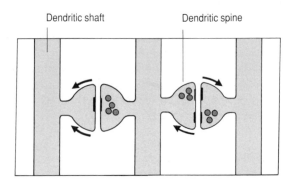

Figure 6.8 Dendrodendritic excitation. The dendrites belong to three separate neurons. On the right is a reciprocal synapse. Arrows indicate direction of electrotonic waves.

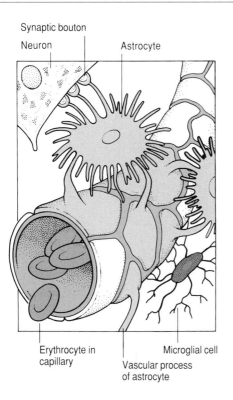

Figure 6.9   Two astrocytes, one microglial cell.

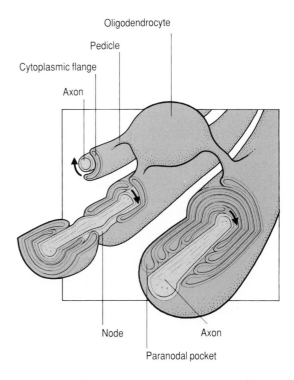

Figure 6.10   Myelination in the CNS. Arrows indicate movement of the growing edge of the cytoplasmic flange of the oligodendrocyte.

cesses are wrapped around capillaries and help to maintain the specialized structure of capillary endothelium in the CNS. Still other processes invest synaptic contacts between neurons.

As well as maintaining the capillary endothelium, three further functions of astrocytes may be mentioned: they are engaged in mopping up K^+ ions during periods of intense neuronal activity; in recycling certain neurotransmitter substances following release (notably the excitatory transmitter, glutamate); and in phagocytosis of decaying synaptic boutons.

Unlike neurons, whose multiplication has ceased around the time of birth, astrocytes can multiply at any time. As part of the healing process following CNS injury, proliferation of astrocytes and their processes results in dense glial scar tissue *(gliosis)*. More importantly, spontaneous local proliferation of astrocytes may give rise to a brain tumor *(Panel 6.2)*.

OLIGODENDROCYTES

Oligodendrocytes are responsible for wrapping myelin sheaths around axons in the white matter

(Figure 6.10). In the gray matter they form **satellite cells** which seem to participate in ion exchange with neurons.

Myelination

Myelination commences during the middle period of gestation, and continues well into the second decade. A single oligodendrocyte lays myelin on upwards of three dozen axons by means of a spiraling process whereby the inner and outer faces of the plasma membrane form the alternating **major** and **minor dense lines** seen in transverse sections of the myelin sheath. Some cytoplasm remains in **paranodal pockets** at the ends of each myelin segment. In the intervals between the glial wrappings the axon is exposed, at **nodes.**

Myelination greatly increases the speed of impulse conduction because the depolarization process jumps from node to node (see Chapter 7). During myelination, K+ ion channels are deleted from the underlying axolemma. For this reason, demyelinating diseases such as multiple sclerosis *(Panel 6.3)* are accompanied by failure of impulse conduction.

CLINICAL PANEL 6.2

GLIOMAS

Brain tumors most commonly originate from neuroglial cells, especially astrocytes.

General symptoms produced by brain tumors are those of *raised intracranial pressure*. They include headache, drowsiness, and vomiting. Radiological investigation may reveal displacement of midline structures to the opposite side. Tumors below the tentorium (usually cerebellar) are likely to block the exit of cerebrospinal fluid from the fourth ventricle, in which case ballooning of the ventricular system will add to the intracranial pressure.

Local symptoms depend upon the position of the tumor. For example, clumsiness of an arm or leg may be caused by a cerebellar tumor on the same side; and motor weakness of an arm or leg may be caused by a cerebral tumor on the opposite side.

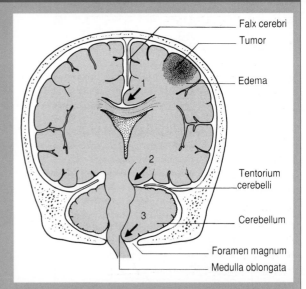

Figure CP 6.2.1 Brain herniations. For numbers, see text.

Progression

Expansion of a tumor may cause one or more brain hernias to develop, as shown in *Figure CP 6.2.1*:

1 *Subfalcal herniation* (in the interval between falx cerebri and corpus callosum) seldom causes specific symptoms.
2 *Uncal herniation* is the term used to denote displacement of the uncus of the temporal lobe into the tentorial notch. Compression of the ipsilateral crus cerebri by the uncus may give rise to *contralateral* motor weakness. Alternatively, compression of the contralateral crus against the sharp edge of the tentorium cerebelli may cause *ipsilateral* motor weakness.
3 *Pressure coning*: a cone of cerebellar tissue (the tonsil) may descend into the foramen magnum, squeezing the medulla oblongata and causing death from respiratory/cardiovascular failure by inactivation of *vital centers* in the reticular formation (Chapter 19).

Unmyelinated axons abound in the gray matter. They are fine (0.2 μm in diameter or less) and not individually ensheathed.

MICROGLIA (*FIGURE 6.9*)

Microglia develop from the neuroepithelium where they have the same percentage as ependymal cells. They are the chief phagocytes of the CNS. Many are close to the blood–brain barrier where they function as immunologically competent cells.

EPENDYMA

Ependymal cells line the ventricular system of the brain. Cilia on their free surface help the propulsion of cerebrospinal fluid through the ventricles.

CLINICAL PANEL 6.3

MULTIPLE SCLEROSIS

Multiple sclerosis (MS) is the commonest neurological disorder of young adults in the temperate latitudes north and south of the equator. It is more prevalent in women, with a female:male ratio of 3:2. The peak age of onset is around 30 years, the range being 15 to 45.

MS is a *primary demyelinating disease:* the initial feature is the development of plaques (patches) of demyelination in the white matter while the axons remain intact. The denuded axons are unable to conduct impulses because K$^+$ channels are normally deleted from the axolemmal membrane when myelin sheaths are initially laid down. Impulse conduction in neighboring myelinated fibers is also compromised by edema (inflammatory exudate). Over time, the plaques are progressively replaced by glial scar tissue and the trapped axons degenerate as well. Old plaques feel firm (sclerotic) in postmortem slices of the brain.

Common locations of early plaques are the cervical spinal cord, upper brainstem, optic nerve, and periventricular white matter including that of the cerebellum. MS is not a systems disease: it is not anatomically selective, and a plaque may involve parts of adjacent motor and sensory pathways.

Presenting symptoms can be correlated with lesion sites, as follows:

- *Motor weakness*, usually in one or both legs, signifies a lesion involving the corticospinal tract.
- *Clumsiness* in reaching and grasping usually accompanies a lesion in the cerebellar white matter.
- *Numbness/tingling*, often spreading up from the legs to the trunk, may be caused by a lesion in the posterior white matter of the spinal cord.
- *Diplopia* (double vision) may be produced by a plaque within the pons or midbrain affecting the function of one of the ocular motor nerves.
- A *scotoma* (patch of blindness in the visual field of one eye) is produced by a plaque within the optic nerve.
- *Urinary retention* (failure of the bladder to empty) can be caused by interruption of the central autonomic pathway descending from the brainstem to the lower part of the cord.

The usual course of the disease is one of remissions and relapses, with an overall slow progression and development of multiple disabilities.

CORE INFORMATION

Neurons

The multipolar neuron of the CNS comprises soma, dendrites, and axon; the axon gives off collateral and terminal branches. The soma contains rough and smooth ER, Golgi complexes, neurofilaments, and microtubules. Microtubules pervade the entire neuron; they are involved in anterograde transport of synaptic vesicles, mitochondria, and membranous replacement material; and in retrograde transport of marker molecules and degraded organelles.

Anatomical varieties of chemical synapse include axodendritic, axosomatic, axo–axonic, and dendrodendritic. Structure includes pre- and postsynaptic membranes, synaptic cleft and subsynaptic web. Synaptic vesicles are synthesized in the soma, from terminal SER, and by endocytosis.

Neuroglia

Astrocytes have supportive, nutritive and retrieval functions, and they maintain integrity of the blood–brain barrier. They are the main source of brain tumors. Oligodendrocytes form CNS myelin sheaths, which are subject to destruction in demyelinating diseases. Microglia are phagocytes.

SELF TEST

Match features on the left with the functions on the right:

1	Microtubules	A	Protein synthesis
2	Nissl bodies	B	Rapid transport
3	Neurofilaments	C	Neurotransmission
4	Synaptic vesicles	D	Skeletal stability
5	Axodendritic synapses	A	Mostly excitatory
6	Axosomatic synapses	B	Mostly inhibitory
7	Axoaxonic synapses	C	Sometimes reciprocal
8	Dendrodendritic synapses	D	Presynaptic inhibition
9	Astrocytes	A	Assist CSF movement
10	Oligodendrocyte	B	Lay down myelin
11	Microglia	C	Retrieve transmitters
12	Ependymal cells	D	Are phagocytes

REFERENCES

Federoff, S. (1995) Development of microglia. In *Neuroglia* (Kettenmann, H. and Ransom, B.R., eds), pp. 163–184. New York: Oxford University Press.

Gehrmann, J., Matsumoto, Y. and Kreutzberg, D.W. (1995) Microglia: intrinsic immunoeffector cells of the brain. *Brain Res. Rev.* **20**: 269-267.

Golding, D.W. (1994) Synaptic, non-synaptic and parasynaptic exocytosis. *BioEssays* **16**: 503-508.

Graftstein B. (1995) Axonal transport: function and mechanisms. In *The Axon* (Waxman, S. Kocsis, J.D. and Stys, P.K., eds), pp. 185–199. New York: Oxford University Press.

Lee, R.M.K.W. (1995) Morphology of cerebral arteries. *Pharmacol. Therap.* **66**: 149-173.

Mercer, J.A. Albanesi, J.P. and Brady, S.T. (1994) Molecular motors and cell motility in the brain. *Brain Path.* **4**: 167-179.

Morell, P. and Quarles, R.H. (1989) Formation, structure, and biochemistry of myelin. In *Basic Neurochemistry: Molecular, Cellular, and Medical Aspects*, 4th edn (Siegel, G.J. *et al.*, eds), pp.109-138. New York: Raven Press.

Norenberg, M.D. (1994) Astrocyte responses to injury. *J. Neuropath. Exp. Neurol.* **53**: 213-220.

Privat, A., Giminez-Robotta, M., and Ridet, J–L. (1995) Morphology of astrocytes. In *Neuroglia* (Kettenmann, H. and Ransom, B.R., eds), pp. 3–22. New York: Oxford University Press.

Raine, C.S. (1989) Neurocellular anatomy. In *Basic Neurochemistry: Molecular, Cellular, and Medical Aspects*, 4th edn (Siegel, G.J. *et al.*, eds), pp. 3-33. New York: Raven Press.

Sano, Y. (1989) Morphological aspects of neurons as secretory cells. *Arch. Histol. Cytol.* **52**: 107-112.

Volknandt, W. (1995) The synaptic vesicle and its targets. *Neurosci.* **64**: 277-300.

Waxman, S.G. (1987) Molecular neurobiology of the myelinated nerve fiber: ion-channel distributions and their implications for demyelinating diseases. In *Molecular Neurobiology in Neurology and Psychiatry* (Kandel E.R., ed.), pp. 7-37. New York: Raven Press.

7

PERIPHERAL NERVES

Chapter Summary

General features

Microscopic structure

Degeneration and regeneration
Wallerian degeneration of peripheral nerves
Regeneration of peripheral nerves
Degeneration in the CNS
Regeneration in the CNS

Study Guidelines

1 Understand where the limb plexuses fit into the general scheme of the spinal nerves.
2 Identify the sheath covering a nerve trunk; a fascicle; a fiber.
3 Be able to draw and label a myelinated fiber.
4 Understand how myelin sheaths are composed of cell membranes.
5 Appreciate the functional significance of the nodes of Ranvier, and why thicker fibers conduct faster.
6 Understand why nerves regenerate better after a crush injury than after a cut.
7 Recognize the two kinds of transneuronal atrophy.
8 Learn more about CNS transplants from review articles!

GENERAL FEATURES

The peripheral nerves comprise the cranial and spinal nerves linking the brain and spinal cord to the peripheral tissues. The neurons contributing to peripheral nerves are partly contained within the central nervous system. The cells giving rise to the motor (*efferent*) nerves to skeletal muscles occupy the CNS gray matter, and the central processes of peripheral sensory (*afferent*) neurons enter the white matter before making contact with other neurons (*Figure 7.1*).

The spinal nerves supply *somatic efferent fibers* to the skeletal muscles of the trunk and limbs, and *somatic afferent fibers* to the skin, muscles and joints. They all carry *visceral efferent,* autonomic fibers and some carry visceral afferent fibers as well. The cranial nerves are more diverse, and collectively also include *branchial efferent fibers* for the supply of muscles that originated from the branchial arches in embryonic life, and *special sense afferents* serving smell, taste, hearing and balance.

The spinal nerves are formed by the union of **anterior** and **posterior nerve roots** at their points of exit from the vertebral canal. The **spinal nerve**

proper is only 1 cm long and occupies an intervertebral foramen. Upon emerging from the foramen it divides into **anterior** and **posterior rami**. Posterior rami supply the erector spinae muscles and the overlying skin. Anterior rami supply the muscles and skin of the side and front of the trunk, including the limbs; they also supply sensory fibers to the parietal pleura and parietal peritoneum.

The cervical, brachial and lumbosacral plexuses are derived from anterior rami, which form the roots of the plexuses. The term 'root' therefore has two different meanings, depending on the context.

MICROSCOPIC STRUCTURE

Figure 7.2 illustrates the structure of a typical peripheral nerve. It is not possible to designate individual nerve fibers as motor or sensory on the basis of structural features alone.

Peripheral nerves are invested with **epineurium,** a loose, vascular connective tissue sheath surrounding the fascicles (bundles of fibers) that make up the nerve. Nerve fibers are exchanged between fascicles along the course of the nerve.

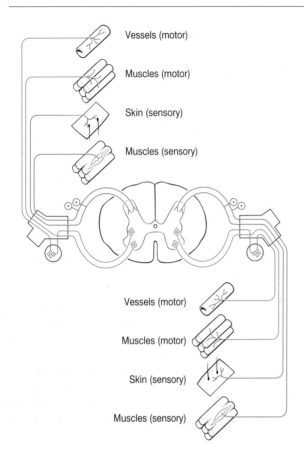

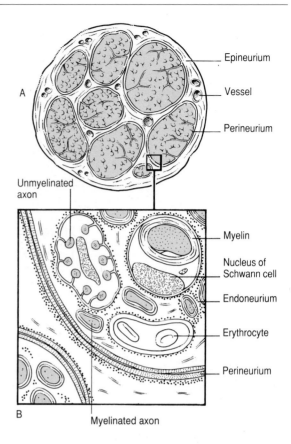

Figure 7.1 Fiber composition of a thoracic spinal nerve. *Left:* components of a posterior ramus. *Right:* components of an anterior ramus.

Figure 7.2 Transverse section of a nerve trunk. **(A)** Light microscopy; **(B)** electron microscopy.

Each fascicle is covered by **perineurium,** composed of several layers of pavement epithelium bonded by tight junctions. Surrounding the individual Schwann cells is a network of reticular collagenous fibers, the **endoneurium.**

Less than half of the nerve fibers are enclosed in myelin sheaths. The remaining, unmyelinated fibers travel in deep gutters along the surface of Schwann cells.

The term 'nerve fiber' is usually used in the context of nerve impulse conduction, where it is equivalent to 'axon'. An anatomical definition is possible for a myelinated fiber: it comprises axon, myelin and neurolemmal sheaths, and endoneurium. A definition is not possible for unmyelinated axons because they share neurolemmal and endoneurial sheaths.

MYELIN FORMATION

The **Schwann cell** is the representative neuroglial cell of the peripheral nervous system. It forms chains of **neurolemmal cells** along the nerves. Modified Schwann cells form **satellite cells** in posterior root ganglia (Chapter 12) and **teloglia** at encapsulated sensory nerve endings (Chapter 9).

If an axon is to be myelinated, it receives the simultaneous attention of a sequence of Schwann cells along its length. Each one encloses the axon completely, creating a 'mesentery' of plasma membrane, the **mesaxon** (Figure 7.3). The mesaxon is displaced progressively, being rotated around the axon. Successive layers of plasma membrane come into apposition to form the **major** and **minor dense lines** (see histology texts for myelin ultrastructure).

Paranodal pockets of cytoplasm persist at the ends of the myelin segments, on each side of the nodes of Ranvier. (Louis Ranvier discovered them 80 years before CNS nodes were seen in the electron microscope in the early 1960s.) The paranodal pockets may be responsible for maintaining the dense population (about 10^5) of Na^+ channels in the nodal plasma membrane.

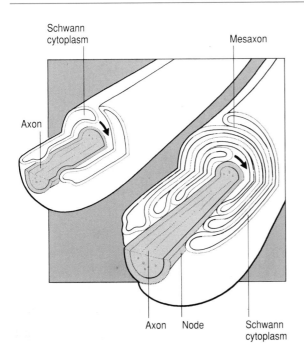

Schwann cytoplasm

Mesaxon

Axon

Axon Node Schwann cytoplasm

Figure 7.3 Myelination in peripheral nervous system. Arrows indicate movement of flange of Schwann cytoplasm.

Myelin expedites conduction

Along unmyelinated fibers impulse conduction is *continuous* (uninterrupted). Its maximum speed is 15 m/s (meters per second). Along myelinated fibers excitable membrane is confined to the nodes of Ranvier because myelin is an electrical insulator. Impulse conduction is called *saltatory* ('jumping') because it jumps from node to node. Speed of conduction is much greater along myelinated fibers, with a maximum of 120 m/s. The number of impulses that can be conducted by myelinated fibers is also much greater.

The larger the myelinated fiber the more rapid the conduction, because larger fibers have longer internodal segments and the nerve impulses take longer 'strides' between nodes. A 'rule of six' can be used to express the ratio between size and speed: a fiber of 10 µm external diameter will conduct at 60 meters per second, one of 15 µm at 90 m/s, and so on.

In physiological recordings, peripheral nerve fibers are classified in accordance with conduction velocities and other criteria. Motor fibers are classified into Groups A, B, and C in descending order. Sensory fibers are classified into Types I–IV. In practice, there is some interchange of usages: for example, unmyelinated sensory fibers are usually called C fibers rather than Type IV.

DEGENERATION AND REGENERATION

When nerves are cut or crushed, their axons degenerate distal to the lesion, because axons are pseudopodial outgrowths and depend on their parent cells for survival. In the peripheral nervous system regeneration is vigorous and it is often complete. In the CNS, on the other hand, it is neither vigorous nor complete.

WALLERIAN DEGENERATION OF PERIPHERAL NERVES (WALLER, 1816–1870)

The principal events in peripheral nerve degeneration are represented in *Figure 7.4* and described in the caption. Following a crush or cut injury to a nerve, the axons and myelin sheaths distal to the cut break up to form 'ellipsoids' during the first 48 hours—mainly because of lysosomal activity by Schwann cells. The debris is cleared by monocytes which enter the damaged endoneurial sheaths from the blood and become macrophages. The end result of degeneration is a shrunken nerve skeleton with intact connective tissue and perineurial sheaths, and a core of intact Schwann cells.

REGENERATION OF PERIPHERAL NERVES

The principal events in regeneration of a peripheral nerve are summarized in *Figure 7.5*. Following a clean cut, axons begin to sprout from the face of the proximal stump within a few hours, but in the more common crush or tear injuries seen clinically, the axons die back for 1 cm or more and sprouting may be delayed for a week. Successful regeneration requires that the axons make contact with Schwann cells of the distal stump (or at least with their basement membranes). Failure to make contact leads to production of a *neuroma* consisting of whorls of regenerating axons trapped in scar tissue at the site of the initial injury. Following amputation of a limb, an *amputation neuroma* can be a source of severe pain.

Successful nerve tips exhibit swellings called **growth cones**, from which fine **filopodia** extend along Schwann cell basement membranes. The filopodia develop surface receptors which become anchored temporarily to complementary molecules in the basement membrane. Filaments of actin within the filopodia become attached to the surface receptors; from these points of anchorage they are able to exert onward traction on the growth cones.

Degeneration

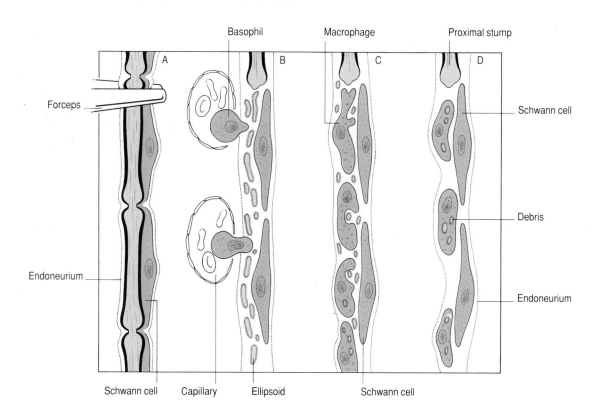

Figure 7.4 Events in degeneration of a single myelinated nerve fiber. **(A)** Intact fiber, showing its four components. The fiber is being pinched at its upper end. **(B)** The myelin and axon have broken up into 'ellipsoids' and droplets. Monocytes are entering the endoneurial tube from the blood. **(C)** The droplets are being engulfed by monocytes. **(D)** Clearance of debris is almost complete. Schwann cells and endoneurium remain intact.

Growth cones are mitogenic to Schwann cells, which complete a single mitotic cycle before wrapping the larger axons with myelin lamellae.

Regeneration proceeds at about 5 mm per day in the larger nerve trunks, slowing down to 2 mm per day in the finer branches. If appropriate endoneurial tubes have been entered, complete functional recovery is likely. Good recovery depends on accurate alignment of proximal and distal stumps, because sensory axons are quite capable of growing along former motor tubes, and motor sprouts along sensory ones. For this reason the outlook is better following a crush injury (endoneurium preserved) than a cut.

When nerve trunks have been completely severed, it is common practice to wait about 3 weeks before attempting repair. By that time, the con-nective tissue sheaths will have thickened a little and will be better able to hold suture material than are freshly injured, edematous sheaths. Moreover, the trimming of the nerves required before insertion of sutures creates a second axotomy, on the axons emerging from the proximal stump. In animal experiments, a second axotomy induces a more vigorous and sustained regenerative response.

Upstream effects of nerve section

■ Within a few days of axotomy, Nissl bodies can no longer be identified by cationic dyes in parent cells in the dorsal root ganglia and spinal gray matter (*Figure 7.6*). The phenomenon is known as *chromatolysis* ('loss of color'). Electron microscopy reveals that the

Regeneration

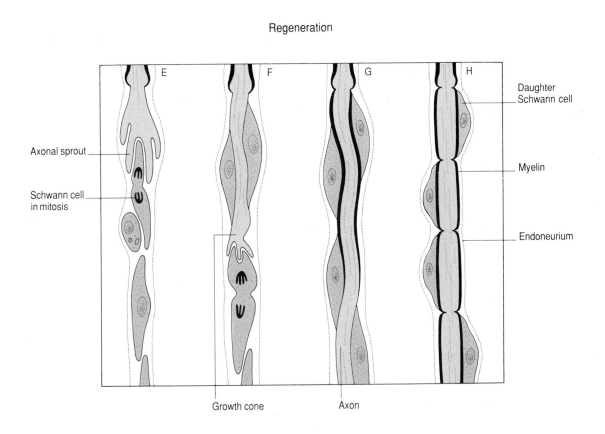

Figure 7.5 Events in regeneration. **(E)** An axonal sprout has entered the distal stump. The sprout is mitogenetic to each Schwann cell it encounters. **(F)** The growth cone is extending distally along the surface of Schwann cells. **(G)** Myelination is commencing along the proximal part of the regenerating axon. **(H)** When regeneration is complete the fiber has a normal appearance but the myelin segments are shorter than the originals.

granular endoplasmic reticulum is in fact increased in amount. Instead of being in clumps it is dispersed throughout the perikaryon, with accumulations deep to the plasma membrane.

■ The nucleus becomes eccentric due to osmotic changes in the perikaryon.

■ Parent motoneurons become isolated from synaptic contacts by the intrusion of neuroglial cells into all of the synaptic clefts.

DEGENERATION IN THE CNS

Following injury to the white matter, distal degeneration occurs after the manner of peripheral nerves. However, clearance of debris by microglial cells and fresh monocytes is much slower. Debris can still be identified after 6

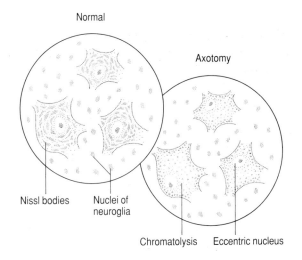

Figure 7.6 Reaction of motoneurons to injury. (Nissl stain; the axon is below, for each cell.)

months in the CNS, whereas in peripheral nerves it is virtually cleared in 6 days.

Chromatolysis is unusual in the CNS. Instead, large-scale necrosis (death) of injured neurons is the rule. Neurons that survive may appear wasted, with permanent isolation from synaptic contacts.

Transneuronal atrophy

CNS neurons have a trophic (sustaining) effect upon one another. If the main input to a group of neurons is destroyed, the group is likely to waste away and die. This is known as *orthograde transneuronal atrophy*. It is comparable to the atrophy that occurs in skeletal muscle when its motor nerve is cut. In some situations *retrograde transneuronal degeneration* takes place, in neurons upstream to those destroyed by the lesion.

End result of CNS injury

If the lesion has been small, the neuronal debris is ultimately replaced by a glial scar composed of astrocyte processes. A large lesion may result in cystic cavities walled by scar tissue, containing cerebrospinal fluid and hemolyzed blood.

REGENERATION IN THE CNS

Remarkable degrees of functional recovery are often observed after CNS lesions. However, injured motor and sensory pathways do not re-establish their original connections. They regenerate for a few millimeters at most, and such synapses as develop are upon other neurons close to the site of injury.

One of the most active areas in neurobiological research is the use of embryonic nervous tissue to replace neurons that have been lost due to injury or disease. The mammalian CNS in general seems to be lacking in *trophic factors* required for successful regeneration. Such factors are evidently present in embryonic neurons because when these are transplanted (with immunological precautions) into adult brain they grow well. This approach is beginning to be applied to patients having restricted areas of brain pathology—notably Parkinson's disease (Chapter 25).

CORE INFORMATION

Structure
Spinal nerves occupy intervertebral foramina. They are formed by union of anterior (motor) and posterior (sensory) nerve roots and they divide into (mixed) anterior and posterior rami. The roots of the limb plexuses are in fact anterior rami. Peripheral nerves have an outer, epineurial connective tissue sheath, a fascicular perineurial sheath, and an endoneurial collagenous sheath investing Schwann cells. A myelinated fiber comprises axon, myelin sheath, Schwann cytoplasm (neurolemma), and endoneurium. Myelin sheaths are derived from chains of Schwann cells; they give rise to saltatory conduction of nerve impulses, at a rate proportionate to fiber diameter.

Degeneration and regeneration
Separation of fibers from parent somas causes axons and myelin sheaths to break down, the debris being removed by phagocytes. Neurolemmal and connective tissue sheaths survive. Axons regenerate by sprouting along vacated neurolemmal sheaths while exhibiting growth cones with filopodia. Motor and sensory end organs may be successfully reinnervated, and fresh myelin sheaths formed.

SELF TEST

Select the best response:

1 Somatic efferent nerve fibers occupy:

A Anterior nerve roots
B Spinal nerves
C Anterior rami
D Posterior rami
E All of the above

2 The lumbosacral plexus is composed of:
A Anterior nerve roots
B Posterior nerve roots
C Anterior rami
D Posterior rami
E All of the above

3 The territory of posterior rami includes:
A Erector spinae muscles
B Limb muscles
C Parietal pleura
D Skin of hand
E None of the above

4 Unmyelinated axons are also called:
A A fibers
B B fibers
C C fibers
D Type 1 fibers
E None of the above

5 Structure(s) degenerating in the distal stump of a cut nerve include:
A Axons
B Myelin sheaths
C Schwann cells
D Connective tissue
E A and B only

6 Structure(s) surviving in the distal stump of a cut nerve include:
A Axons
B Myelin sheaths
C Schwann cells
D Connective tissue
E C and D only

REFERENCES

Berthold, C.H. and Rydmark, M. (1995) Morphology of normal peripheral axons. In *The Axon* (Waxman, S. Kocsis, J.D. and Stys, P.K., eds), pp. 13–48. New York: Oxford University Press.

Birch, R., Bonney, G., Payan, J., Wynn Parry, C.B., and Iggo, A. (1986) Peripheral nerve injuries. *J. Bone Joint Surg.* **68B:** 2–21.

Bisby, M.A. Regeneration of peripheral nervous system axons. In *The Axon* (Waxman, S., Kocsis, J.D. and Stys, P.K., eds), pp. 355–374. New York: Oxford University Press.

Boyer, K.L. and Bakay, R.A.E. (1995) The history, theory and present status of brain transplantation. *Neurosurg. Clin. N. Am.* **6:** 113–125.

Gag, F.H. and Fisher, L.J. (1991) Intracerebral grafting: a tool for the neurobiologist. *Neuron* **6:** 1–12.

Goldberg, D.J. and Burmeister, D.W. (1989) Looking into growth cones. *Trends Neurosci.* **12:** 503–506.

Ide, C. and Kato, S. (1990) Peripheral nerve regeneration. *Neurosci. Res. Suppl.* **13:** S157–S164.

Koutouzis, T.K., Emerich, D.F., Bourlongan, C.V., Freeman, T.B., Cahill, D.W., and Sanberg, P.R. (1944) Cell transplantation for central nervous disorders. *Crit. Rev. Neurobiol.* **8:** 125–162.

McQuarry, I.G. (1988) Cytoskeleton of the regenerating axon. In *Current Issues in Neural Regeneration Research*, pp. 23–32. New York: Alan R. Liss.

O'Reilly, P.M.R. and FitzGerald, M.J.T. (1985) Internodal segments in human laryngeal nerves. *J. Anat.* **140:** 645–650.

Stoll, G., Griffin, J.W., Li, C.Y., and Trapp, R.D. (1989) Wallerian degeneration in the peripheral nervous system: participation of both Schwann cells and macrophages in myelin degradation. *J. Neurocytol.* **18:** 671–683.

Tetzlaff, W., Graeber, M.B., and Kreutzberg, G.W. (1986). Reaction of motoneurons and their microenvironment to axotomy. *Exp. Brain Res. Suppl.* **13:** S3–8.

8

INNERVATION OF MUSCLES AND JOINTS

<table>
<tr><td>

Chapter Summary

Motor innervation of skeletal muscle
Motor end plates
Motor units in old age

Sensory innervation of skeletal muscle
Neuromuscular spindles
Tendon endings
Free nerve endings

Innervation of joints

CLINICAL PANEL
Myasthenia gravis

</td><td>

Study Guidelines

1 Try to appreciate the vast significance of motor units with respect to movements of all kinds; and to appreciate the functional significance of their sizes and muscle chemistries.
2 Learn to sketch a motor end plate indicating locations of transmitter, receptors and hydrolytic enzyme.
3 Sketch an intrafusal muscle fiber indicating location of two motor and two sensory nerve endings.
4 Explain how spindles in quadriceps may/may not be unloaded during extension of the knee.
5 Draw a section of spinal cord; on one side show the segmental connections of a 1a fiber; on the other, those of a 1b fiber.

</td></tr>
</table>

In gross anatomy, the nerves to skeletal muscles are branches of mixed peripheral nerves. The branches enter the muscles about one-third of the way along their length, at *motor points* (*Figure 8.1*). Motor points have been identified for all major muscle groups, for the purpose of *functional electrical stimulation* by physical therapists, in order to increase muscle power.

Only 60% of the axons in the nerve to a given muscle are motor to the muscle fibers that make up the bulk of the muscle. The rest are sensory in nature although the largest sensory receptors—the neuromuscular spindles—have a motor supply of their own.

MOTOR INNERVATION OF SKELETAL MUSCLE

The nerve of supply branches within the muscle belly, forming a plexus from which groups of axons emerge to supply the muscle fibers (*Figure 8.1*). The axons supply single motor end plates placed about half way along the muscle fibers (*Figure 8.2A*).

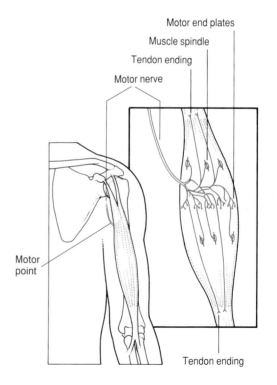

Figure 8.1 Pattern of innervation of skeletal muscle.

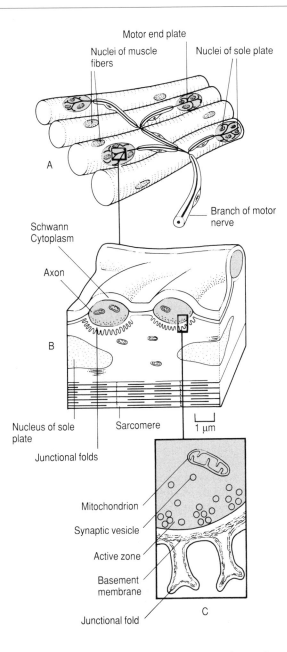

Figure 8.2 Motor nerve supply to skeletal muscle. **(A)** Four motor end plates supplied from a single axon; **(B)** enlargement from **(A)**; **(C)** enlargement from **(B)** showing active zones.

A *motor unit* comprises a motor neuron in the spinal cord or brainstem together with the *squad* of muscle fibers it innervates. In large muscles (e.g. the flexors of the hip or knee) each motor unit contains 1000 muscle fibers or more. In small muscles (e.g. the intrinsic muscles of the hand) each unit contains ten muscle fibers or less. Small units contribute to the finely graded contractions used for delicate manipulations.

There are three different types of skeletal muscle fiber:

1 *Slow-twitch, oxidative (SO) fibers* are small, rich in mitochondria and blood capillaries (hence, they are red). They exert small forces and are fatigue resistant. They are deeply placed and suited to sustained postural activities, including standing.
2 *Fast, glycolytic (FG) fibers* are large, mitochondria poor, and capillary poor (hence, white). They produce brief, powerful contractions. They predominate in superficial muscles.
3 *Intermediate (fast, oxidative-glycolytic, FOG)* fibers have properties intermediate between the other two. Every muscle contains all three kinds of fiber, but a given motor unit contains only one kind. The fibers of each unit interdigitate with those of other units.

MOTOR END PLATES

At the **myoneural junction** the axon forms a handful of branchlets which groove the surface of the muscle fiber (*Figure 8.2B*). The underlying sarcolemma is thrown into **junctional folds**. The basement membrane of the muscle fiber traverses the synaptic cleft and lines the folds. The underlying sarcoplasm shows an accumulation of nuclei, mitochondria and ribosomes known as a **sole plate**.

Each axonal branchlet forms an elongated terminal bouton, containing thousands of synaptic vesicles loaded with acetylcholine (ACh). Synaptic transmission takes place at **active zones** facing the crests of the junctional folds (*Figure 8.2C*). ACh is extruded by exocytosis into the synaptic cleft. It diffuses through the basement membrane to reach ACh receptors in the sarcolemma. Activation of the receptors leads to depolarization of the sarcolemma. The depolarization is led into the interior of the muscle fiber by T-tubules. The sarcoplasmic reticulum liberates $Ca2^+$ ions which initiate contraction of the sarcomeres (see biochemistry texts for details).

Cholinesterase enzyme is concentrated in the basement membrane, and about 30% of released ACh is hydrolyzed without reaching the postsynaptic membrane. After hydrolysis, the choline moiety is returned to the axoplasm.

MOTOR UNITS IN OLD AGE

The progressive wasting of muscles seen in the

elderly is due to loss of motoneurons from the spinal cord and brainstem, and to low-grade peripheral neuropathy arising from vascular disease and often from nutritional deficiency. Electromyographic (EMG) records taken from contracting muscles show *giant motor unit potentials* during the seventh and eighth decades. The extra-large potentials result from takeover of vacated motor end plates of lost motoneurons, by collateral sprouts from the axons of adjacent healthy motor units.

The commonest disorder of the myoneural junction is *myasthenia gravis (Panel 8.1)*.

SENSORY INNERVATION OF SKELETAL MUSCLE

NEUROMUSCULAR SPINDLES

Muscle spindles are up to l cm in length and vary in number from a dozen to several hundred in different muscles. They are abundant (a) in the antigravity muscles along the vertebral column, femur and tibia; (b) in the muscles of the neck; and (c) in the intrinsic muscles of the hand. All of these muscles are rich in slow, oxidative muscle fibers. Spindles are scarce where FG or FOG fibers predominate.

Muscle spindles contain up to a dozen **intrafusal muscle fibers** (*Figure 8.3*). (Ordinary muscle

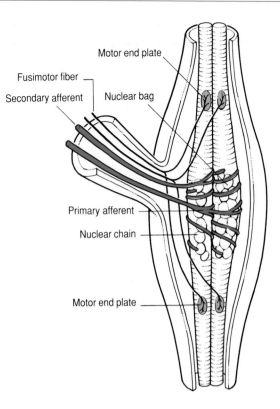

Figure 8.3 Representative pattern of innervation of a neuromuscular spindle. One bag muscle fiber and one chain muscle fiber are shown. The primary afferent is supplying both, the secondary afferent is supplying the chain fiber. Fusimotor fibers are supplying the striated segments of both.

MYASTHENIA GRAVIS

The ACh receptors of skeletal muscle normally undergo turnover with a half-life (i.e. a 50% loss) of 10 days. New receptors are constantly synthesized in Golgi complexes located around the nuclei of the sole plate and inserted into the sarcolemma of the junctional folds. Old receptors are removed by endocytosis and degraded by lysosomes.

In myasthenia gravis, the immune system produces antibodies to the ACh receptor. The antigen-antibody complex has a half–life of only 2 days, leading to a progressive loss of receptors and of junctional folds. Muscles most affected are those supplied by cranial nerves.

Clinically, myasthenia gravis is characterized by weakness and easy fatigue of the muscles of the orbit, face, and mouth. The limbs are sometimes affected as well. In severe cases, weakness of the muscles of swallowing and respiration may be life-threatening.

Administration of an anticholinesterase drug such as neostigmine can be both diagnostic and therapeutic. By prolonging the binding time of ACh with the remaining receptors, it usually causes prompt improvement in muscle power.

The abnormal antibodies seem to originate in the thymus gland, which is usually hyperplastic in these cases and contains a lymphoid tumor in 10% of patients. Removal of the thymus may be beneficial if symptoms cannot be otherwise controlled.

fibers are extrafusal in this context.) The larger intrafusal fibers emerge from the **poles** (ends) of the spindle and are anchored to connective tissue (perimysium). The smaller ones are anchored to the collagenous spindle capsule. At the spindle **equator** (middle), the sarcomeres are replaced almost entirely by nuclei, in the form of 'bags' (in large fibers) or 'chains' (in small fibers).

Innervation

Spindles have a motor as well as a sensory nerve supply. The motor fibers, called *fusimotor*, are in the Aγ size range, in contrast to the Aα fibers supplying extrafusal muscle. The fusimotor axons divide to supply the striated segments at both ends of the intrafusal muscles (*Figure 8.3*). A single *primary* sensory fiber of Type Ia caliber forms *annulospiral* wrappings around the bag/chain segments of the intrafusal muscle fibers. *Secondary* sensory endings are found on one or both sides of the primary; they are supplied by Type II fibers.

Activation

Muscle spindles are *stretch receptors*. Ion channels in the surface membrane of the sensory terminals are opened by stretch, creating positive electrotonic waves which summate close to the final heminode of the parent sensory fiber. Summation produces a *receptor potential* which will fire off nerve impulses when it reaches threshold.

Muscle spindles may be stretched either *passively* or *actively*.

Passive Stretch

Passive stretch of muscle spindles occurs when an entire muscle belly is passively lengthened. For example, in eliciting a tendon reflex such as the *knee jerk*, the spindles in the belly of the muscle are passively stretched when the tendon is struck. The Type Ia and Type II fibers discharge to the spinal cord, where they synapse upon the dendrites of α motoneurons (*Figure 8.4*). (α motoneurons are so called because they give rise to axons of Aα diameter.) The response to the *positive feedback* from spindles is a twitch of contraction in the extrafusal muscle fibers. The spindles, because they lie in parallel with the extrafusal muscle, are passively shortened; they are described as being *unloaded*.

Tendon reflexes are mainly *monosynaptic*

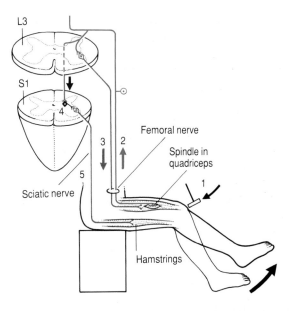

Figure 8.4 Patellar reflex, including reciprocal inhibition. Arrows indicate nerve impulses. **(1)** A tap to the patellar ligament stretches the spindles in quadriceps femoris. **(2)** Spindles discharge excitatory impulses to the spinal cord. **(3)** α motoneurons respond by eliciting a twitch in quadriceps, with extension of the knee. **(4,5)** Ia inhibitory internuncials respond by suppressing any activity in the hamstrings.

reflexes. They have a *latency* (stimulus-response interval) of about 15-25 msec.

In addition to exciting homonymous motoneurons (that is, motoneurons supplying the same muscles), the spindle afferents *inhibit* the α motoneurons supplying the antagonist muscles, through the medium of inhibitory internuncial (interposed) neurons (*Figure 8.4*). This effect is called *reciprocal inhibition*. The inhibitory neurons involved are called *Ia internuncials*.

Information Coding

Spindle primary afferents are most active *during* the stretching process. The more rapid the stretch, the more impulses they fire off. They therefore encode the *rate* of stretch.

Spindle secondary afferents are more active than the primaries when a given position is held. The greater the degree of *maintained* stretch, the more impulses they fire off. They therefore encode the *degree* of muscle stretch.

Active Stretch

Active stretch is produced by the fusimotor

neurons, which elicit contraction of the striated segments of the intrafusal muscle fibers. The connective tissue attachments being relatively fixed, the intrafusal fibers *stretch the spindle equators* by pulling them in the direction of the spindle poles. (This could be called a Christmas-cracker effect.)

During voluntary movements, alpha and gamma motoneurons are *coactivated* by the corticospinal (pyramidal) tract. As a result, the spindles are *not* unloaded by extrafusal muscle contraction. Through ascending connections, the spindle afferents on both sides of the relevant joints are able to keep the brain informed about contractions and relaxations during any given movement.

TENDON ENDINGS

Golgi tendon organs are found at muscle-tendon junctions (*Figure 8.5*). A single Ib caliber nerve fiber forms elaborate sprays which intertwine with tendon fiber bundles enclosed within a connective tissue capsule.

A dozen or more muscle fibers insert into the intracapsular tendon fibers, which are *in series* with the muscle fibers. The nerve endings are activated by the tension that develops during muscle contraction. Because the rate of impulse discharge along the parent fiber is related to the applied tension, tendon endings signal the *force* of muscle contraction.

The Ib afferents exert *negative feedback* on to the homonymous motoneurons, in contrast to the positive feedback exerted by muscle spindle afferents. The effect is called *autogenetic inhibition,* and the reflex arc is disynaptic because of the interpolation of an inhibitory neuron (*Figure 8.6*). There is an accompanying *reciprocal excitation* of motoneurons supplying antagonist muscles.

FREE NERVE ENDINGS

Muscles are rich in freely ending nerve fibers, distributed to the intramuscular connective tissue and investing fascial envelopes. They are responsible

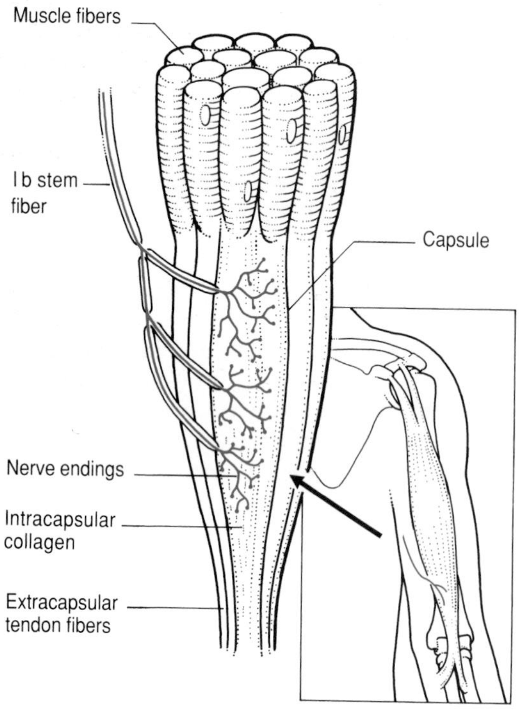

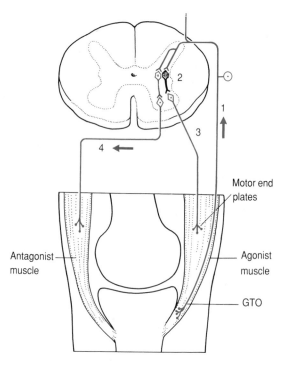

Figure 8.5 Golgi tendon organ.

Figure 8.6 Reflex effects of Golgi tendon organ (GTO) stimulation. **(1)** Agonist contraction excites GTO afferent which **(2)** excites inhibitory internuncial synapsing on **(3)** homonymous motoneuron and excites excitatory internuncial synapsing on **(4)** motoneuron supplying antagonist.

for pain sensation caused by direct injury or by accumulation of metabolites including lactic acid.

INNERVATION OF JOINTS

Freely ending unmyelinated nerve fibers are abundant in joint ligaments and capsules, and in the outer parts of intra-articular menisci. They mediate pain when a joint is strained, and they operate an excitatory reflex to protect the capsule. For example, the anterior wrist capsule is supplied by the median and ulnar nerves; if it is suddenly stretched by forced extension, motor fibers in these nerves are reflexly activated and cause wrist flexion.

Animal experiments have shown that when a joint is inflamed, more freely ending nerve fibers are excited than is the case when a healthy joint capsule is stretched. It seems that some nerve endings are *only* stimulated by inflammation.

Encapsulated nerve endings in and around joint capsules include Ruffini endings which signal tension, lamellated endings responsive to pressure, and Pacinian corpuscles responsive to vibration (see Chapter 9).

CORE INFORMATION

Muscle

A motor unit comprises a motoneuron and the group of muscle fibers it supplies. Each unit contains only one histochemical type of muscle fiber. At the myoneural synapse the terminal bouton (containing vesicular acetylcholine quanta) is separated from sarcolemmal junctional folds (containing ACh receptors) by basement membrane containing acetylcholinesterase.

Muscle spindles contain intrafusal muscle fibers supplied at each end by gamma fusimotor neurons. Sensory fibers of Ia diameter provide primary annulospiral endings at the equator and fibers of Type II diameter provide secondary endings nearby; both kinds are stretch receptors. Stretch may be passive, e.g. by a tendon reflex, or active during fusimotor activity. Homonymous motoneurons are monosynaptically excited; antagonists are reciprocally inhibited via Ia internuncials. Spindle primaries signal the rate of muscle stretch; secondaries signal the degree. During voluntary movements α and γ motoneurons are coactivated.

Golgi tendon organs signal the force of muscle contraction. They comprise encapsulated tendon tissue innervated by Ib diameter afferents, which exert disynaptic inhibition on homonymous motoneurons and reciprocal excitation of antagonists.

Free intramuscular nerve endings subserve pain sensation.

Joints

Free nerve endings abound in ligaments and capsules and in the outer part of menisci. They mediate pain, and operate an articular protective reflex. Encapsulated endings signal joint movement.

SELF TEST

Select the best response:

1 In a motor nerve to a muscle the proportion of afferent fibers is approximately:

- A 10%
- B 20%
- C 30%
- D 40%
- E 50%

2 Component(s) of a motor end plate include:

- A Presynaptic membrane
- B Basement membrane
- C Junctional folds
- D All of the above
- E A and B only

3 Fusimotor activity causes:

- A Direct shortening of extrafusal muscle fibers
- B Direct shortening of intrafusal fibers
- C Passive stretch of intrafusal muscle fibers
- D A and B only
- E None of the above

4 Which of the following signal the force of muscle contraction?

- A Spindle primary endings
- B Spindle secondary endings
- C Golgi tendon endings
- D Fusimotor endings
- E Free nerve endings

5 In a reflex arc:

- A Knee jerk is monosynaptic
- B Ankle jerk is monosynaptic
- C 'Reciprocal inhibition' refers to the antagonist
- D 'Autogenetic inhibition' refers to the prime mover
- E All of the above are correct

6 Interneurons serving reciprocal inhibition are called:

- A Ia
- B Ib
- C $A\alpha$
- D $A\beta$
- E $A\gamma$

REFERENCES

Buchthal, F. and Schmalbruch, H. (1980) Motor units of mammalian muscle. *Physiol. Rev.* **60**: 90–125.

Burke, D. and Gandevia, S.C. (1990) Peripheral motor system. In *The Human Nervous System* (Paxinos, G., ed.), pp. 125–148. San Diego: Academic Press.

McCloskey, D.I. (1994) Human proprioceptive sensation. *J. Clin. Neurosci.* **1**: 173–177.

McCloskey, D.I. and Gandevia, S.C. (1993) Aspects of proprioception. In *Science and Practice in Clinical Neurology* (Gandevia, S.C., Burke, D., and Anthony, M., eds), pp. 3–19. Cambridge: University Press.

Salpeter, M.M. (1987) Vertebrate neuromuscular junctions: general morphology, molecular organization, and functional consequences. In *The Vertebrate Neuromuscular Junction* (Salpeter, M.M., ed.), pp. 55–116. New York: Alan R. Liss.

Wyke, B. (1981) The neurology of joints: a review of general principles. *Clin. Rheum. Dis.* **7**: 223—239.

9
INNERVATION OF SKIN

Chapter Summary

Sensory units

Nerve endings
Free nerve endings
Follicular nerve endings
Merkel cell–neurite complexes
Encapsulated nerve endings
Peripheral neuropathies

CLINICAL PANELS
Axon reflex
Peripheral neuropathies

Study Guidelines

1 Learn to define: sensory unit, sensory overlap, receptive field, receptor adaptation.
2 State locations and response properties of three kinds of encapsulated receptors.
3 Learn to sketch a hair follicle and insert palisade nerve endings.
4 Try to appreciate the huge numbers of mechanoreceptors that are deployed in each hand. Name two kinds of receptors used to discriminate textures, e.g. to read Braille.

From the cutaneous branches of the spinal nerves, innumerable fine twigs enter a **dermal nerve plexus** located in the base of the dermis (*Figure 9.1*). Within the plexus, individual nerve fibers divide and overlap extensively with others before terminating at higher levels of the skin. Because of overlap, the area of anesthesia resulting from injury to a cutaneous nerve (e.g. superficial radial, saphenous) is smaller than its anatomical territory.

SENSORY UNITS

A given stem fiber forms the same kind of nerve ending at all of its terminals. In physiological recordings the stem fiber and its family of endings constitute a *sensory unit*. Together with its parent unipolar nerve cell, the sensory unit is analogous to the motor unit described in Chapter 8.

The territory from which a sensory unit can be excited is its *receptive field*. There is an inverse relationship between the size of receptive fields and sensory acuity. For example, fields measure about 2 cm^2 on the arm, 1 cm^2 at the wrist, and 5 mm^2 on the finger pads.

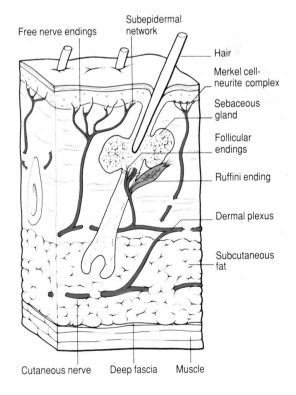

Figure 9.1 Innervation of hairy skin.

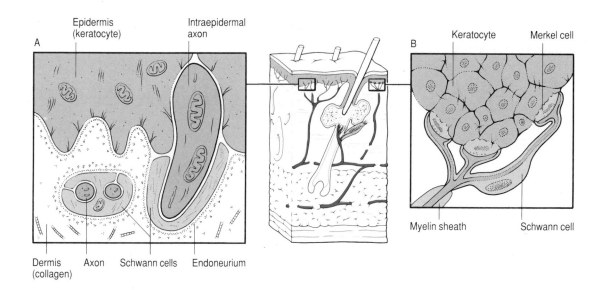

Figure 9.2 **(A)** Unmyelinated axons in dermis (left) and epidermis (right). **(B)** Merkel cell–neurite complex.

Sensory units interdigitate so that different *modalities* of sensation can be perceived from a given patch of skin.

NERVE ENDINGS

FREE NERVE ENDINGS

As they run toward the skin surface, sensory fibers shed their perineurial sheaths and then their myelin sheaths (if any) before branching further in a subepidermal network (*Figure 9.1*). The Schwann cell sheaths open to permit naked axons to terminate between collagen bundles (**dermal nerve endings**) or within the epidermis (**intraepidermal nerve endings**, *Figure 9.2A*).

Functions

Some sensory units with free nerve endings are *thermoreceptive;* they supply either 'warm spots' or 'cold spots' scattered over the skin. Two kinds of *nociceptive* ('painful') units with free endings are also found. One responds to severe mechanical deformation of the skin, such as pinching with a forceps. The parent fibers are finely myelinated (Aδ). The other consists of 'polymodal nociceptors'; these are C fiber units responding to mechanical deformation, to intense heat (sometimes to intense cold as well), and to irritant chemicals.

C fiber units are responsible for the axon reflex (*Panel 9.1*).

FOLLICULAR NERVE ENDINGS

Just below the level of the sebaceous glands, myelinated fibers apply a *palisade* of terminals along the outer root sheath epithelium of the hair follicles (*Figure 9.1*). Outside this, a set of *circumferential* terminals encircles the follicle at the same level.

Each follicular unit supplies many follicles and there is much territorial overlap. Follicular units are 'rapidly adapting': they fire when the hairs are being bent, but not when the bent position is held. Rapid adaptation accounts for our being largely unaware of our clothing except when putting it on or taking it off.

MERKEL CELL–NEURITE COMPLEXES

Expanded nerve terminals are applied to **Merkel cells (tactile menisci)** in the basal epithelium of epidermal pegs and ridges (*Figure 9.2B*). These Merkel cell-neurite complexes are 'slowly adapting' (SA). They discharge continuously in response to sustained pressure (for example, when holding a pen or wearing spectacles), and they are markedly sensitive to the *edges* of objects held in the hand.

ENCAPSULATED NERVE ENDINGS

The capsules of the three nerve endings to be described below are composed of an outer coat

NEUROGENIC INFLAMMATION: THE AXON REFLEX

When the skin is stroked with a sharp object, a red line appears in seconds due to capillary dilatation in direct response to the injury. A few minutes later a red *flare* spreads into the surrounding skin, due to arteriolar dilatation, followed by a white wheal due to exudation of plasma from the capillaries. These phenomena constitute the *triple response*. The wheal and flare responses are produced by *axon reflexes* in the local sensory cutaneous nerves. The sequence of events is shown by the numbers in *Figure CP 9.1.1*.

1 The noxious stimulus is transduced (converted to nerve impulses) by polymodal nociceptors.

2 As well as transmitting impulses to the CNS in the normal, orthodromic direction, the axons send impulses in an *antidromic* direction from points of bifurcation into the neighboring skin. The nociceptive endings respond to antidromic stimulation by releasing one or more peptide substances, notably substance P.

3 Substance P binds with receptors on the walls of arterioles, leading to arteriolar dilatation—the flare response.

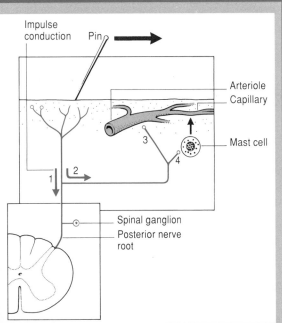

Figure CP 9.1.1 The axon reflex. For the numbers, see text.

4 Substance P also binds with receptors on the surface of mast cells, stimulating them to release *histamine*. The histamine increases capillary permeability and leads to local accumulation of tissue fluid—the wheal response.

---

of connective tissue, a middle coat of perineural epithelium, and an inner coat of modified Schwann cells (**teloglia**). All three are mechanoreceptors, responding to mechanical stimulation.

- **Meissner's corpuscles** are most numerous in the finger pads, where they lie beside the intermediate ridges of the epidermis (Figures 9.3 and 9.4A). In these ovoid receptors, several axons run a zig-zag course among stacks of teloglial lamellae. Meissner's corpuscles are rapidly adapting (RA) receptors. Together with the slowly adapting Merkel cell–neurite complexes, they provide the tools for delicate detective work on textured surfaces such as cloth or wood, or on embossed surfaces such as Braille text (*Figure 9.5*). Elevations as little as 5 μm in height can be detected.
- **Ruffini endings** are found in both hairy and glabrous skin (Figures 9.1 and 9.3). They respond to drag (shearing stress) and are slow-

ly adapting (SA) receptors. Their structure resembles that of Golgi tendon organs, having a collagenous core in which one or more axons branch liberally (Figure 9.4B).

- **Pacinian corpuscles** are the size of grains of rice. They are subcutaneous (Figure 9.3), and are numerous along the sides of the fingers and in the palm. Inside a thin connective sheath are onion-like layers of perineural epithelium containing some blood capillaries. Innermost are several teloglial lamellae surrounding a single central axon which has shed its myelin sheath at its point of entry (Figure 9.4C). Pacinian corpuscles are rapidly adapting (RA) and are especially responsive to *vibration*—particularly to bony vibration. In the limbs many corpuscles are embedded in the periosteum of the long bones.

Pacinian corpuscles discharge one or two impulses when compressed, and again when

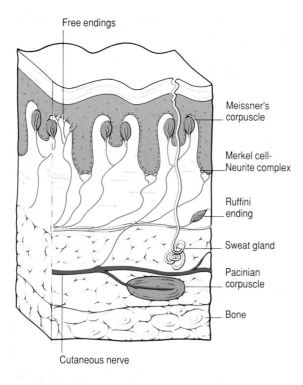

Figure 9.3   Innervation of finger pad.

released. In the hands, they seem to function in group mode: when an object such as an orange is picked up, as many as 500 Pacinian corpuscles are activated momentarily, with a repetition when the object is released. For this reason they have been called 'event detectors' during object manipulation.

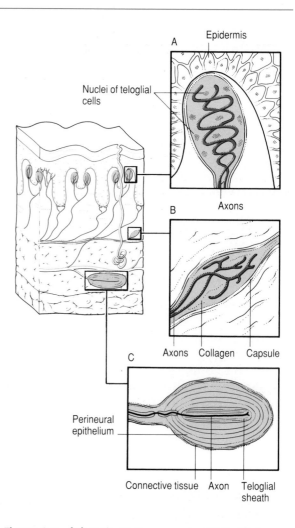
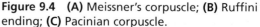

Figure 9.4   **(A)** Meissner's corpuscle; **(B)** Ruffini ending; **(C)** Pacinian corpuscle.

CLINICAL PANEL 9.2

PERIPHERAL NEUROPATHIES: LEPROSY

Diseases of peripheral nerves (*peripheral neuropathies*) have a wide variety of causes which include inherited and acquired metabolic disorders, nutritional deficiencies, reaction to drugs, and infections. The most common peripheral neuropathy in demographic terms is leprosy. Leprosy is prevalent in India and central Africa and is endemic in pockets elsewhere.

The leprosy bacillus enters the skin through minor abrasions. It travels proximally within the perineurium of the cutaneous nerves and kills off the Schwann cells. Loss of myelin segments ('segmental demyelination') blocks impulse conduction in the larger nerve fibers. Later, the inflammatory response to the bacillus compresses all of the axons, leading to Wallerian degeneration of entire nerves and gross thickening of the connective tissue sheaths. Patches of anesthetic skin develop on the fingers, toes, nose, and ears. The protective function of skin sensation is lost and the affected parts suffer injury and loss of tissue. Motor paralyses occur later on, as a consequence of invasion of mixed nerve trunks proximal to the points of origin of their cutaneous branches.

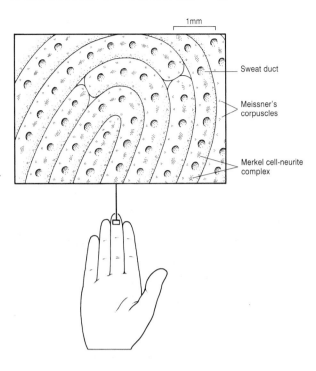

1mm

Sweat duct

Meissner's corpuscles

Merkel cell-neurite complex

Figure 9.5 Finger pad skin, showing distribution of Meissner's corpuscles and Merkel cell-neurite complexes.

The digital receptors are classified as follows by sensory physiologists:

- Merkel cell-neurite complexes = SA I
- Meissner's corpuscles = RA I
- Ruffini endings = SA II
- Pacinian corpuscles = RA II

When three-dimensional objects are being manipulated out of sight, significant contributions to perceptual evaluation are made by muscle afferents (especially from muscle spindles) and articular afferents from joint capsules. The cutaneous, muscular, and articular afferents relay information independently to the contralateral somatic sensory cortex. The three kinds of information are integrated (brought together at cellular level) in the posterior part of the parietal lobe, which is specialized for *spatial sense*. The tactile dimension of spatial sense is called *stereognosis*. In the clinic, this faculty is tested by asking the patient to identify an object such as a key without looking at it.

Panel 9.2 gives a short account of *peripheral neuropathies*, with special reference to leprosy.

CORE INFORMATION

Cutaneous nerves branch to form a dermal nerve plexus through which individual afferent fibers branch and overlap. Each stem fiber and its terminal sensory receptors constitute a sensory unit; the territory of a stem fiber is its receptive field.

Sensory units with free nerve endings include thermoreceptors and both mechanical and thermal nociceptors. Follicular units are rapidly adapting touch receptors, active only when hairs are in motion. Merkel cell–neurite complexes belong to slowly adapting edge detectors.

Encapsulated endings are mechanoreceptors. Meissner's corpuscles lie beside intermediate ridges in glabrous skin and are rapidly adapting. Ruffini endings lie near hair follicles and fingernails; they are slowly adapting drag receptors. Pacinian corpuscles are subcutaneous, rapidly adapting vibration receptors.

Coded information from skin, muscles and joints is integrated at the level of the parietal lobe of the brain, yielding the capacity for stereognosis (identification of an object felt but not seen).

SELF TEST

Answer A if 1, 2 and 3 only are correct
       B if 1 and 3 only are correct
       C if 2 and 4 only are correct
       D if 4 only is correct
       E if all four are correct

1 The following are sensory receptors comprising nerve endings applied to epithelial cells:

  1 Pacinian corpuscles
  2 Merkel cell–neurite complexes
  3 Ruffini endings
  4 Follicular receptors

2 The following are examples of encapsulated sensory receptors:

  1 Pacinian corpuscles
  2 Polymodal receptors
  3 Meissner's corpuscles
  4 Follicular receptors

3 The following are examples of rapidly adapting receptors:

  1 Meissner's corpuscles

  2 Pacininan corpuscles
  3 Follicular receptors
  4 Ruffini endings

4 Follicular nerve endings

  1 Are absent from glabrous skin
  2 Discharge impulses continuously
  3 Are absent from hair bulbs
  4 Are mainly circumferential

5 Purely nociceptive cutaneous neurons:

  1 Signal pain
  2 Have mostly C caliber fibers
  3 Are unipolar
  4 Overlap by branching within the dermal plexus

6 The following are edge detectors:

  1 Meissner's corpuscles
  2 Pacinian corpuscles
  3 Ruffini endings
  4 Merkel cell–neurite complexes

REFERENCES

Bannister, L.H. (1976) Sensory terminals of peripheral nerves. In *The Peripheral Nerve* (Landon, D.N., ed.). London: Chapman & Hall.

Cunningham, F.O. and FitzGerald, M.J.T. (1972) Encapsulated nerve endings in hairy skin. *J. Anat.* 112: 93-97.

Foreman, J.C. (1987) Peptides and neurogenic inflammation. *Br. Med. Bull.* 43: 386-400.

Iggo, A. (1985) Sensory receptors in the skin of mammals and their sensory functions. *Rev. Neurol.* **141:** 599-615.

James, L.A. (1994) Peripheral mechanisms for touch and proprioception. *Can. J. Physiol. Pharm.* **72:** 484-487.

Johansson, R.S. (1991) How is grasping modified by somatosensory input? In *Motor Control: Concepts and Issues* (Humphrey, D.R. and Freund, H.-J., eds.), pp. 331-355.

Mitsumoto, H. and Wilburn, A.J. (1994) Causes and diagnosis of sensory neuropathies: a review. *J.Clin. Neurohysiol.* **11:** 553-567.

Torebjork, A.B., Vallbo, A.B. and Ochoa, J.L. (1987) Intraneural microstimulation in man: its relation to specificity of tactile sensations. *Brain* **110:** 1509-1529.

10

AUTONOMIC NERVOUS SYSTEM AND VISCERAL AFFERENTS

Chapter Summary

Components of the autonomic nervous system

Sympathetic nervous system

Parasympathetic nervous system
Cranial parasympathetic system
Sacral parasympathetic system

Neurotransmitters in the autonomic nervous system
Ganglionic transmission
Junctional transmission
Other types of neurons
Interaction of the autonomic and immune systems

Visceral afferents
Visceral pain
Tenderness
Pain and the mind

CLINICAL PANELS
Sympathetic interruption
Drugs and the sympathetic system
Drugs and the parasympathetic system

Study Guidelines

1 Try to match up *Figure 10.1* with atlas pictures showing the sympathetic chain in place in dissections.
2 Resolve the paradox that despite an outflow restricted to 14 or 15 ventral roots, all 31 spinal nerve trunks acquire sympathetic fibers.
3 Appreciate that the sympathetic ganglia along the abdominal aorta are activated by preganglionic fibers, as is the adrenal medulla.
4 Pay special attention to the autonomic innervation of the eye.
5 Appreciate that the four parasympathetic ganglia in the head are functionally similar to intramural ganglia elsewhere.
6 The pelvic ganglia are mixed autonomic ganglia.
7 Realize that the preganglionic neurons of both divisions are cholinergic and that the target receptors in all of the autonomic ganglia are nicotinic.
8 Note that at tissue level, synapses are replaced by looser 'junctions' which permit diffusion of transmitter to outlying receptors.
9 You should focus on four kinds of junctional receptors of the sympathetic system, and on four actions initiated by muscarinic receptors in the parasympathetic system.
10 Learn from *Panel 10.2.1* how pharmacologists intercept the recycling and degradation sequence at sympathetic nerve endings. The same principles apply to CNS drug therapy, notably in psychiatric disorders.
11 Follow *Panel 10.3* to contrast the effects of cholinergic and anticholinergic drugs.
12 *Visceral afferents* utilize autonomic pathways to gain access to the nervous system. They are especially important in the context of thoracic and abdominal pain.

COMPONENTS OF THE AUTONOMIC NERVOUS SYSTEM

The **autonomic** ('self-regulating') **nervous system** is distributed to the peripheral tissues and organs by way of outlying autonomic ganglia. Controlling centers in the hypothalamus and brainstem send **central autonomic fibers** to synapse upon **preganglionic neurons** located in the gray matter of the brainstem and spinal cord. From these neurons **preganglionic fibers** (mostly myelinated) project out of the CNS to synapse upon multipolar neurons in the autonomic ganglia. Unmyelinated **postganglionic fibers** emerge and form terminal networks in the target tissues. Both anatomically and functionally, the autonomic system is composed of **sympathetic** and **parasympathetic divisions.**

SYMPATHETIC NERVOUS SYSTEM

The sympathetic system is so called because it acts in sympathy with the emotions. In association with rage or fear, the sympathetic system prepares the body for 'fight or flight': the heart rate is increased, the pupils dilate and the skin sweats. Blood is diverted from the skin and intestinal tract to the skeletal muscles, and the sphincters of the alimentary and urinary tracts are closed.

The sympathetic outflow from the nervous system is *thoracolumbar,* the preganglionic neurons being located in the lateral gray horn of the spinal cord at thoracic and upper two (or three) lumbar segmental levels. From these neurons, preganglionic fibers emerge in the corresponding anterior nerve roots and enter the sympathetic chain. The fibers do one of four things (*Figure 10.1*):

1 Some fibers synapse in the nearest ganglion. Postganglionic fibers enter spinal nerves T1–L2 and supply blood vessels and sweat glands in the territory of these nerves.
2 Some fibers *ascend* the sympathetic chain and synapse in the **superior** or **middle cervical ganglion,** or in the **stellate ganglion**. (The stellate consists of the fused inferior cervical and first thoracic ganglia; it lies in front of the neck of the first rib.) Postganglionic fibers supply the

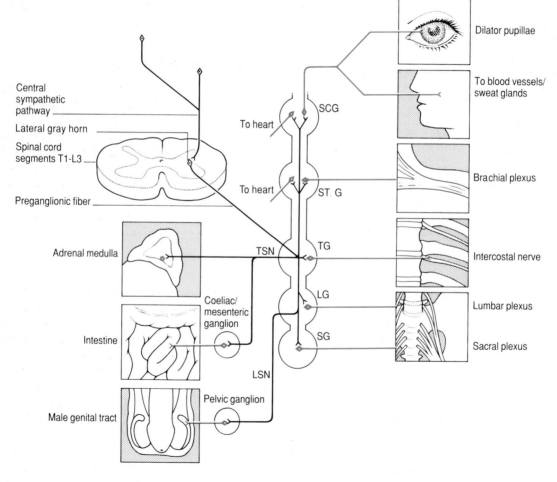

Figure 10.1 General plan of the sympathetic system. Ganglionic neurons and postganglionic fibers are shown in red. LG, lumbar ganglia; LSN, lumbar splanchnic nerve; SCG, superior cervical ganglion; SG, sacral ganglia; ST.G, stellate ganglion; TG, thoracic ganglia; TSN, thoracic splanchnic nerve.

CLINICAL PANEL 10.1

SYMPATHETIC INTERRUPTION

Stellate block

Injection of local anesthetic around the stellate ganglion—stellate block—is a procedure used in order to test the effects of sympathetic interruption on blood flow to the hand. Both pre- and postganglionic fibers are inactivated, producing sympathetic paralysis in the head and neck on that side, as well as in the upper limb. A successful stellate block is demonstrated by (a) *a warm, dry hand*, and (b) *Horner's syndrome*, which consists of a constricted pupil due to unopposed action of the pupillary constrictor, and *ptosis* (drooping) of the upper eyelid due to paralysis of smooth muscle fibers contained in the levator muscle of the upper eyelid (*Figure CP 10.1.1*).

Functional sympathectomy of the upper limb may be carried out by cutting the sympathetic chain below the stellate ganglion. This is not an anatomical sympathectomy because the ganglionic supply to the limb from the middle cervical and stellate ganglia remains intact. It is a functional one because the ganglionic neurons for the limb are deprived of tonic sympathetic drive. Horner's syndrome is avoided by making the cut at the level of the second rib: the preganglionic fibers for the head and neck enter the stellate direct from the first thoracic spinal nerve.

Two indications for interruption of the sympathetic supply to one or both upper limbs are painful blanching of the fingers in cold weath-

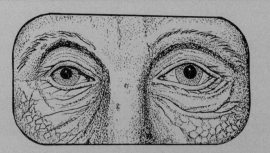

Figure CP 10.1.1 Horner's syndrome, patient's right side. Note the moderate ptosis of the eyelid, and the moderate miosis (pupillary constriction). The affected pupil reacts to light but recovers very slowly. (Drawn from a photograph kindly provided by Dr David Russel).

er (*Raynaud phenomenon*), and *hyperhidrosis* (excessive sweating) of the hands—usually an embarrassing affliction of teenage girls.

The sympathetic supply to the eye is considered further in Chapter 18.

Lumbar sympathectomy

In order to improve blood flow in the lower limb, the preganglionic nerve supply may be interrupted by cutting the upper end of the lumbar sympathetic chain. The usual procedure is to remove the second and and third lumbar sympathetic ganglia. In males, bilateral lumbar sympathectomy may result in persistent, painful erections (*priapism*) because of interruption of a pathway that maintains the resting, flaccid state of the penis.

head, neck, and upper limbs; also the heart. Of particular importance is the supply to the dilator muscle of the pupil (*Panel 10.1*).

3 Some fibers *descend* to synapse in lumbar or sacral ganglia of the sympathetic chain. Postganglionic fibers enter the lumbosacral plexus for distribution to the blood vessels and skin of the lower limbs.

4 Some fibers *traverse* the chain and emerge as the (preganglionic) thoracic and lumbar splanchnic nerves. The thoracic splanchnic nerves (usually called, simply, the splanchnic nerves) pass through the lower eight thoracic ganglia, pierce the diaphragm, and synapse in celiac, mesenteric, and renal ganglia within the abdomen. Postganglionic fibers accompany branches of the aorta to reach the gastrointestinal tract, liver, pancreas, and kidneys. **Lumbar splanchnic nerves** pass through the upper three lumbar ganglia and meet in front of the bifurcation of the abdominal aorta. They enter the pelvis as the **hypogastric nerves** before ending in pelvic ganglia, from which the genitourinary tract is supplied.

The medulla of the adrenal gland is the homolog of a sympathetic ganglion, being derived from the neural crest. It receives a direct input from fibers of the thoracic splanchnic nerve of its own side (see later).

The sympathetic system exerts tonic (continuous) constrictor activity on blood vessels in the limbs. In order to improve the blood flow to the hands or feet, impulse traffic along the sympathetic system can be interrupted surgically (*Panel 10.1*).

THE PARASYMPATHETIC NERVOUS SYSTEM

The parasympathetic system generally has the effect of counterbalancing the sympathetic system. It adapts the eyes for close-up viewing, slows the heart, promotes secretion of salivary and intestinal juices, and accelerates intestinal peristalsis.

The parasympathetic outflow from the CNS is craniosacral (*Figure 10.2*). Preganglionic fibers emerge from the brainstem in four cranial nerves—the oculomotor, facial, glossopharyngeal, and vagus—and from sacral segments of the spinal cord.

CRANIAL PARASYMPATHETIC SYSTEM

Preganglionic parasympathetic fibers emerge in four cranial nerves:

1 In the oculomotor nerve, to synapse in the **ciliary ganglion**. Postganglionic fibers innervate the sphincter of the pupil and the ciliary muscle. Both muscles act to produce the *accommodation reflex.*

2 In the facial nerve, to synapse in the **pterygopalatine ganglion,** which innervates the lacrimal and nasal glands; and in the submandibular ganglion, which innervates the submandibular and sublingual glands.

3 In the glossopharyngeal nerve, to synapse in the **otic ganglion,** which innervates the parotid gland.

4 In the vagus nerve, to synapse in parasympathetic ganglia close to the heart and lungs; and to synapse upon ganglion cells in the wall of the stomach and small intestine, and in the ascending and transverse parts of the colon.

SACRAL PARASYMPATHETIC SYSTEM

The sacral segments of the spinal cord occupy the conus medullaris (conus terminalis) at the lower extremity of the spinal cord, behind the body of the first lumbar vertebra. From the lateral gray matter of segments S2, S3 and S4, preganglionic

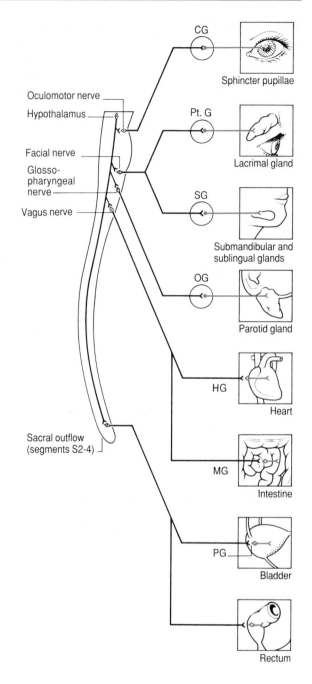

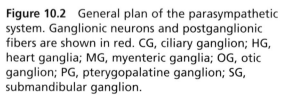

Figure 10.2 General plan of the parasympathetic system. Ganglionic neurons and postganglionic fibers are shown in red. CG, ciliary ganglion; HG, heart ganglia; MG, myenteric ganglia; OG, otic ganglion; PG, pterygopalatine ganglion; SG, submandibular ganglion.

fibers descend in the cauda equina within ventral nerve roots. Upon emerging from the pelvic sacral foramina the fibers separate out as the **pelvic splanchnic nerves.** Some fibers of the left and right pelvic splanchnic nerves synapse on ganglion cells in the wall of the distal colon and rectum. The rest synapse in **pelvic ganglia,** which contain sympathetic as well as parasympathetic neurons. Postganglionic parasympathetic fibers supply the detrusor muscle of the bladder; also the tunica media of the internal pudendal artery and of its branches to the trabecular tissue of the penis/clitoris (see later).

NEUROTRANSMISSION IN THE AUTONOMIC SYSTEM

GANGLIONIC TRANSMISSION

The preganglionic neurons of the sympathetic

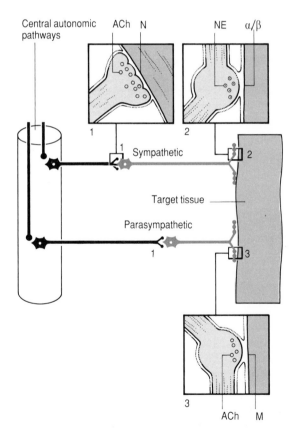

Figure 10.3 Autonomic transmitters and receptors. Ganglionic neurons and postganglionic fibers are shown in red. ACh, acetylcholine; M, muscarinic receptors; N, nicotinic receptors; NE, norepinephrine.

and parasympathetic systems are *cholinergic:* the neurons liberate acetylcholine (ACh) on to the ganglion cells at axodendritic synapses (*Figure 10.3*). The receptors on the ganglion cells are *nicotinic*—so named because the excitatory effect can be imitated by locally applied nicotine.

JUNCTIONAL TRANSMISSION

Postganglionic fibers of the sympathetic and parasympathetic systems form *neuroeffector junctions* with target tissues (*Figure 10.3*). Transmitter substances are liberated from innumerable varicosities strung along the course of the nerve fibers.

The chief transmitter at sympathetic neuroeffector junctions is *norepinephrine (noradrenalin)*, which is liberated from dense-cored vesicles. The postganglionic sympathetic system in general is described as *adrenergic*. An exception to the adrenergic rule is the *cholinergic* sympathetic supply to the eccrine sweat glands over the body surface.

The chief transmitter at parasympathetic neuroeffector junctions is acetylcholine. The postganglionic parasympathetic system in general is *cholinergic*.

Junctional receptors

The physiological effects of autonomic stimulation depend upon the nature of the *postjunctional receptors* inserted by target cells into their own plasma membranes. In addition, transmitter release is influenced by *prejunctional receptors* in the axolemmal membrane of the nerve terminals.

Sympathetic Junctional Receptors (Adrenoceptors) (Figure 10.4)

Two kinds of *alpha adrenoceptor* and two kinds of *beta adrenoceptor* have been identified for norepinephrine:

1 *Postjunctional, α_1 adrenoceptors* initiate contraction of smooth muscle in: peripheral small arteries and large arterioles; the dilator pupillae; the sphincters of the alimentary tract and bladder neck; and the vas deferens.

2 *Prejunctional, α_2 adrenoceptors* are present on parasympathetic as well as on sympathetic terminals. They inhibit transmitter release in both cases. On sympathetic terminals, they are called *autoreceptors*.

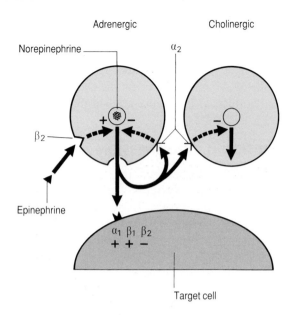

Figure 10.4 Adrenergic activity at a neuroeffector junction. Release of norepinephrine is promoted by epinephrine and inhibited by prejunctional a2 receptors, which also inhibit transmitter release from neighboring parasympathetic varicosities.

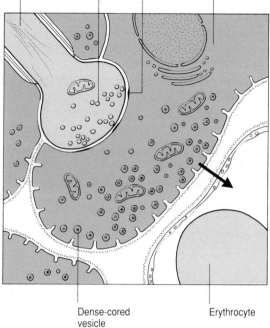

Figure 10.5 Chromaffin cell of the adrenal medulla receiving a synaptic contact from a preganglionic fiber of the thoracic splanchnic nerve. Acetylcholine (ACh) activates nicotinic receptors. 80% of the dense-cored vesicles are large and contain epinephrine; 20% are small and contain norepinephrine. Arrow indicates release into capillary bed.

3 *Postjunctional, β_1 adrenoceptors* increase pacemaker activity in the heart and increase the force of ventricular contraction. In response to a severe fall of blood pressure, sympathetic activation of β_1 receptors on the juxtaglomerular cells of the kidney causes secretion of renin. Renin initiates production of the powerful vasoconstrictor, angiotensin II.

4 *β_2 receptors* respond to circulating epinephrine (adrenalin) (*Figure 10.5*) as well as to locally released norepinephrine.

Postjunctional β_1 receptors relax smooth muscle, notably in the tracheobronchial tree and in the accommodatory muscles of the eye. Some postjunctional β_2 receptors are on the surface of hepatocytes in the liver, where they initiate glycogen breakdown to provide glucose for immediate energy needs.

Prejunctional β_2 receptors on adrenergic terminals promote release of norepinephrine.

Most of the norepinephrine liberated at sympathetic terminals is retrieved by an *amine uptake pump*. Some of it is degraded after uptake by a mitochondrial enzyme, *monoamine oxidase*.

The effects of drugs on the sympathetic system are considered in *Panel 10.2*.

Parasympathetic junctional receptors

Parasympathetic junctional receptors are called *muscarinic* because they can be mimicked by application of the drug muscarine. Parasympathetic stimulation produces the following muscarinic effects (*Figure 10.6*):

■ slowing of the heart in response to vagal stimulation, and diminished force of ventricular contraction

■ contraction of smooth muscle, with the following effects: intestinal peristalsis, bladder emptying, accommodation of the eye for 'near vision'

■ glandular secretion

In addition to the above postjunctional effects, prejunctional muscarinic receptors located on sympathetic varicosities inhibit release of norepinephrine.

The effects of *drugs* on the parasympathetic system are considered in *Panel 10.3*. Drugs hav-

CLINICAL PANEL 10.2

DRUGS AND THE SYMPATHETIC SYSTEM

Considerable scope is offered for pharmacological interference at sympathetic nerve endings. Drugs which cross the blood-brain barrier (Chapter 5) may exert their effects upon central rather than peripheral adrenoceptors. Potential sites of drug action are numbered in Figure *CP 10.2.1*.

1 Norepinephrine (NE) is loosely bound to a protein in the dense-cored vesicles. It can be unbound by specific drugs, whereupon it diffuses into the axoplasm and is degraded by monoamine oxidase.

2 Exocytosis into the synaptic cleft can be accelerated. Amphetamine, for example, exerts its central stimulant effect by flooding the extracellular space with expelled NE.

3 α or β receptors can be selectively either stimulated or blocked. As was mentioned in Chapter 7, a receptor can be likened to a lock, and a drug which operates the lock is an *agonist*. A drug which 'jams' the lock without operating it is a *blocker*. 'Beta agonists' are used to relax the bronchial musculature in asthmatic patients. Cardioselective 'beta blockers' are used to limit access of NE to b1 receptors.

4 The amine uptake mechanism can be blocked in the CNS by the tricyclic antidepressant drugs, or by cocaine. As a result, NE accumulates in the brain extracellular fluid.

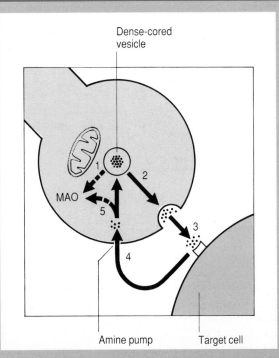

Figure CP 10.2.1 Transmitter release and recycling at adrenergic nerve endings. MAO, monoamine oxidase. For numbers, see text.

5 Some antidepressant drugs increase the NE content of synaptic vesicles by inhibiting monoamine oxidase, which normally degrades some of the transmitter after retrieval.

---

ing muscarinic effects are described as *cholinergic*. Drugs that prevent access of ACh to junctional receptors are *anticholinergic*.

A major consideration in the use of drugs either to imitate or to suppress sympathetic or parasympathetic activity, is the existence of α, β, and muscarinic receptors in the *central* nervous system. In psychiatric practice, in particular, drugs are often chosen for their action at central rather than their peripheral receptors.

OTHER TYPES OF NEURONS

Non-adrenergic, non-cholinergic (NANC) neu-

rons are found in both divisions of the autonomic system. In sympathetic ganglia, small internuncial neurons liberate *dopamine*—a precursor of noradrenaline. Some of the dopamine is secreted into capillaries, the rest binds with dopamine receptors on the main (adrenergic) neurons and exerts a mild inhibitory effect.

NANC neurons are especially numerous among the ganglion cells in the wall of the alimentary tract, and in the pelvic ganglia. More than 50 different *peptide* substances have been identified, either singly or in various combinations, in these neurons. For the most part, they act as *modulators*, acting either pre- or postjunc-

CLINICAL PANEL 10.3

DRUGS AND THE PARASYMPATHETIC SYSTEM

Possible peripheral effects of cholinergic and anticholinergic drugs are listed in *Figure CP 10.3.1*. Some success has been achieved in the search for organ- or tissue-specific drugs. For example, the contribution of the vagus nerve to acid secretion in the stomach involves activation of a muscarinic receptor (M_1) which is distinct from the receptor type (M_2) found in the heart or on smooth muscle. An M_1 receptor blocker is now available for patients suffering from peptic ulcer, for the specific purpose of reducing gastric acidity.

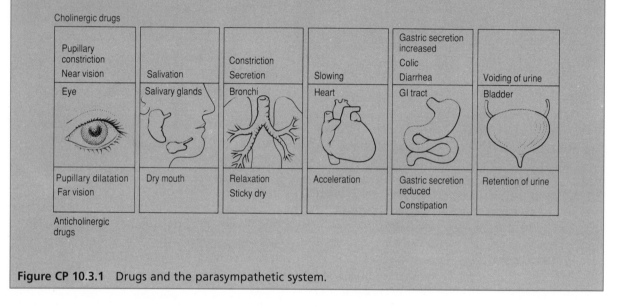

Figure CP 10.3.1 Drugs and the parasympathetic system.

tionally to influence the duration of action of classical transmitters. Some are *cotransmitters*, i.e. released in combination along with acetylcholine.

Vasoactive intestinal polypeptide (VIP) is a cotransmitter in the cholinergic supply to the salivary glands and to sweat glands. VIP is a powerful vasodilator and conveniently opens the local vascular bed (through specific VIP receptors on arterioles) just when the muscarinic ACh receptors are raising glandular metabolism.

Nitric oxide (NO) is well established as a transmitter in the parasympathetic system. It is a powerful smooth muscle relaxant (see below).

Penile/clitoral erection

The *nervi erigentes* ('erectile nerves') are postganglionic pelvic splanchnic nerve fibers supplying the smooth muscle of the internal pudendal arteries and of the trabecular erectile tissue of the phallus. ACh, VIP and NO have been identified in the nervi, and in some neurons all three transmitters act synergistically. The nervi are

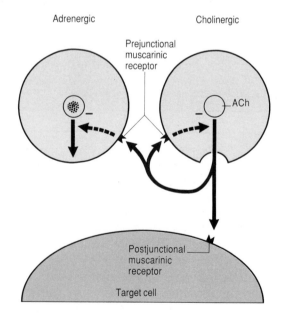

Figure 10.6 Cholinergic activity at a neuroeffector junction. Release of excess acetylcholine (ACh) is inhibited by prejunctional muscarinic receptors, which also inhibit transmitter release from neighboring sympathetic varicosities.

activated by central parasympathetic neurons following psychic stimulation of the anterior hypothalamus; and/or through a spinal reflex arc in response to direct genital stimulation. Activation produces smooth muscle relaxation, with flooding of the cavernous spaces. Resistance provided by the investing fibrous sheaths of the corpora cavernosa is sufficient to maintain tumescence.

Notes on seminal emission and ejaculation

The mature sperm are stored in the lower end of the vas deferens and in the tail of the epididymis. The entire length of the vas is intensely rich in adrenergic nerve endings and α receptors. So too is the smooth muscle of the bladder neck, prostate, and seminal vesicles. The fibers are relayed by sympathetic ganglion cells in the pelvic plexuses.

Emission occurs at the male climax: peristaltic waves milk the sperm rapidly into the prostatic urethra. The secretions of the prostate and seminal vesicles are squeezed into the urethra as well, to complete the semen, and the bladder neck is sealed off.

Contact of the propelled semen with the urethral mucous membrane triggers reflex contractions of the bulbospongiosus muscle, to *ejaculate* ('throw out') the semen from the urethra. The pudendal nerve provides both limbs of this reflex arc.

The sympathetic system and psychogenic impotence

In addition to the 'prevertebral' supply of the vas deferens mentioned above, a second, 'paravertebral' sympathetic pathway relays in the sacral part of the sympathetic chain and supplies the trabecular tissue, which is rich in α receptors. The resting, flaccid state of the penis depends upon tonic activity in this pathway; in this context, the corpus cavernosum resembles a well-muscled artery. For erection to take place, the sympathetic supply must be switched off while the parasympathetic, relaxant supply is switched on. Both events may be co-ordinated at the level of the hypothalamus (Chapter 21). Failure to switch off tonic sympathetic activity is regarded as the commonest immediate cause of *psychogenic impotence*, which is defined as impotence in the presence of intact anatomical pathways. Damage to reflex arcs, e.g. by spinal cord injury (Chapter 13) may cause *reflexive impotence*.

INTERACTION OF THE AUTONOMIC AND IMMUNE SYSTEMS

The lymphatic tissues of the thymus, lymph nodes, and respiratory and alimentary mucous membranes receive adrenergic and cholinergic nerve fibers. They also receive fibers containing various neuronal peptide substances, many of these fibers having their cell bodies in spinal and cranial sensory ganglia. Attempts to incorporate these findings into concepts of normal and disordered immune function are only tentative as yet.

VISCERAL AFFERENTS

Afferents from thoracic and abdominal viscera utilize autonomic pathways to reach the central nervous system. They participate in important reflexes involved in the control of circulation, respiration, digestion, micturition, and coition. Details on visceral reflexes are to be found in textbooks of physiology.

Visceral activities are not normally perceived, but they do reach conscious levels in a variety of disease states. Visceral pain is of immense importance in the context of clinical diagnosis.

VISCERAL PAIN

There are three fundamental types of visceral pain:

1 *Pure visceral pain*, felt in the region of the affected organ
2 *Visceral referred pain*, projected subjectively into the territory of the corresponding nerves
3 *Viscerosomatic pain*, caused by spread of disease to somatic structures.

Pure visceral pain

Pure visceral pain is characteristically vague and deep-seated. It is often accompanied by sweating or nausea. It is experienced as the initial pain in association with inflammation and/or ulceration in the alimentary tract; with obstruction of the intestine, bile duct, or ureter; or when the capsule of a solid organ (liver, kidney, pancreas) is stretched by underlying disease. In marked contrast, the viscera are completely insensitive to cutting or burning.

Visceral referred pain

As its severity increases, visceral pain is 'referred'

to somatic structures innervated from the same segmental levels of the spinal cord. For example, the pain of myocardial ischemia is referred to the chest wall ('angina pectoris'), pains of biliary or intestinal origin are referred to the anterior abdominal wall, and labor pains are referred to the sacral area of the back.

According to the generally accepted 'convergence–projection' theory of referred pain, the brain falsely interprets the source of noxious stimulation because visceral and somatic nociceptors have some spinothalalamic neurons in common; in previous experience, these neurons habitually signaled somatic pain.

Viscerosomatic pain

The parietal serous membranes (pleura and peritoneum) receive a rich sensory supply from the overlying intercostal nerves, and they are exquisitely sensitive to acute inflammatory exudates. In the abdomen, extension of an inflammatory process to the surface of stomach, intestine, appendix or gallbladder gives rise to a severe, steady pain in the abdominal wall directly overlying the inflamed organ. With the onset of acute peritonitis, the abdominal wall is 'splinted' by the muscles in a protective reflex.

TENDERNESS

Tenderness is *pain elicited by palpation*. In the abdomen, it is sought by pressing the hand and fingers against the abdominal wall. The clinician is, in effect, clothing the finger pads with the patient's parietal peritoneum and using this to seek out an inflamed organ. If the organ is mobile, like the appendix, 'shifting tenderness' may be elicited if the patient is willing to roll from one side to the other.

PAIN AND THE MIND

Although visceral pain has well-established causative mechanisms (inflammation, spasm of smooth muscle, ischemia, distension), thoracic or abdominal pain may be experienced in the complete absence of visceral disease. Pain that recurs or persists over a long period (months) and is not accounted for by standard investigational procedures, is more likely to have a *psychological* rather than a physical explanation. This is not to deny that the pain is real, but to imply that it originates within the brain itself. An example is the abused child whose abdominal pains represent a cry for help. In adults, recurrent and rather ill-defined pains are a common manifestation of *major depression* (see Chapter 21).

CORE INFORMATION

The ANS contains three chains of effector neurons: central neurons project from hypothalamus/brainstem to brainstem/spinal cord preganglionic neurons. These send preganglionic fibers to autonomic ganglion cells which in turn send postganglionic fibers to target tissues.

Sympathetic preganglionic outflow to the sympathetic chain of ganglia is thoracolumbar. Some fibers synapse in nearest ganglia. Some ascend to the superior cervical, middle cervical, or stellate ganglion whence postganglionic fibers innervate head, neck, upper limbs, and heart. Some descend to synapse in lumbar or sacral ganglia whence postganglionic fibers enter the lumbosacral plexus to supply lower limb vessels. Some pass through the chain and synapse instead in central abdominal ganglia (for the supply of gastrointestinal and genitourinary tracts) or in the adrenal medulla.

Parasympathetic preganglionic outflow is craniosacral. Cranial nerve distributions are: oculomotor n. → ciliary g. → sphincter pupillae and ciliaris; facial n. → pterygopalatine g. → lacrimal and nasal glands; facial n. → submandibular g. → submandibular and sublingual glands; glossopharyngeal n. → otic g. → parotid gland; vagus n. → intramural ganglia of heart, bronchi and alimentary tract → muscle and glands. Sacral nerves 2-4 deliver preganglionic fibers to intramural ganglia of distal colon and rectum, and to pelvic ganglia for supply of bladder and internal pudendal artery.

All preganglionic neurons are cholinergic. They activate nicotinic receptors in the ganglia. All postganglionic fibers end at neuroeffector junctions. In the sympathetic system they are generally adrenergic, liberating norepinephrine which may activate postjunctional α_1 adrenoceptors on smooth muscle, prejunctional α_2 on local nerve endings, postjunctional β_1 on cardiac muscle, or postjunctional β_2 which are more responsive to epinephrine. Epinephrine is liberated by adrenomedullary chromaffin cells; β_2 receptors on smooth muscle cause relaxation when activated.

Parasympathetic postganglionic fibers are cholinergic. The cholinoceptive receptors on cardiac and smooth muscle and glands are muscarinic.

Visceral afferents

Nociceptive afferents from thoracic and abdominal viscera use autonomic pathways to reach the CNS. Pure visceral pain is vague and deep-seated. Visceral referred pain is experienced in somatic structures innervated from the same segmental levels. Viscerosomatic pain arises from chemical/thermal irritation of one the serous membranes: the pain is severe and steady and accompanied by protective contraction of body wall muscles.

SELF TEST

Answer **A** if the item is associated with A only
        B if associated with B only
        C if associated with both A and B
        D if associated with neither A nor B

A Sympathetic structure(s)
B Parasympathetic structure(s)
C Both
D Neither

1 Ciliary ganglion
2 Submandibular ganglion
3 Stellate ganglion
4 Pelvic ganglia
5 Chromaffin cells

A Sympathetic function
B Parasympathetic function
C Both
D Neither

6 Dilatation of pupil
7 Intestinal peristalsis
8 Visceral pain

9 Erection of penis/clitoris
10 Voiding of urine

A Adrenergic fibers
B Cholinergic fibers
C Both
D Neither

11 To stellate ganglion
12 From stellate ganglion
13 To eccrine sweat glands
14 From pelvic ganglia
15 Referred pain

A Mediated via α receptors
B Mediated via muscarinic receptors
C Both
D Neither

16 Constriction of pupil
17 Arteriolar constriction
18 Bronchial relaxation
19 Penile/clitoral erection
20 Voiding of urine

REFERENCES

Andersson, K.E. and Wagner, D. (1995) Physiology of penile erection. *Physiol. Rev.* **75**: 191-236.

Appenzeller, D. (1982) *The Autonomic Nervous System: An Introduction to Basic and clinical Concepts, 3rd edn.* Amsterdam: Elsevier Biomedical Press.

Coupland, R.E. (1989) The natural history of the chromaffin cell. *Arch. Histol. Cytol.* **52**: 331-341.

Drummond, P.D. (1993) Autonomic innervation of the face. In *Science and Practice of Clinical Neurology* (Gandevia, S.C., Burke, D. and Anthony, M., eds.), pp. 223-242. Cambridge: University Press.

Kinder, M.V., Bastiaanssen, E.H.C., Janknegt, R.A. and Marani, E. (1995) Neuronal circuitry of the lower urinary tract. *Anat. Embryol.* **192**: 195-209.

Martinotti, E. (1991) Adrenergic subtypes on vascular smooth muscle. *Pharmacol. Res.* **24** 297-306.

McLeod, J.G. (1993) Disorders of the autonomic system. In *Science and Practice in Clinical Neurology* (Gandevia, S.C., Burke, D. and Anthony, M., eds.), pp. 205-222. Cambridge: University Press.

McMahon, S.B., Dmitrieva, N. and Kolzenburg, M. (1995) Visceral pain. *Brit. J. Anaesth.* **75**: 132-144.

Paintal, A.S. (1986) The visceral sensations—some basic mechanisms. *Prog. Brain Res.* **67**: 3-18.

Procacci, P., Zoppi, M. and Maresca, M. (1986). Clinical approach to visceral sensation. *Prog. Brain Res.* **67**: 21-28.

Weihe, E., Nohr, D., Michel, S., Muller, S., Zentel, H.-J., Fink, T. and Krekel, J. (1991) Molecular anatomy of the neuro-immune connection. *Int. J. Neurosci.* **59**: 1-23.

Watson, C. and Vijayan, N. (1995) The sympathetic innervation of the eyes and face - a clinicoanatomical review. *Clin. Anat.* **8**: 262-272.

11

NERVE ROOTS

Chapter Summary

Development of the spinal cord
Cellular differentiation
Ascent of the cord
Neural arches

Adult anatomy

Distribution of spinal nerves
Segmental sensory distribution
Segmental motor distribution
Nerve root compression
   syndromes
Lumbar puncture
Anesthetic procedures

CLINICAL PANELS
Spina bifida
Nerve root compression

Study Guidelines

1 During development, some immature neurons send out ventral roots while others project along the marginal zone to form tracts. Sensory fibers come in from the neural crest.
2 In the mature vertebral canal, note the disparities of levels, e.g. a collapsed T11 vertebra would crush cord segment L1.
3 Recall that ventral roots S2–4 of cauda equina contain preganglionic parasympathetic fibers vital for bladder and bowel emptying and that the corresponding posterior roots contain visceral afferents vital for reflexes.
4 Do remember the extradural venous plexus and the harm it can do.
5 It is clinically important to appreciate that a sense of numbness/tingling in the fingers in later life may result from compression of posterior nerve roots!
6 For the commonest and lowest two levels of disc prolapse, the *next* spinal nerve is the likely one to be caught.
7 Be sure that you understand the anatomy of lumbar puncture.

DEVELOPMENT OF THE SPINAL CORD

CELLULAR DIFFERENTIATION

The neural tube of the embryo consists of a pseudostratified epithelium surrounding the neural canal (*Figure 11.1A*). Dorsal to the sulcus limitans the epithelium forms the **alar plate;** ventral to the sulcus it forms the **basal plate.** (The terms 'ventral' and 'dorsal' correspond to 'anterior' and 'posterior' in postnatal anatomy.)

The neuroepithelium contains germinal cells which synthesize DNA before retracting to the innermost, **ventricular zone,** where they divide. The daughter nuclei move outward, synthesize fresh DNA, then retreat and divide again. After several such cycles, postmitotic cells round up in the **intermediate zone.** Some of the postmitotic cells are immature neurons; the rest are **glioblasts** which after further division become astrocytes or oligodendrocytes. Some of the glioblasts form an ependymal lining for the neural canal.

The microglial cells of the CNS are derived from the same parents as ependymal cells.

Enlargement of the intermediate zone of the alar plate creates the dorsal horn of gray matter. The dorsal horn receives the central processes of dorsal root ganglion cells (*Figure 11.1B*). As explained in Chapter 1, the ganglion cells are derived from the neural crest.

Partial occlusion of the neural canal by the developing dorsal gray horn gives rise to the dorsal median septum and to the definitive central canal of the cord (Figure 11.1C).

Enlargement of the intermediate zone of the basal plate creates the ventral gray horn and the ventral median fissure (*Figure 11.1C*). Axons emerge from the ventral horn and form the ventral nerve roots.

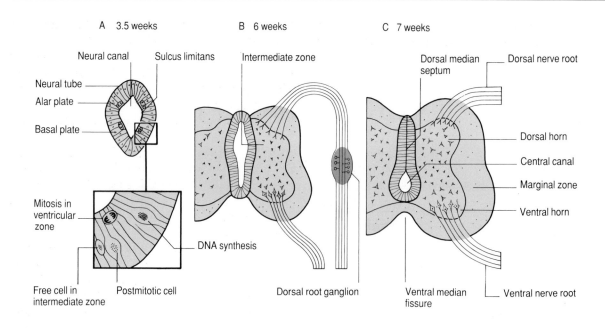

Figure 11.1 Cellular differentiation in the embryonic spinal cord.

In the outermost, **marginal zone** of the cord, axons run from spinal cord to brain and vice versa.

Caudal cell mass

The neural tube reaches caudally only to the level of the second lumbar mesodermal somites. Following closure of the posterior neuropore, the ectoderm and mesoderm at the level of the more caudal lumbar and sacral somites blend to form a **caudal cell mass**. This ribbon of cells becomes canalized and links up with the neural tube; it gives rise to the lower end of the spinal cord.

ASCENT OF THE CORD (*FIGURE 11.2*)

The spinal cord occupies the full length of the vertebral canal until the end of the 12th postconceptual week. The sixth to eighth weeks are marked by regression of the tail: the number of coccygeal vertebrae is reduced from six to three, and the enclosed part of the neural tube shrivels to become a neuroglial thread, the filum terminale.

After the 12th week the vertebral column grows more rapidly than the spinal cord, and the cord is forced to ascend the vertebral canal. The tip of the cord reaches the second or third lumbar level at the time of birth. The adult level (first or second lumbar) is reached three weeks later.

As a consequence of greater ascent of the lower part of the cord compared to the upper part, the spinal nerve roots show an increasing disparity

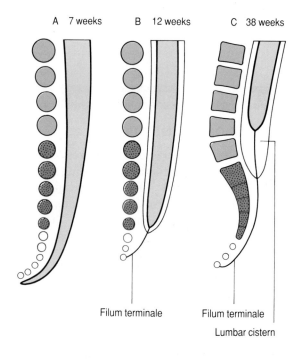

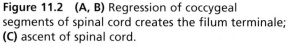

Figure 11.2 (A, B) Regression of coccygeal segments of spinal cord creates the filum terminale; **(C)** ascent of spinal cord.

between their segmental levels of attachment to the cord, and the corresponding vertebral levels (*Figure 11.3*).

NEURAL ARCHES

During the fifth week, the mesenchymal vertebrae surrounding the notochord give rise to **neural arches** for protection of the spinal cord (*Figure 11.4*). The arches are initially bifid (split). Later, they fuse in the midline and form the vertebral spines.

Conditions in which the two halves of the neural arches fail to unite are collectively known as spina bifida (*Panel 11.1*).

ADULT ANATOMY

The spinal cord and nerve roots are sheathed by pia mater and float in cerebrospinal fluid con-

tained in the subarachnoid space. The **denticulate ligament** pierces the arachnoid so that the cord is anchored to the dura mater on each side. Outside the dura is the **extradural (epidural) venous plexus** (*Figure 11.5*) which harvests the vertebral red marrow and empties into the segmental veins (deep cervical, intercostal, lumbar, sacral). These veins are without valves, and reflux of blood from the territory of segmental veins is a notorious cause of cancer spread from the prostate, lung, breast, and thyroid gland. In fact, nerve root compression from collapse of an invaded vertebra may be the presenting sign of cancer in one of these organs.

The respective anterior and posterior nerve roots join at the intervertebral foramina, where the posterior root ganglia are located (*Figure 11.5*). The arachnoid mater blends with the perineurium of the spinal nerve, and the dura mater blends with the epineurium. The nerve roots carry extensions of the subarachnoid space into the intervertebral foramina.

Below the level of the spinal cord, the nerve roots passing to the lower lumbar and sacral intervertebral foramina constitute the **cauda equina** ('horse's tail'). The cauda equina floats in the lumbar subarachnoid cistern (*Figures 11.6, 11.7*), which reaches to the level of the second

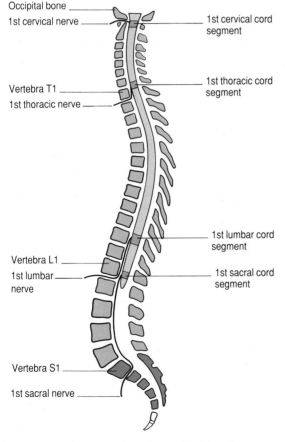

Figure 11.3 Segmental and vertebral levels compared. Spinal nerves 1–7 emerge above the corresponding vertebrae, the remaining spinal nerves emerge below.

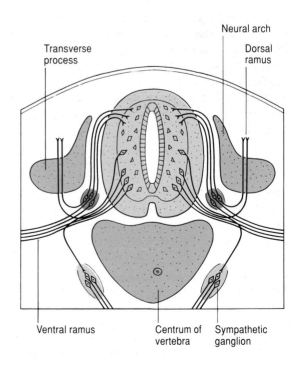

Figure 11.4 Normal, bifid stage of neural arch development in an embryo of 8 weeks.

CLINICAL PANEL 11.1

SPINA BIFIDA

Among the more common congenital malformations of the CNS are several conditions included under the general heading, *spina bifida*. The 'bifid' effect is produced by failure of union of the two halves of the neural arches, usually in the lumbosacral region (*Figure CP 11.1.1*)

Spina bifida occulta (A) is usually symptom-free, being detected incidentally in lumbosacral radiographs.

In *spina bifida cystica* a meningeal cyst protrudes through the vertebral defect. In 10% of these cases the cyst is a meningocele containing no nervous elements (B). In 90%, unfortunately, the cyst is a *meningomyelocele*, containing either spinal cord or cauda equina (C); the lower limbs, bladder and rectum are para-

lyzed, as in the case illustrated in Figure *CP 11.1.2*, and meningitis is likely to supervene sooner or later. To make matters worse, an Arnold–Chiari malformation (Chapter 4) is almost always present as well.

The most severe form of spina bifida is *myelocele* (D), where the neural folds have remained open and CSF leaks on to the surrounding skin. The clinical outlook is very poor.

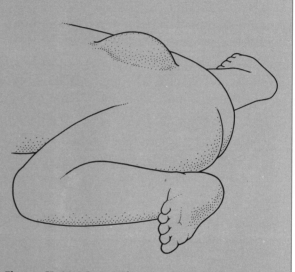

Figure CP 11.1.2 Lumbar meningomyelocele (from a photograph). The 'frog leg' posture is characteristic of combined femoral and sciatic nerve paralysis, with preservation of hip flexion by the iliopsoas.

Figure CP 11.1.1 Varieties of spina bifida. **(A)** Spina bifida occulta; **(B)** meningocele; **(C)** meningomyelocele; **(D)** myelocele.

sacral vertebra. At its upper end the cauda comprises nerve roots L3–S5 of both sides—a total of 32 roots.

In the center of the cauda equina is the unimportant filum terminale, which pierces the meninges to become attached to the coccyx.

DISTRIBUTION OF SPINAL NERVES

Each spinal nerve gives off a recurrent branch which provides mechanoreceptors and pain receptors for the dura mater, posterior longitudinal ligament, and intervertebral disc. The synovial 'facet' joints between successive articular

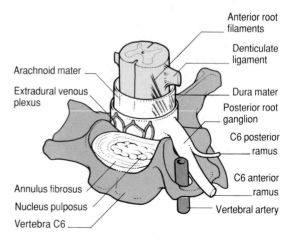

Figure 11.5 Relationships of the sixth cervical spinal nerve.

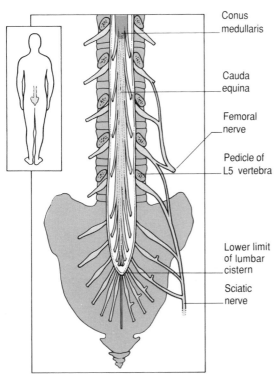

Figure 11.6 The cauda equina in the lumbar cistern. Contributions to the femoral and sciatic nerves are shown on the right side.

processes are each supplied by the nearest three spinal nerves. Pain caused by injury or disease of any of the above structures is referred to the cutaneous territory of the corresponding posterior rami (*Figure 11.8*).

SEGMENTAL SENSORY DISTRIBUTION: THE DERMATOMES

A **dermatome** is the strip of skin supplied by an individual spinal nerve. The dermatomes are orderly in the embryo (*Figure 11.9*) but they are distorted by the outgrowth of the limbs (*Figure 11.10*). Spinal nerves C5, C6, C7, C8 and T1 are drawn into the upper limb, so that C4 abuts on T2 at the level of the sternal angle. Nerves L2, L3, L4, L5, S1 and S2 are drawn into the lower limb, so that L2 abuts on S3 over the buttock. Maps like those in Figure 11.10 fail to portray *overlap* in the cutaneous distribution of successive dorsal nerve roots. On the trunk, for example, the skin over an intercostal space is supplied by the nerves immediately above and below as well as by the proper nerve.

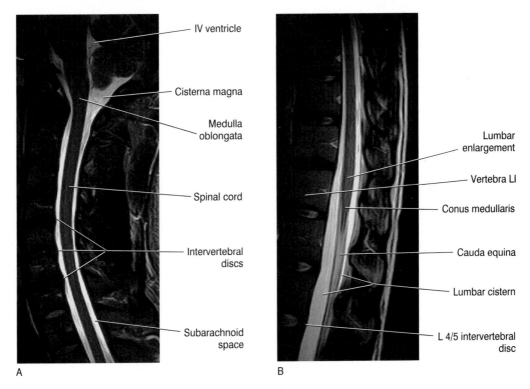

Figure 11.7 Sagittal MRI scans of the vertebral canal, weighted so as to enhance cerebrospinal fluid. **(A)** Brainstem, cerebellum and cervical spinal cord are outlined. **(B)** Lumbosacral spinal cord and cauda are outlined. (From a series kindly provided by Dr J. Paul Finn, Director, MR research and Development, Siemens MedicalSystems Inc., Iselin, New Jersey)

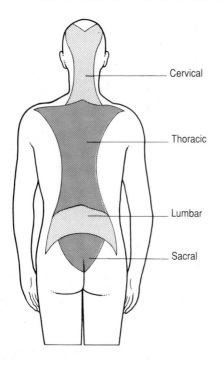

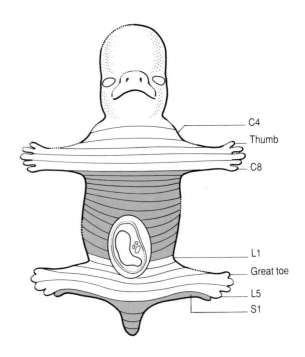

Figure 11.8 Cutaneous distribution of posterior rami of spinal nerves.

Figure 11.9 Embryonic dermatome pattern.

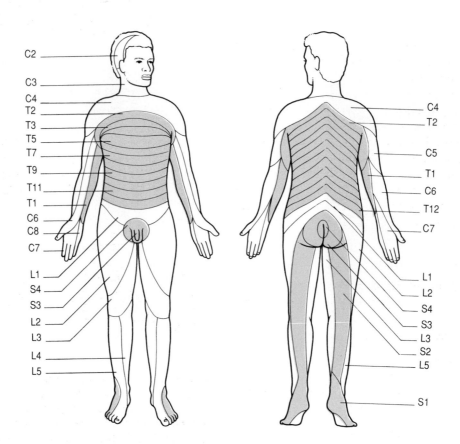

Figure 11.10 Adult dermatome pattern.

SEGMENTAL MOTOR DISTRIBUTION

In the limbs, the individual muscles are supplied by more than one spinal nerve because of interchange in the limb nerve plexuses. The segmental supply of the limbs is expressed in terms of *movements* in *Figure 11.11*.

NERVE ROOT COMPRESSION SYNDROMES

Nerve root compression within the vertebral canal is most frequent where the spine is most mobile, namely at lower cervical and lower lumbar levels (*Panel 11.2*). The effects of root compression may be expressed in five different ways:

1. Pain perceived in the muscles supplied by the corresponding spinal nerve(s)
2. Paresthesia (numbness or tingling) along the respective dermatome(s)
3. Cutaneous sensory loss—more likely if two successive dermatomes are involved, because of overlap
4. Motor weakness
5. Loss of a tendon reflex if the segmental level is appropriate (*Table 11.1*).

LUMBAR PUNCTURE (SPINAL TAP)

To obtain a sample of cerebrospinal fluid, a needle is passed forward and upward between the spines of vertebrae L3 and L4 or between L4 and L5. The patient lies curled up on one side during the procedure; aseptic precautions are observed and the skin and interspinous ligaments are anesthetized before the needle is inserted. A slight 'give' is felt when the fused dura-arachnoid layer has been penetrated.

A lumbar puncture is not performed if there is any reason to suspect the presence of raised intracranial pressure (see Panel 2 in Chapter 6).

ANESTHETIC PROCEDURES

A so-called *spinal anesthetic* is often given in preference to a general anesthetic, prior to surgi-

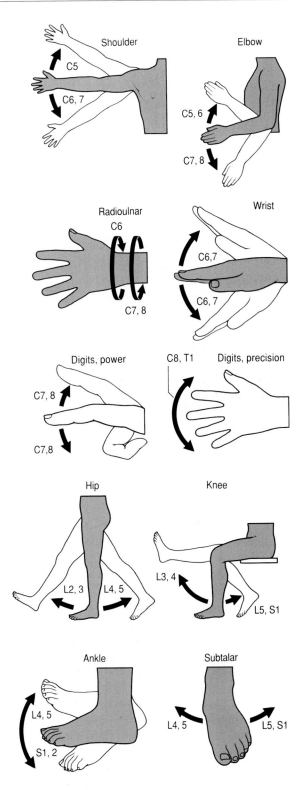

Figure 11.11 Segmental control of limb movements. (Adapted from Last, R.J. (1973) *Anatomy: Regional and Applied*, 5th edn. Edinburgh: Churchill Livingstone; and Rosse, C. and Clawson, D.K. (1980) *The Musculoskeletal System in Health and Disease*. Hagerstown: Harper & Row.)

Table 11.1 Segmental levels of tendon reflexes

Segmental level	Reflex
C5,6	Biceps
C5,6	Brachioradialis ('supinator reflex')
C7	Triceps
L3,4	Knee jerk
S1	Ankle jerk

NERVE ROOT COMPRESSION

Cervical roots

The intervertebral discs and synovial joints of the neck are subject to degenerative disease (*cervical spondylosis*) in 50% of 50-year-old people and in 70% of 70 year olds. Although any or all of the joints may deteriorate, problems are most frequent in relation to vertebra C6, which provides the fulcrum for flexion/extension movements of the neck. Spinal nerve C6 (above) or C7 (below) may be pinched by extruded disc material or by bony excrescences around the synovial joints (*Figure CP 11.2.1*). Sensory, motor, and reflex disturbances may result in accordance with the data in *Figures 11.9* and *11.10* and *Table 11.1*.

Lumbosacral roots

One important cause of low-back pain is a *prolapsed intervertebral disc (herniated nucleus pulposus)*. Fully 95% of all disc prolapses occur immediately above or below the last lumbar vertebra. The typical herniation is *posterolat-eral*, with compression of the nerve roots passing to the next intervertebral foramen (*Figure CP 11.2.2*). Symptoms include backache caused by rupture of the annulus fibrosus, and pain in the buttock/thigh/leg caused by pressure on posterior root fibers contributing to the sciatic nerve. The pain is increased by stretching the affected root, e.g. by having the straightened leg raised by the examiner.

An L4/5 disc prolapse produces pain/paresthesia over the L5 dermatome. Motor weakness may be detected during dorsiflexion of the great toe (later, of all toes and of the ankle), and during eversion of the foot. Abduction of the hip may also be weak; this movement is tested with the patient lying on one side.

With an L5/S1 prolapse (the commonest of all), symptoms are felt in the back of the leg/sole of foot (S1 dermatome). Plantar flexion may be weak and the ankle jerk reduced or absent.

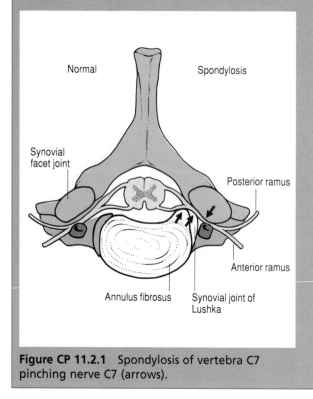

Figure CP 11.2.1   Spondylosis of vertebra C7 pinching nerve C7 (arrows).

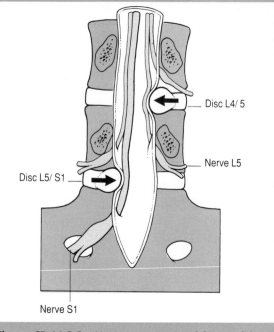
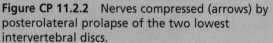

Figure CP 11.2.2   Nerves compressed (arrows) by posterolateral prolapse of the two lowest intervertebral discs.

cal procedures on the prostate in the elderly. A local anesthetic is injected into the lumbar cistern in order to block impulse conduction in the lumbar and sacral nerve roots. Care is taken that the anesthetic does not reach a high level in the subarachnoid space, for fear of paralyzing the intercostal and phrenic nerve root fibers serving respiration.

ANESTHESIA AND CHILDBIRTH

In skilled hands, pain-free labor can be assured by blocking the lumbar and sacral nerve roots extradurally. For *epidural anesthesia*, local anesthetic is carefully introduced into the extradural space by the lumbar route. For *caudal anesthesia* the extradural space is approached in an upward direction, through the sacral hiatus. In both procedures, the anesthetic diffuses through the dural sheath of the nerve roots where they leave the vertebral canal. Labor may be prolonged because of interruption of excitatory reflex arcs linking perineum to uterus through the lower end of the spinal cord. However, avoidance of general anesthesia is valuable in allowing immediate bonding to take place between mother and child.

CORE INFORMATION

The neuroepithelium of the embryonic cord undergoes mitotic activity in the inner, ventricular zone. Daughter cells move into the intermediate zone and become either neuroblasts or glioblasts. The developing dorsal horn receives central processes of neural crest-derived spinal ganglion cells. The ventral horn issues axons that form ventral nerve roots. The outer, marginal zone contains the axons of developing nerve pathways. The caudal end of the cord develops separately from the caudal cell mass, which links up with the neural tube. After the 12th week, rapid growth of the vertebral column causes the cord to ascend the vertebral canal; its lower tip is at L2–L3 level at birth and at L1–L2 level three weeks later. The result is a progressive disparity between segmental levels of nerve root attachment to the cord and intervertebral levels of exit of spinal nerves. The neural arches are dorsal projections of vertebral mesenchyme; the initial bifid arrangement is normally lost by fusion of the projections to form spines.

The mature cord and nerve roots are sheathed by pia mater and float in the subarachnoid space, anchored to dura by the denticulate ligament. The extradural space contains valveless veins which drain vertebral bone marrow into segmental veins and provide potential avenues for spread of cancer cells. Below the level of the cord, the cauda equina comprises paired nerve roots L3–S5 of both sides. As it emerges from the intervertebral foramen (occupied by the posterior root ganglion), each spinal nerve gives a recurrent branch supplying ligaments and dura mater.

Segmental sensory distribution is shown by the regular dermatomal pattern of skin innervation by the posterior roots (via the mixed peripheral nerves). Segmental motor supply is expressed in the form of movements peformed by specific muscle groups. Nerve root compression, e.g. by a prolapsed disc, may be expressed segmentally by muscle pain, dermatomal paresthesia/anesthesia, motor weakness, loss of a tendon reflex.

Lumbar puncture (spinal tap) is performed by passing a needle between spines at L3/L4 or L4/5 — but not if raised intracranial pressure is suspected. A spinal anesthetic is given by injecting local anesthetic into the lumbar cistern. An epidural anesthetic is given into the lumbar epidural space. A caudal anesthetic is given through the sacral hiatus.

SELF TEST

Answer **A if 1, 2, and 3 only are correct**
         B if 1 and 3 only are correct
         C if 2 and 4 only are correct
         D if 4 only is correct
         E if all four are correct

1 Ascent of the spinal cord during fetal life causes elongation of the:

  1 Vertebral canal
  2 Spinal nerve roots
  3 Vertebral column
  4 Filum terminale

2 The term 'spina bifida' implies failure of union of:

  1 Vertebral bodies
  2 Pedicles
  3 Transverse processes
  4 Neural arches

3 The following are characteristic(s) of epidural veins:

  1 No valves
  2 Drain vertebral bone marrow
  3 Empty into segmental veins
  4 Communicate with pelvic veins

4 The cauda equina comprises:

  1 Anterior nerve roots
  2 Anterior rami
  3 Posterior nerve roots
  4 Posterior rami

5 Supplied by posterior rami of spinal nerves:

  1 Intervertebral discs
  2 Skin of the back
  3 Dura mater
  4 Erector spinae muscles

6 Compression of S1 nerve root by a prolapsed intervertebral disc may lead to:

  1 Paresthesia in the the sole of the foot
  2 Pain in the calf muscles
  3 Loss of the ankle jerk
  4 Weakness of ankle dorsiflexion

REFERENCES

Adams, C.B.T. and Logue, V. (1971) Studies in cervical spondylitic myelopathy. 1. Movement of the cervical roots, dura, and cord, and their relation to the course of extrathecal roots. *Brain* **94**: 557–568.

Auteroche, P. (1983) Innervation of the zygapophyseal joints of the lumbar spine. *Anat. Clin.* **5**: 17–28

Barson, A.J. and Logue, V. (1970) The vertebral level of termination of the spinal cord during normal and abnormal development. *J. Anat.* **106**: 489-497.

Bogduk, N. (1993) Spinal pain: backache and neck pain. In *Science and Practice in Clinical Neurology* (Gandevia, S.C. Burke, D. and Anthony, M., eds), pp. 39–60. Cambridge: University Press.

Groen, D.J., Baljet, R., and Drukker, J. (1990) Nerves and nerve plexuses of the human vertebral column. *Am. J. Anat.* **188**: 282–296.

Holsheimer, J., den Boer, J.A., Strujik, J.J., and Rozeboom, A.R. (1994) MR assessment of the normal position of the spinal cord in the spinal canal. *Am. J. Neuroradiol.* **15**: 951–959.

Russell, E.J. (1990) Cervical disc disease. *Radiology* **177**: 313–325.

Sunderland, S. (1974) Meningeal-dural relationships in the intervertebral foramen. *J. Neurosurg.* **40**: 756–763.

12

SPINAL CORD: ASCENDING PATHWAYS

Chapter Summary

General features
Types of spinal neurons
Spinal ganglia

Ascending sensory pathways
Categories of sensation
Sensory testing

Somatic sensory pathways
Posterior column-medial
   lemniscal pathway
Spinothalamic pathway
Spinoreticular tracts
Spinocerebellar pathways

Other ascending pathways

CLINICAL PANEL
Syringomyelia

Study Guidelines

1 Confirm that the mature spinal cord is not segmented internally.
2 Confirm that anterior horn cells take the form of columns rather than laminae.
3 Appreciate that 'unconscious sensation' simply means that the ascending afferent impulse activity concerned does not generate any kind of perception.
4 Remember that conscious proprioception is more sensitive than either vision or vestibular labyrinth in telling us when we are going off balance.
5 Get used to the idea that muscles tell us more than joints do about the position of our limbs in space.
6 It is clinically important to appreciate that one of the two 'conscious' pathways crosses the midline at all levels of the spinal cord, whereas the other crosses all at once, within the brainstem.
7 Appreciate the meaning of the term 'dissociated sensory loss.'

GENERAL FEATURES

The arrangement of gray and white matter at different levels of the spinal cord is shown in *Figure 12.1*. The cervical and lumbosacral enlargements are produced by expansions of the gray matter required to service the limbs. White matter is most abundant in the upper reaches of the cord, which contain the sensory and motor pathways serving all four limbs. In the posterior funiculus, for example, the gracile fasciculus carries information from the lower limb and is present at cervical as well as lumbosacral segmental levels, whereas the cuneate fasciculus carries information from the upper limb and is not seen at lumbar level.

Although it is convenient to refer to different levels of the spinal cord in terms of numbered segments, corresponding to the sites of attachment of the paired nerve roots, the cord shows no evidence of segmentation internally. The nuclear groups seen in transverse sections are in reality cell columns, most of them spanning several segments (*Figure 12.2*).

TYPES OF SPINAL NEURONS

The smallest neurons (soma diameters 5-20 μm) are *propriospinal*, being entirely contained within the cord. Some are confined within a single segment; others span two or more segments by way of the neighboring **propriospinal tract** (*Figure 12.3*). Many of the smallest neurons participate in spinal reflexes. Others are intermediate cell stations interposed between fiber tracts descending from the brain and motor neurons projecting to the locomotor apparatus. Others again are so placed as to influence sensory transmission from lower to higher levels of the CNS.

Medium-sized neurons (soma diameters

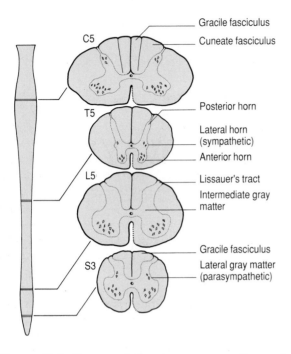

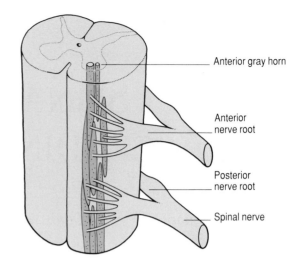

Figure 12.1 Representative transverse sections of the spinal cord.

Figure 12.2 Two segments of the spinal cord, showing cell columns in the anterior gray horn.

20–50 μm) are found in all parts of the gray matter except the substantia gelatinosa. Most are *relay (projection) cells* receiving synaptic boutons from posterior root afferents and projecting their axons to the brain. The projections are in the form of *tracts,* a tract being defined as a functionally homogeneous group of fibers. As will be seen, the term 'tract' is often used loosely because many projections originally thought to be 'pure' contain more than one functional class of fiber.

The largest neurons of all are the **alpha motoneurons** (soma 50-100 μm) for the supply of skeletal muscles. Scattered among them are small, **gamma motoneurons** supplying muscle spindles. In the medial part of the anterior horn are **Renshaw cells,** which exert tonic inhibition upon alpha motoneurons.

Spinal reflex arcs originating in muscle spindles and tendon organs have been described in Chapter 8. Originating in the skin is the *flexor reflex,* whereby the lower limb flexes in response to a noxious stimulus applied to the sole. The reflex is polysynaptic, with propriospinal spread over several segments. The full response involves a *crossed extensor reflex* designed to support the body weight on the opposite leg; the internuncials responsible cross the midline (*Figure 12.3*).

Laminae of Rexed

In thick sections of the spinal cord, the nerve cells exhibit a laminar (layered) arrangement. True lamination is confined to the posterior horn (*Figure 12.4*), but 10 laminae of Rexed have been defined in the gray matter as a whole in order to correlate findings from animal research in different laboratories.

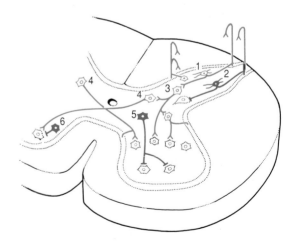

Figure 12.3 Propriospinal internuncial neurons. **(1)** Excitatory substantia gelatinosa neuron; **(2)** inhibitory substantia gelatinosa neuron; **(3)** flexor reflex internuncial; **(4)** neuron serving crossed extensor reflex; **(5)** Ia inhibitory internuncial; **(6)** Renshaw cell.

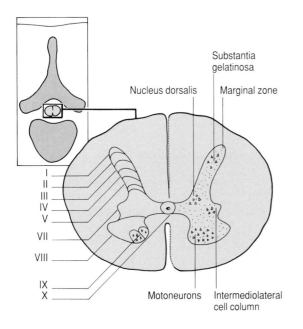

Figure 12.4 Laminae (I–X) and named cell groups at mid-thoracic level.

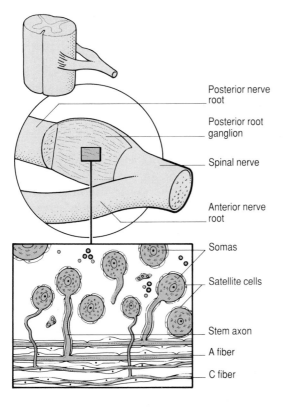

Figure 12.5 Posterior root ganglion. In bottom figure note T-shaped bifurcation of stem fibers.

SPINAL GANGLIA

The spinal or posterior root ganglia are located in the intervertebral foramina, where the anterior and posterior roots come together to form the spinal nerves. Thoracic ganglia contain about 50 000 unipolar neurons, and those serving the limbs contain about 100 000. The individual ganglion cells are invested with modified Schwann cells called **satellite cells** (*Figure 12.5*). The common stem axon of each cell bifurcates, sending a centrifugal process into one or other ramus of the spinal nerve (or into the recurrent branch) and a centripetal ('center-seeking') process into the spinal cord. Following stimulation of the peripheral sensory receptors, trains of nerve impulses traverse the point of bifurcation without interruption, although the cell body is also depolarized. The initial segment of the stem axon does not normally generate impulses but it may do so if the adjacent part of the posterior root is compressed, for example by a prolapsed intervertebral disc.

Traditionally, the centripetal axons of all spinal ganglion cells have been thought to enter posterior nerve roots. It is now known that many visceral afferents (in particular) enter the cord by way of ventral roots and work their way to the posterior gray horn. This feature accounts for the frequent failure of *posterior rhizotomy* (surgical section of posterior roots) to relieve pain originating from intra-abdominal cancer.

Central terminations of posterior root afferents (*Figure 12.6*)

In the *dorsal root entry zone* close to the surface of the cord, the afferent fibers become segregated into medial and lateral streams. The medial stream comprises medium and large fibers which divide within the posterior funiculus into ascending and descending branches. The branches swing into the posterior gray horn and synapse in laminae II, III, and IV. The largest ascending fibers run all the way to the posterior column nuclei (gracilis/cuneatus) in the medulla oblongata. These long fibers form the bulk of the gracile and cuneate fasciculi.

The lateral stream comprises small (Aδ and C) fibers which, upon entry, divide into short ascending and descending branches within the **posterolateral tract** *of Lissauer*. They synapse upon neurons in the marginal zone (lamina I) and in the substantia gelatinosa (lamina II); some fibers synapse upon dendrites of cells belonging to laminae III–V.

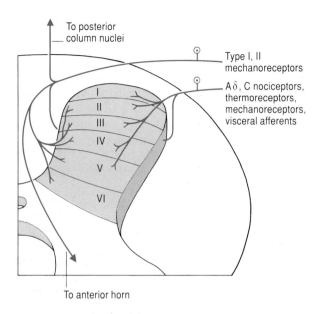

To posterior column nuclei

Type I, II mechanoreceptors

Aδ, C nociceptors, thermoreceptors, mechanoreceptors, visceral afferents

To anterior horn

Figure 12.6 Terminations of primary afferent neurons in the posterior gray horn.

ASCENDING SENSORY PATHWAYS

CATEGORIES OF SENSATION

In accordance with the flowchart in *Table 12.1*, neurologists speak of two kinds of sensation, conscious and unconscious. Conscious sensations are perceived, at the level of the cerebral cortex. Unconscious sensations are not perceived; they have reference to the cerebellum (see later).

Conscious sensations

These are of two kinds of conscious sensation: *exteroceptive* and *proprioceptive*. Exteroceptive sensations come from the external world; they impinge either on somatic receptors on the body surface or on telereceptors serving vision and hearing. Somatic sensations include touch, pressure, heat, cold, and pain.

Conscious proprioceptive sensations arise within the body. The receptors concerned are those of the locomotor system (muscles, joints, bones) and of the vestibular labyrinth. The pathways to the cerebral cortex form the substrate for position sense when the body is stationary, and for kinesthetic sense during movement.

Unconscious sensations

These also are of two kinds. *Unconscious proprioception* is the term used to describe afferent information reaching the cerebellum through the spinocerebellar pathways and their brainstem equivalents. This information is essential for smooth motor co-ordination.

Secondly, *enteroception* (Greek, enteron, gut) is a little-used term referring to unconscious afferent signals involved in visceral reflexes.

SENSORY TESTING

Routine assessment of *somatic exteroceptive sensation* includes tests for:

■ touch, by grazing the skin with the finger tip or a cotton swab
■ pain, by applying the point of a pin
■ thermal sense, by applying warm or cold test tubes to the skin.

In alert and co-operative patients, active and passive tests of conscious proprioception can be performed. Active tests examine the patient's ability to execute set-piece activities with the eyes closed:

■ in the erect position, to stand still, and to 'toe the line', without swaying
■ in the seated position, to bring the index finger to the nose from the extended position of the arm (finger-to-nose test)
■ in the recumbent position, to place the heel of the foot on the opposite knee (heel-to-knee test)

Table 12.1 Categories of sensation

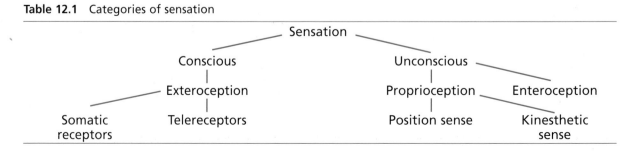

Passive tests of conscious proprioception include:

■ Joint sense. The clinician grasps the thumb or great toe by the sides and moves it while asking the patient to name the direction of movement ('up' or 'down'). Joint sense is mediated in part by articular receptors but mainly by passive stretching of neuromuscular spindles. (If the nerves supplying a joint are anesthetized, or if the joint is completely replaced by a prosthesis, joint sense is only slightly impaired. Alternatively, activation of spindles by means of a vibrator creates the illusion of movement when the relevant joint is stationary.)

■ Vibration sense. The clinician assesses the patient's ability to detect the vibrations of a tuning fork applied to the radial styloid process or to the shin.

SOMATIC SENSORY PATHWAYS

Two major pathways are involved in somatic sensory perception. They are the *posterior column-medial lemniscal pathway* and the *spinothalamic pathway*. They have the following features in common (*Figure 12.7*):

■ Both comprise first-order, second-order, and third-order sets of sensory neurons.
■ The somas of the first-order neurons, or *primary afferents*, occupy posterior root ganglia.
■ The somas of the second-order neurons occupy CNS gray matter on the same side as the first-order neurons.
■ The second-order axons *cross the midline* and then ascend to terminate in the thalamus.
■ The third-order neurons project from the thalamus to the somatic sensory cortex.

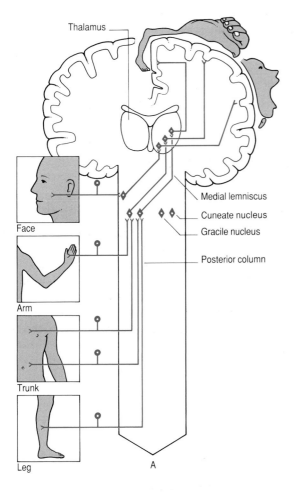
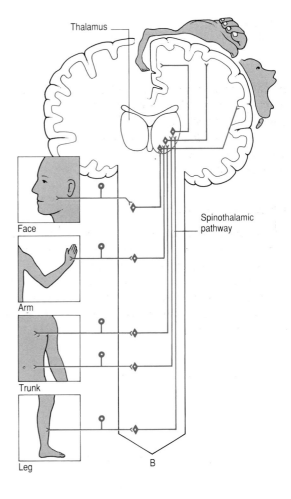

Figure 12.7   Basic plans of: **(A)** posterior column–medial lemniscal pathway; **(B)** spinothalamic pathway.

- Both pathways are *somatotopic:* an orderly map of body parts can be identified experimentally in the gray matter at each of the three loci of fiber termination.
- Synaptic transmission from primary to secondary neurons, and from secondary to tertiary, can be modulated (inhibited or enhanced) by other neurons.

POSTERIOR COLUMN-MEDIAL LEMNISCAL PATHWAY

The first-order afferents include the largest somas in the posterior root ganglia. Their peripheral processes receive information from the largest sensory receptors: Meissner's and Pacinian corpuscles, Ruffini endings and Merkel cell–neurite complexes, neuromuscular spindles, and Golgi tendon organs. The centripetal processes from cells supplying the lower limb and lower trunk send long collaterals in the **gracile fasciculus (fasciculus gracilis)** to reach the gracile nucleus in the medulla oblongata (*Figure 12.8*). The corresponding collaterals from the upper limb and upper trunk run in the **cuneate fasciculus (fasciculus cuneatus)** to reach the cuneate nucleus.

The second-order afferents commence in the posterior column nuclei, namely the **nucleus gracilis** and **nucleus cuneatus**. They pass ventrally in the tegmentum of the medulla oblongata before intersecting their opposite numbers in the great **sensory decussation**. Having crossed the midline, the fibers turn rostrally in the **medial lemniscus.**

The medial lemniscus diverges from the midline as it ascends through the tegmentum of the pons and midbrain. It terminates in the lateral part of the ventral posterior nucleus of the thalamus (**ventral posterolateral nucleus**).

Terminating in the medial part of the same nucleus (**ventral posteromedial nucleus**) is the trigeminal lemniscus, which serves the head region.

The third-order afferents project from the thalamus to the somatic sensory cortex (See Chapter 24 for details).

Functions

The chief functions of the posterior column-medial lemniscal pathway are those of *conscious proprioception* and *discriminative touch.* Together, these attributes provide the parietal lobe with an instantaneous body image so that

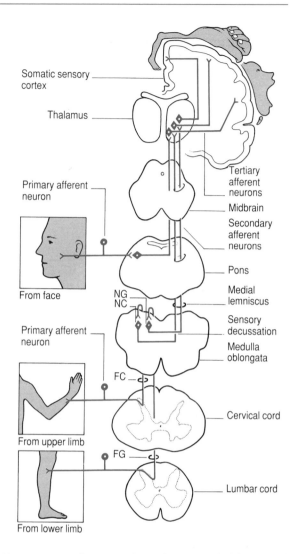

Figure 12.8 The posterior column–medial lemniscal pathway. FC, fasciculus cuneatus; FG, fasciculus gracilis; NC, nucleus cuneatus; NG, nucleus gracilis.

we are constantly aware of the position of body parts both at rest and during movement. Without this informational background, the execution of movements is severely impaired. For example, if the posterior columns are sectioned on both sides in a monkey, the animal tends to miss its target when swinging from one bar to another even though its entire motor apparatus remains intact.

In humans, disturbance of posterior column function is most often observed in association with demyelinating diseases such as multiple sclerosis. The classical symptom is known as *sensory ataxia.* This term signifies a movement disorder resulting from sensory impairment, in contrast to *cerebellar ataxia,* in which a movement disorder results from a lesion within the motor system.

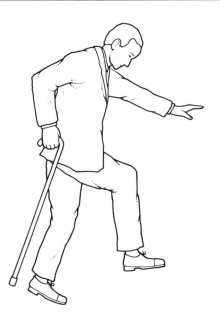

Figure 12.9 The 'stamp and stick' gait of sensory ataxia.

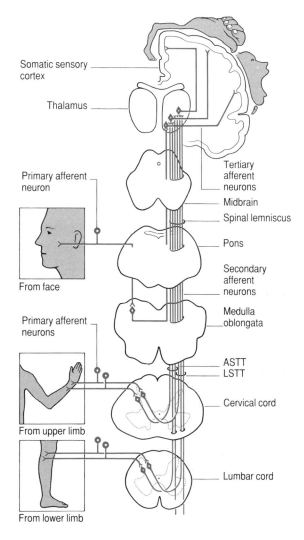

Figure 12.10 The spinothalamic pathway. ASTT, anterior spinothalamic tract; LSTT, lateral spinothalamic tract.

The patient with a severe sensory ataxia can stand unsupported only with the feet well apart and with the gaze directed downward to include the feet. The gait is broad-based, with a stamping action that maximizes any conscious proprioceptive function that remains (*Figure 12.9*).

Sensory testing in posterior column disease reveals severe swaying when the patient stands with the feet together and the eyes closed. This is *Romberg's sign*. (Inability to 'toe the line' with the eyes closed is tandem Romberg's sign.) The finger-to-nose and/or heel-to-knee tests may reveal loss of kinesthetic sense. Joint sense and vibration sense may also be impaired. (*Note:* Romberg's sign may also be elicited in patients suffering from vestibular disorders (Chapter 16); in cerebellar disorders there may be instability of station whether the eyes are open or closed (Chapter 20).)

Tactile, painful and thermal sensations are preserved, but there is impairment of *tactile discrimination*. The patient has difficulty in discriminating between single and paired stimuli applied to the skin; in identifying numbers traced on to the skin by the examiner's finger; and in distinguishing between objects of similar shape but of different textures.

A difficulty in assigning specific functional deficits to posterior column disease is the rarity of pathology affecting the posterior funiculi *alone*. In particular, the posterior part of the lateral funiculus is likely to be involved as well. Postmortem findings from patients having different degrees of pathology in the posterior and lateral funiculi, suggest that kinesthetic sense from the lower limb may be mediated in part by fibers that leave the gracile fasciculus at thoracic level and relay rostrally in the posterior part of the lateral funiculus.

SPINOTHALAMIC PATHWAY

The spinothalamic pathway consists of second-order sensory neurons projecting from laminae I, III, IV, and V of the posterior gray horn to the contralateral thalamus (*Figure 12.10*). The cells of origin receive excitatory and inhibitory synapses from neurons of the substantia gelatinosa; these have important 'gating' (modulatory) effects on sensory transmission, as explained in Chapter 19.

The axons of the spinothalamic pathway cross the midline in the anterior commissure at all segmental levels. Having crossed, they run upward in the anterolateral part of the cord. This 'anterolateral pathway' (as it is sometimes called) is divisible into an **anterior spinothalamic tract** located in the anterior funiculus and a **lateral spinothalamic tract** located in the lateral funiculus. The two tracts merge in the brainstem as the **spinal lemniscus**. The spinal lemniscus is joined by trigeminal afferents from the head region, and it accompanies the medial lemniscus to the ventral posterior nucleus of the thalamus, terminating immediately behind the medial lemniscus. Third-order sensory neurons project from the thalamus to the somatic sensory cortex (Chapter 24).

Functions

The functions of the spinothalamic pathway have been elucidated by the procedure known as *cordotomy*, whereby the spinothalamic pathway is interrupted on one or both sides for the relief of intractable pain. For a *percutaneous cordotomy*, the patient is sedated and a needle is passed between the atlas and the axis, into the subarachnoid space. Under radiological guidance, the needle tip is advanced into the anterolateral region of the cord.

A stimulating electrode is passed through the needle. If the placement is correct a mild current will elicit paresthesia (tingling) on the opposite side of the body. The anterolateral pathway is then destroyed electrolytically. Afterwards, the patient is insensitive to *pinprick*, *heat*, or *cold* applied to the opposite side (*Figure 12.11*). Sensitivity to *touch* is reduced. The effect commences several segments below the level of the procedure because of the oblique passage of spinothalamic fibers across the white commissure.

Cordotomy is sometimes performed for patients terminally ill with cancer. It is not used for benign conditions because the analgesic (pain-relieving) effect wears off after about a year. This functional recovery may be due to nociceptive transmission either in uncrossed fibers of the spinoreticular system (see later) or in C fiber collaterals sent to the posterior column nuclei by some axons of the lateral root entry stream.

The internal anatomy of the human spinothalamic pathway has been worked out from postoperative sensory testing and is shown in

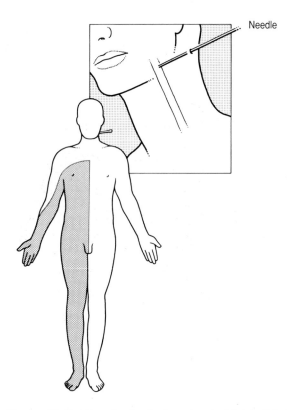

Figure 12.11 Usual extent of analgesia (shaded) following cordotomy at C1/2 segmental level.

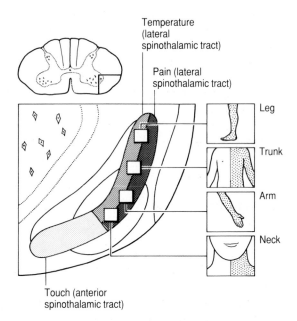

Figure 12.12 Sensory modalities in spinothalamic pathway at upper cervical level.

Figure 12.12. The picture is one of *modality segregation*. The lateral spinothalamic tract mediates noxious and thermal sensations separately, and the anterior spinothalamic tract mediates touch. The lateral tract is somatotopically arranged, the neck being represented at the front and the leg at the back. The anterior tract is likely (though not proven) to be somatotopic also.

A rare but classical condition illustrating dissociated sensory loss is illustrated in *Panel 12.1.*

SPINORETICULAR TRACTS

The spinoreticular tracts are the most antique somatosensory pathways. The reticular formation of the brainstem has scant regard for the midline, being essentially bilaterally distributed in terms of its ascending and descending connections. Spinoreticular fibers originate in laminae V–VII and accompany the spinothalamic pathway as far as the brainstem (*Figure 12.13*). Postmortem studies of nerve fiber degeneration following cordotomy procedures indicate that at least half of the spinoreticular fibers may be uncrossed. Accurate estimations based on axonal degeneration are difficult because some spinothalamic fibers give off collaterals to the reticular

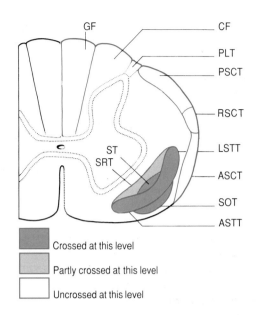

Crossed at this level

Partly crossed at this level

Uncrossed at this level

Figure 12.13 Ascending pathways at upper cervical level. ASCT, anterior spinocerebellar tract; ASTT, anterior spinothalamic tract; CF, cuneate fasciculus; GF, gracile fasciculus; LSTT, lateral spinothalamic tract; PLT, posterolateral tract; PSCT, posterior spinocerebellar tract; RSCT, rostral spinocerebellar tract; SOT, spino-olivary tract; SRT, spinoreticular tract; ST, spinotectal tract.

CLINICAL PANEL 12.1

SYRINGOMYELIA

Syringomyelia is a disorder of uncertain etiology, characterized by development of a syrinx (fusiform cyst) in or beside the central canal, usually in the cervical region (Figure *CP 12.1.1*). Initial symptoms arise from obliteration of spinothalamic fibers decussating in the white commissure.

The early clinical picture is one of *dissociated sensory loss:* sensitivity is lost to painful and thermal stimuli whereas sensitivity to touch is retained because the posterior column–medial lemniscal pathway is preserved. Typically, the patient develops ulcers on the fingers arising from painless cuts and burns. The joints of the elbow, wrist, and hand may become disorganized over time, or even dislocated, owing to loss of warning sensation from stretched joint capsules.

Progressive expansion of the syrinx may compromise conduction in the long ascending and descending pathways.

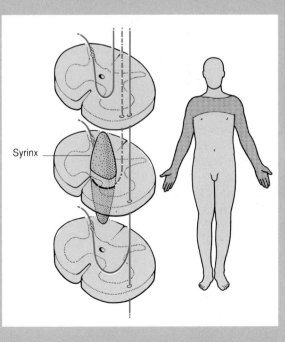

Figure CP 12.1.1 Syringomyelia. Shading shows distribution of analgesia.

formation as they pass by.

The spinoreticular tracts terminate at all levels of the brainstem and they are not somatotopically arranged. Impulse traffic is continued rostrally to the thalamus in the *ascending reticular activating system* (Chapter 19). Briefly, the spinoreticular system has two interrelated functions:

1 To arouse the cerebral cortex, i.e. to induce or maintain the waking state.
2 To report to the limbic cortex (e.g. the cingulate gyrus) about the nature of the stimulus. The emotional response may be pleasurable (e.g. to stroking) or aversive (e.g. to pinprick).

In summary, the phylogenetically old, 'paleospinothalamic' pathways through the reticular formation are concerned with the arousal and affective (emotional) aspects of somatic sensory stimuli. In contrast, the direct, 'neospinothalamic' pathway is analytical, encoding information about modality, intensity, and location.

SPINOCEREBELLAR PATHWAYS

Four fiber tracts run from the spinal cord to the cerebellum. They are:

- posterior spinocerebellar
- cuneocerebellar
- anterior spinocerebellar
- rostral spinocerebellar.

The first two are principally concerned with unconscious proprioception. The second two report continuously about the state of play among the internuncial neurons of the spinal cord.

Unconscious proprioception

Unconscious proprioception is served by the posterior spinocerebellar tract for the lower limb and lower trunk, and by the cuneocerebellar tract for the upper limb and upper trunk. Both are uncrossed, in keeping with the known control by each cerebellar hemisphere of its own side of the body.

The posterior spinocerebellar tract originates in the **nucleus dorsalis** of Clarke (thoracic nucleus) in lamina VII at the base of the posterior gray horn (*Figure 12.4*). The nucleus dorsalis extends from T1 through L1 segmental levels and the primary afferents from the lower limb enter the gracile fasciculus to reach it (*Figure 12.14*). Nucleus dorsalis receives primary afferents of all kinds from the muscles and joints, including an intense input

from muscle spindle primaries. It also receives collaterals from cutaneous sensory neurons. The fibers of the posterior spinocerebellar tract are the largest in the entire CNS, measuring 20 μm in external diameter. Very fast conduction (120 m/s) is required to keep the cerebellum informed about ongoing movements. The tract ascends close to the surface of the cord (*Figure 12.13*) and enters the inferior cerebellar peduncle.

The **cuneocerebellar tract** comes from the **accessory cuneate nucleus,** which lies above and outside the cuneate nucleus. The primary afferent inputs are of the same nature as those for the nucleus dorsalis; they reach it through the cuneate fasciculus. The cuneocerebellar tract enters the inferior cerebellar peduncle.

Information from reflex arcs

Two tracts originate in the intermediate gray matter of the cord. Although they receive some

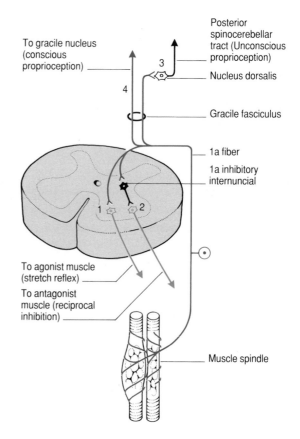

Figure 12.14 Functional anatomy of a spindle primary afferent from the lower limb. (**1**) Stretch reflex; (**2**) Ia internuncial serving reciprocal inhibition; (**3**) unconscious proprioception; (**4**) kinesthesia.

primary afferents of a similar nature to those already mentioned, their main function is to monitor the state of activity of spinal reflex arcs.

From the lower half of the cord, the pathway is the **anterior spinocerebellar tract** (*Figure 12.13*). The component fibers cross initially and run close to the surface as far as the midbrain. They then turn into the *superior* cerebellar peduncle and some of them re-cross within the cerebellar white matter.

From the upper half of the cord, the **rostral spinocerebellar tract** ascends without crossing and enters the superior and inferior cerebellar peduncles.

The **spinotectal tract** (crossed) runs alongside the spinothalamic pathway (*Figure 12.13*), which it resembles in its origin and functional composition. It ends in the superior colliculus, where it joins crossed visual and auditory inputs involved in turning the eyes/head/trunk toward sources of sensory stimulation.

The **spino-olivary tract** (crossed) sends tactile information to the **inferior olivary nucleus** in the medulla oblongata. The inferior olivary nucleus has an important function in *motor learning* through its action on the contralateral cerebellar cortex (Chapter 20). The spino-olivary tract may have a role in modifying olivary discharge when a moving part encounters an obstacle (for example, if the toe is stubbed while climbing a stairway).

A *spinocervical tract* is well developed in the cat, where the spinothalamic pathways are small. It seems to be vestigial or absent in humans.

CORE INFORMATION

The unipolar neurons of the spinal ganglia are first-order (primary) sensory neurons. They send a centrifugal process to peripheral tissues and a centripetal process into the cord. They serve all categories of somatic and visceral sensation, conscious and unconscious.

Conscious proprioception and discriminative touch are served by large centripetal processes that ascend to the posterior column nuclei in the medulla where second-order neurons project via the sensory decussation to the contralateral thalamus; third-order neurons project to the somatic sensory cortex.

Painful, thermal, and cruder tactile sensations are served by fine processes that enter Lissauer's tract and end in the posterior gray horn; second order neurons project across the midline at all segmental levels, coalescing as the spinothalamic tract (anterior and lateral) which is similarly relayed by the thalamus. The spinoreticular tract projects to the brainstem reticular formation of both sides; it has an arousal function and is concerned with qualititative aspects of stimuli.

First-order neurons serving unconscious proprioception from the lower body end in the nucleus dorsalis, for relay to the ipsilateral cerebellum by the posterior spinocerebellar tract; from the upper body they run via cuneate fasciculus to accessory cuneate nucleus, for relay by the cuneocerebellar tract.

Information about activity in spinal reflex arcs is relayed (partly crossed) by the anterior and rostral spinocerebellar tracts.

The spinotectal tract (tactile function, crossed) runs to the superior colliculus for integration with visual data. The spino-olivary runs to the inferior olivary nucleus.

SELF TEST

Select the false statement in each case:

1 The following are examples of conscious proprioception:

A Joint sense
B Position sense
C Kinesthetic sense
D Vibration sense
E Tactile discrimination

2 The following are tests of posterior column function:

A Ability to 'toe the line'
B Heel to knee test
C Tuning fork to tibia
D Two point discrimination
E Sensitivity to pinprick

3 Muscle spindle afferents have the following central terminations:

A Lateral gray horn
B Posterior column nuclei
C 1a internuncial neurons
D Alpha motoneurons
E Nucleus dorsalis

4 In the spinothalamic tract:

A The fibers belong to first-order neurons
B The fibers cross in the white commissure
C Crossing occurs at all segmental levels
D Tract terminates in ventral posterior nucleus of thalamus
E Section of right tract at T12 level would result in anesthesia of left leg

5 The fasciculus gracilis:

A Is composed of fibers belong to first-order neurons
B Is composed of uncrossed fibers
C Tract signals position of big toe but not of thumb
D Includes fibers with long internodes
E Terminates in ventral posterior nucleus of thalamus

6 At T12 segmental level the following tracts are uncrossed, *except*:

A Spinothalamic
B Gracile fasciculus
C Posterior spinocerebellar
D Posterolateral
E Rostral spinocerebellar

REFERENCES

Cervero, F. (1986) Dorsal horn neurons and their sensory inputs. In *Spinal Afferent Processing* (Yaksh, T.L., ed), pp. 197–216. New York: Plenum Press.

Coggeshall, R.E. (1990) Unmyelinated primary afferent fibers in the dorsal column, a possible alternate ascending pathway for noxious information. In *Recent Achievements in Restorative Neurology 3: Altered Sensation and Pain* (Dimitrijivic, *et al.*, eds), pp. 128–131. Basel: Karger.

Dykes, R.W. (1983) Parallel processing of somatosensory information: a theory. *Brain Res. Rev.* **6:** 47–115.

Nathan, P.W., Smith, M.C. and Cook, A.W. (1986) Sensory effects in man of lesions of the posterior columns and of some other afferent pathways. *Brain* **109:** 1003–1041.

Smith, M.C. and Deacon, P. (1984) Topographical anatomy of the posterior columns of the spinal cord in man. *Brain* **107:** 671–698.

Willis, W.D. (1985) Ascending somatosensory systems. In *Spinal Afferent Processing* (Yaksh, T.L., ed), pp. 243–274. New York: Plenum Press.

13

SPINAL CORD: DESCENDING PATHWAYS

Chapter Summary

Anatomy of the anterior gray horn
Cell columns
Cell types

Descending motor pathways
Corticospinal tract
Upper and lower motor
  neurons
Reticulospinal tracts
Tectospinal tract
Vestibulospinal tract
Raphespinal tract
Aminergic pathways
Central autonomic pathways

Blood supply of the spinal cord
Arteries
Veins

CLINICAL PANELS
  Strychnine poisoning
  Upper motor neuron disease
  Lower motor neuron disease
  Spinal cord injury

Study Guidelines

1 If you put *Figures 13.1* and *13.6* together while reading this chapter, the location of pathways descending to spinal motoneurons will be seen to make good sense. The *lateral corticospinal tract* passes alongside the motoneurons supplying the muscles of hand and foot, where this tract is uniquely important. The *pontine reticulospinal tract* and the *vestibulospinal tract* are close to extensor motoneurons and the *medullary reticulospinal tract* is close to flexor motoneurons. The *anterior corticospinal tract* and *vestibulospinal tract* are close to motoneurons serving vertebral muscles.
2 Note the six different kinds of target neurons selected by the lateral corticospinal tract, all for good reasons.
3 Note that the reticulospinal tracts are concerned with more automatic kinds of movement and with postural fixation.
4 The Clinical Panels dealing with upper and lower motor neuron disease and spinal cord injury are especially important. Learn to draw up a table comparing the diagnostic features of the two kinds of disorder.

ANATOMY OF THE ANTERIOR GRAY HORN

CELL COLUMNS

Each of the columns of motoneurons in the anterior gray horn supplies a group of muscles having similar functions. The individual muscles are supplied from cell groups (nuclei) within the columns. Axial (trunk) muscles are supplied from medially placed columns, proximal limb segment muscles from the mid-region, and distal limb segment musculature from lateral columns (*Figure 13.1*). Columns supplying extensor muscles lie anterior to columns supplying flexors; hence the presence of ventromedial and dorsomedial columns for the trunk, and ventrolateral and dorsolateral columns for the limbs. A retrodorsolateral nucleus is devoted to the intrinsic muscles of the hand and foot. An isolated, central nucleus supplies the diaphragm.

The segmental levels of the six somatomotor cell columns are listed in *Table 13.1*. The autonomic nervous system is represented by the intermediolateral cell column.

CELL TYPES

Large **alpha motoneurons** supply the extrafusal fibers of the skeletal muscles. Interspersed among

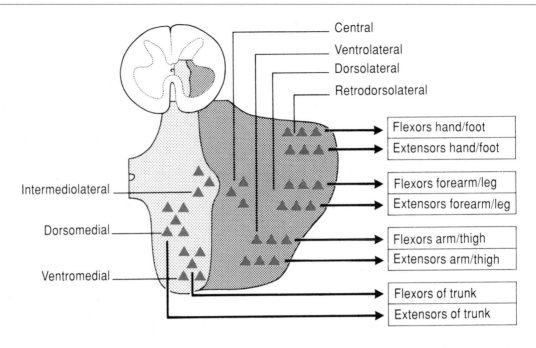

Figure 13.1   Cell columns in the anterior gray horn of the spinal cord: somatotopic organization.

them are small **gamma motoneurons** supplying the intrafusal fibers of neuromuscular spindles.

Tonic and phasic motoneurons

The α motoneurons have large dendritic trees receiving some 10 000 excitatory boutons from propriospinal neurons and from supraspinal pathways descending from the cerebral cortex and brainstem. (The term 'supraspinal' refers to any pathway descending to the cord from a higher level.) The somas of α motoneurons receive some 5 000 inhibitory boutons, mostly from propriospinal sources.

Two principal types of α motoneurons are recognized, tonic and phasic. Tonic α motoneurons innervate squads of slow, oxidative–glycolytic

Table 13.1   The somatomotor cell columns

Cell column	Muscles
Ventromedial (all segments)	Erector spinae
Dorsomedial (T1-L2)	Intercostals, abdominals
Ventrolateral (C5-8, L2-S2)	Arm/thigh
Dorsolateral (C6-8, L3-S3)	Forearm/leg
Retrodorsolateral (C8, T1, S1-2)	Hand/foot
Central (C3-5	Diaphragm

(SOG) muscle fibers; they are readily depolarized and have relatively slowly conducting axons with small spike amplitudes. Phasic α motoneurons innervate squads of fast, oxidative (FO) and fast, oxidative–glycolytic (FOG) muscle fibers. The phasic neurons are larger, have higher thresholds, and have rapidly conducting axons with large spike amplitudes.

Usually tonic neurons are recruited first when voluntary movements are initiated, even if the movement is to be fast.

Renshaw cells

The axons of the α MNs give off recurrent branches which form excitatory, cholinergic synapses upon inhibitory internuncial neurons called **Renshaw cells** in the medial part of the anterior horn. The Renshaw cells form inhibitory, glycinergic synapses upon the α motonerons. This is a classical example of *negative feedback*, or *recurrent inhibition*, through which the discharges of α motoneurons are self-limiting (see *Panel 13.1*).

Segmental-level inputs to α motoneurons

At each segmental level, α motoneurons receive powerful excitatory and inhibitory inputs. Note

CLINICAL PANEL 13.1

STRYCHNINE POISONING

Strychnine is a glycine receptor blocker. The victim of strychnine poisoning suffers agonizing convulsions because of liberation of α motoneurons from the tonic inhibitory control of Renshaw cells. The convulsions resemble those induced by the tetanus toxin, described in Chapter 6. This is no surprise because tetanus toxin prevents the release of glycine from Renshaw cells. Postmortem studies of normal human brain, using radiolabeled strychnine, have shown glycine receptors to be especially abundant in the nucleus of the trigeminal nerve supplying the jaw muscles, and in the nucleus of the facial nerve supplying the muscles of facial expression. These two muscle groups are especially affected in both types of convulsive attack.

that any inhibitory effect produced by activity in dorsal nerve root fibers requires interpolation of inhibitory internuncials, since all primary afferent neurons are excitatory in nature.

Segmental-level inputs to a flexor α motoneuron include the following:

- Type Ia and Type II afferents from spindles in the flexor muscles provide the afferent limb of the monosynaptic stretch reflex (for example, the biceps reflex).
- Type Ia afferents from spindles in extensor muscles exert reciprocal inhibition upon the flexor motoneurons via Ia inhibitory internuncials.
- Type Ib afferents from Golgi tendon organs in the flexor muscles exert autogenetic inhibition upon the flexor motoneurons.
- Type Ib afferents from Golgi tendon organs in extensor muscles exert reciprocal excitation of flexors via excitatory internuncials.
- Afferents from the flexor aspect of relevant synovial joints are stimulated when the capsule becomes taut in extension. They initiate an articular protective reflex, as described in Chapter 9.
- The *flexor reflex* is the withdrawal movement that occurs upon noxious stimulation of skin or muscle. Large numbers of excitatory, 'flexor reflex' internuncials are activated over several spinal segments on the same side as the stimulus, as well as inhibitory internuncials supplying motoneurons to antagonist muscles. In the lower limb, flexion of one leg is accompanied by an *extensor thrust* of the opposite leg, through the activity of excitatory internuncials projecting across the midline.
- Renshaw cells.

A reciprocal list can be drawn up for extensor motoneurons, with substitution of extensor thrust inputs for flexor reflex internuncials.

DESCENDING MOTOR PATHWAYS

Important pathways descending to the spinal cord are the following:

- corticospinal
- reticulospinal
- vestibulospinal
- tectospinal
- raphespinal
- aminergic
- autonomic.

CORTICOSPINAL TRACT

The corticospinal tract is the great voluntary motor pathway. Some 60–80% of its fibers take origin from the primary motor cortex in the precentral gyrus. Other sources are the supplementary motor area on the medial side of the hemisphere, the premotor cortex on the lateral side, the somatic sensory cortex, and the superior parietal lobule (*Figure 13.2*). The contributions from the two sensory areas mentioned terminate in sensory nuclei of the brainstem and spinal cord, where they modulate sensory transmission.

The corticospinal tract descends through the corona radiata and internal capsule to reach the brainstem. It continues through the crus of the midbrain and the basilar pons to reach the medulla oblongata. Here it forms the **pyramid** (hence the synonym, **pyramidal tract**).

During its descent through the brainstem, the

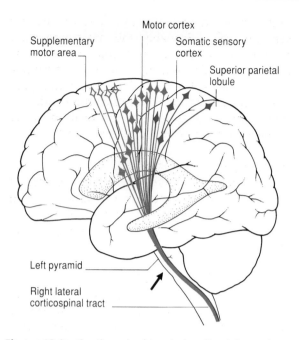

Figure 13.2 Corticospinal tract visualized from the left side. The supplementary motor area is on the medial surface of the hemisphere. Arrow indicates level of pyramidal decussation. Non-motor neurons are shown in blue.

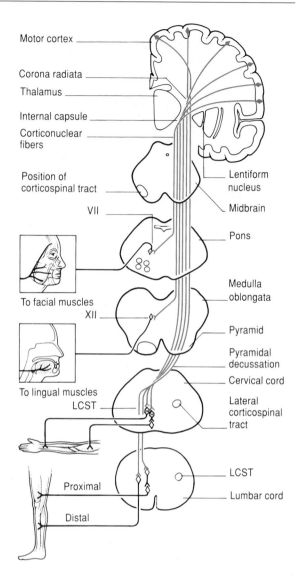

Figure 13.3 Corticospinal tract viewed from the front. At spinal cord level only the lateral corticospinal tract is shown. LCST, lateral corticospinal tract; VII, nucleus of facial nerve; XII, hypoglossal nucleus.

corticospinal tract gives off fibers which activate motor cranial nerve nuclei, notably those serving the muscles of the face, jaw, and tongue. These fibers are called **corticonuclear,** or **corticobulbar** (*Figure 13.3*).

Just above the spinomedullary junction (*Figure 13.4*):

- About 80% of the pyramidal fibers cross the midline in the **pyramidal decussation.**
- These fibers descend on the contralateral side of the spinal cord as the **lateral corticospinal tract** (crossed corticospinal tract).
- About 10% enter the **anterior corticospinal tract,** which occupies the anterior funiculus at cervical and upper thoracic levels. These fibers cross in the white commissure and supply motoneurons serving deep muscles in the neck.
- About 10% of the pyramidal fibers enter the lateral corticospinal tract on the same side.

The corticospinal tract contains about one million nerve fibers. The average conduction velocity is 60 m/s, indicating an average fiber diameter of 10 μm ('rule of six' in Chapter 6). About 3% of the fibers are extra large (up to 20 μm); they

arise from **giant neurons (cells of Betz),** located mainly in the leg area of the motor cortex (Chapter 24). All corticospinal fibers are excitatory and appear to use glutamate as their transmitter substance.

Targets of the lateral corticospinal tract (LCST)

Distal Limb Motoneurons

In the anterior gray horn, LCST axons synapse

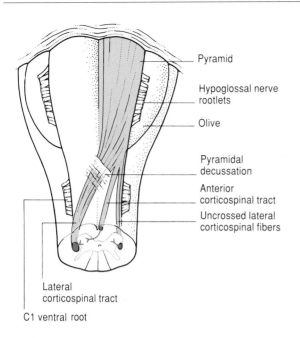

Figure 13.4 Ventral view of medulla oblongata and upper spinal cord, showing the three spinal projections of the left pyramid.

upon the dendrites of α and γ motoneurons supplying distal limb muscles, i.e. the extrinsic and intrinsic muscles of the hands and feet. A unique property of these *corticomotoneuronal fibers* of LCST is that of *fractionation*, whereby small groups of neurons can be selectively activated. This is most obvious in the case of the index finger, which can be flexed or extended quite independently, although three of its long tendons arise from muscle bellies devoted to all four fingers. Fractionation is essential for the execution of skilled movements such as buttoning a coat or tying shoe laces. Skilled movements are lost, and seldom recover, following damage to the corticomotoneuronal system anywhere from the motor cortex to the spinal cord.

As mentioned already in Chapter 8, the α and γ motoneurons are coactivated by the LCST during a given movement, so that spindles in the prime movers are signaling active stretch while those in the antagonists are signaling passive stretch.

Renshaw cells.

The number of possible functions served by LCST synapses on Renshaw cells is large because some of the cells synapse mainly upon Ia inhibitory internuncials, and others upon other Renshaw cells. Probably the most important function is to permit co-contraction of prime movers and their antagonists, in order to fix one or more joints—for example, when a chopping or shoveling action is required of the hand. Co-contraction is achieved by inactivation of Ia inhibitory internuncials by Renshaw cells.

Excitatory internuncials

In the intermediate gray matter and the base of the anterior horn, motoneurons supplying axial (vertebral) and proximal limb muscles are recruited mainly indirectly by the LCST, by way of excitatory internuncials.

Ia inhibitory internuncials

Also located in the intermediate gray matter are the Ia inhibitory internuncials, and these are the *first* neurons to be activated by the LCST during voluntary movements. Activity of the Ia internuncials causes the antagonist muscles to relax before the prime movers (agonists) contract. In addition, it renders the antagonists' motoneurons refractory to stimulation by spindle afferents passively stretched by the movement. The sequence of events is shown in *Figure 13.5* and its caption, for voluntary flexion of the knee.

In ballistic (fast) movement at any of the major joints, EMG records reveal a 'triphasic response' in the form of a momentary interruption of agonist activity by a twitch of the antagonist muscle group.

Presynaptic inhibitory neurons serving the stretch reflex

Consider a marathon runner. At each stride, gravity pulls the body out of the air onto a knee extended by the quadriceps muscle. At the moment of impact, all of the muscle spindles in the contracted quadriceps are thrown into active stretch. The obvious danger is that the quadriceps tendon will rupture. Golgi tendon endings (Chapter 8) offer some protection through autogenetic inhibition, but the main protection seems to be through presynaptic inhibition by the LCST of spindle afferents close to their contact points with motoneurons. At the same time, preservation of the ankle jerk is advantageous in this situation, giving immediate recruitment of calf motoneurons for the next take-off. The extent of suppression of the stretch reflex by the LCST in fact appears to depend upon the particular motor program being executed.

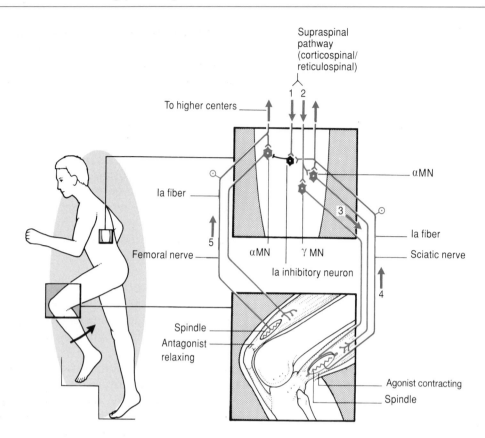

Figure 13.5 Sequence of events in a voluntary movement (flexion of the knee). **(1)** Activation of Ia internuncials to inhibit antagonist α motoneurons; **(2)** activation of agonist α and γ motoneurons; **(3)** activation of extrafusal and intrafusal muscle fibers; **(4)** feedback from actively stretched spindles increases excitation of agonist α motoneurons and inhibition of antagonist α motoneuron; **(5)** Ia fibers from passively stretched antagonist spindles find the respective α motoneurons refractory. *Note:* The sequence γ motoneuron-Ia fiber-α motoneuron is known as the gamma loop.

Presynaptic inhibitory neurons

In the posterior gray horn, there is some suppression of sensory transmission into the spinothalamic pathway during voluntary movement.

Modulation is more subtle at the level of the gracile and cuneate nuclei, where pyramidal tract fibers (after crossing) are capable of either enhancing sensory transmisssion during slow, exploratory movements, or reducing it during rapid movements.

UPPER AND LOWER MOTOR NEURONS

In the context of disease, clinicians refer to the corticospinal (and corticonuclear) neurons as upper motor neurons (*Panel 13.2*), and those of the brain stem and spinal cord as lower motor neurons (*Panel 13.3*).

RETICULOSPINAL TRACTS

The reticulospinal tracts originate in the reticular formation of the pons and medulla oblongata. They are partially crossed.

The **pontine reticulospinal tract** descends in the anterior funiculus, and the **medullary reticulospinal tract** descends in the lateral funiculus (*Figure 13.6*). Both tracts are believed to act upon motoneurons supplying axial (trunk) and proximal limb muscles. Access is indirect, by way of internuncial neurons shared with the corticospinal tract.

Information from animal experiments indicates that the pontine reticulospinal tract acts upon extensor motoneurons and the medullary reticulospinal tract upon flexor motoneurons. Both pathways exert reciprocal inhibition.

The reticulospinal system is involved in two

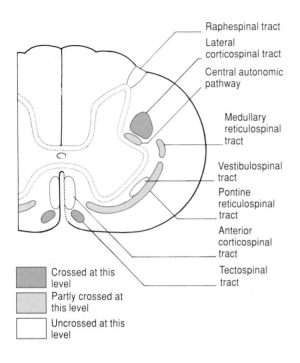

Raphespinal tract

Lateral corticospinal tract

Central autonomic pathway

Medullary reticulospinal tract

Vestibulospinal tract

Pontine reticulospinal tract

Anterior corticospinal tract

Tectospinal tract

■ Crossed at this level

■ Partly crossed at this level

□ Uncrossed at this level

Figure 13.6 Descending pathways at upper cervical level.

different kinds of motor behavior: *locomotion* and *postural control.*

Locomotion

Walking and running are rhythmical events involving all four limbs. Movements of the two sides are reciprocal with respect to flexor and extensor contractions and relaxations. In lower animals, locomotion is regulated by a hierarchical system in which the lowest members are internuncial neurons on both sides at cervical and lumbosacral levels, activating the flexors and extensors of the individual limbs. They are called *pattern generators.* Co-ordinating the pattern generators for the individual limbs is a further generator situated in the intermediate gray matter at the upper end of the spinal cord; it is capable of initiating rhythmical movements after section of the neuraxis at the spinomedullary junction. Locomotion is initiated from a *locomotor center* stretched across the midbrain at the level of the inferior colliculi. In anesthetized animals, electrical stimulation of the mesencephalic locomotor center with pulses of increasing frequency produces walking movements, then trotting, and finally, galloping.

Although the basic locomotor patterns are inbuilt, they are modulated by sensory feedback from the terrain. Overall control of the motor output resides in the premotor cortex, which has direct projections to the pontine and medullary neurons that give rise to the reticulospinal tracts. The tracts are used to steer the animal as it walks or runs, and to override the spinal generators, for example in scaling a wall.

Human locomotion is less 'spinal' than that of quadrupeds. However, the general neuroanatomical framework has been conserved during higher evolution, and the basic physiology seems to be in place as well. In particular, a bilaterally organized motor system controlling proximal and axial muscles *must* exist to account for the return of near-perfect locomotor function following removal of an entire cerebral hemisphere during childhood or adolescence. Such people never recover manual skill on the contralateral side, and this reinforces the belief among physical therapists that two distinct pathways are involved in motor control: *pyramidal* and *'extrapyramidal.'* The latter term denotes the reticulospinal pathway and its controls upstream in the cerebral cortex and basal ganglia.

Posture

Definitions of posture vary with the context in which the term is used. In the general context of standing, sitting, and recumbency, posture may be defined as the position held between movements. In the local context of a single hand or foot, the term denotes *postural fixation*—the immobilization of proximal limb joints by co-contraction of the surrounding muscles, leaving the distal limb parts free to do voluntary business. As will be noted in Chapter 24, there is reason to believe that the human premotor cortex is programmed to select appropriate proximal muscle groups by way of the reticulospinal tracts, to set the stage for any particular movement of the hand or foot.

The interpolation of internuncial neurons between the two main motor pathways acting upon motoneurons serving axial and proximal limb muscles, means that either pathway may be in command for a particular movement sequence—the extrapyramidal (reticulospinal) pathway for routine tasks, the pyramidal pathway for tasks requiring close attention—for example, picking one's way along a path strewn with rubble.

CLINICAL PANEL 13.2

UPPER MOTOR NEURON DISEASE

Upper motor neuron disease is a clinical term used to denote interruption of the cortico-spinal tract somewhere along its course. If the lesion occurs above the level of the pyramidal decussation, the signs will be detected on the opposite side of the body; if it occurs below the decussation, the signs will be detected on the same side.

Sudden interruption of the corticospinal tract is characterized by the following features:

1 The affected limb(s) show an initial flaccid (floppy) paralysis with loss of tendon reflexes. Normal muscle tone—defined as the resistance to passive movement (e.g. flexion/extension of the knee by the examiner)—is lost.

2 After several days or weeks, some return of voluntary motor function can be expected. At the same time, muscle tone increases progressively. The typical long-term effect on muscle tone is one of *spasticity*, with abnormally brisk reflexes (*hyperreflexia*). Classically, spasticity in the leg is 'clasp-knife' in character: after initial strong resistance to passive flexion of the knee, the joint gives way.

3 *Clonus* can often be elicited at the ankle/wrist. It consists of rhythmic contraction of the flexor muscles 5–10 times per second in response to sudden passive dorsiflexion.

4 *Babinski sign (extensor plantar response)* consists of dorsiflexion of the great toe and fanning of the other toes in response to a scraping stimulus applied to the sole of the foot. The normal response is flexion of the toes (see Figure CP 13.2.1).

5 *The abdominal reflexes are absent* on the affected side. A normal abdominal reflex consists of brief contraction of the abdominal muscles when the overlying skin is scraped.

The above features are most commonly observed after a vascular *stroke* interrupting the corticospinal tract on one side of the cerebrum or brainstem. The usual picture here is one of initial flaccid *hemiplegia* ('half-paralysis'), followed by a permanent spastic *hemi-*

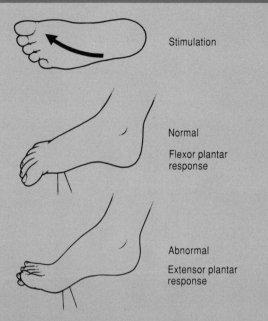

Stimulation

Normal
Flexor plantar response

Abnormal
Extensor plantar response

Figure CP 13.2.1   The plantar reflex.

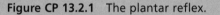

paresis ('half-weakness'). As illustrated in Chapter 27, *Panel 27.2*, the spasticity following a stroke characteristically affects the antigravity muscles. In the lower limb these are the extensors of the knee and the plantar flexors of the foot; in the upper limb, they are the flexors of the elbow and of the wrist and fingers. Following complete transection of the spinal cord, on the other hand, there may be a *paraplegia in flexion* of the lower limbs, owing to concurrent interruption of the vestibulospinal tract *(Panel 13.4)*.

The 'positive' signs listed under **2**, **3**, and **4** cannot be explained on the basis of interruption of the corticospinal tract alone. In the rare cases in which the human pyramid has been transected surgically, spasticity and hyperreflexia have not been prominent later on, although a Babinski sign has been present.

Spasticity and hyperreflexia are largely explained by the fact that stretch reflexes in spastic muscle groups are hyperactive. EMG records of spastic muscles show enhanced motor unit activity in response to relatively slow rates of stretch, e.g. slow passive elbow extension. However, this is not the sole basis of explanation. In patients with spastic hemi-

PANEL 13.2 (continued)

paresis, the ankle flexors show increased tone (resistance to passive dorsiflexion) even with very slow rates of stretch—too slow to elicit any EMG response. The resistance takes several weeks to become pronounced. It is called 'passive stiffness' and may be caused by progressive accumulation of collagen within the muscles affected.

Why are motoneurons hyperexcitable?
In paraplegic patients, spasticity and hyper-reflexia are often accompanied by increased cutaneomuscular reflex excitability, through polysynaptic propriospinal pathways. Pulling on a pair of trousers may be enough to produce spasms of the hip and knee flexors, sometimes accompanied by autonomic effects (sweating, hypertension, emptying of the bladder). Where the requisite technical facilities exist, the situation can be dramatically improved by perfusion of the lumbar CSF cistern with minute amounts of *baclofen,* a GABA mimetic (imitative) drug. The first inference is that the drug diffuses through the pia–glial membrane of the spinal cord, activates GABA receptors located on the surface of primary afferent nerve terminals, and dampens impulse traffic by means of pre-synaptic inhibition. The second inference is that the resident population of GABA neurons in the substantia gelatinosa has fallen silent in these cases through loss of tonic supraspinal 'drive'. The normal source of supraspinal drive seems to derive in part from the corticospinal tract, and in part from corticoreticulospinal fibers that reach the spinal cord via the tegmentum of the brainstem rather than via the pyramids.

How do voluntary movements recover?
The simplest explanation for the return of voluntary movement on the affected side would be a progressive increase in influence of the *ipsilateral* (unaffected) motor cortex on the 10% of *uncrossed* fibers in the pyramidal tract. Radiological studies of cortical metabolic activity (Chapter 24) indicate that ipsilateral motor areas do in fact become more active. It is of interest in this context that in righthanded individuals i.e. where the left hemisphere is dominant (a) right hemiplegias are usually more disabling than left hemiplegias; and (b) patients with right hemiplegia more often report some clumsiness of skilled movement on the *left* side. The inference seems to be that in righthanders the left cortical motor areas normally make a significant contribution to motor function on the ipsilateral side.

TECTOSPINAL TRACT

The tectospinal tract is a crossed pathway descending from the tectum of the midbrain to the medial part of the anterior gray horn at cervical and upper thoracic levels. It is strategically placed for access to axial motoneurons (*Figure 13.6*).

The tectospinal tract is an important motor pathway in the reptilian brain, being responsible for orienting the head/trunk toward sources of visual stimulation (superior colliculus) or auditory stimulation (inferior colliculus). It is likely to have similar automatic functions in humans.

VESTIBULOSPINAL TRACT

The vestibulospinal tract is an important uncrossed pathway whereby the tone of anti-gravity muscles is automatically increased when the head is tilted to one side. It descends in the anterior funiculus (*Figure 13.6*) and its function is to keep the center of gravity between the feet. It originates in the vestibular nucleus in the medulla oblongata. (*Note:* As explained in Chapter 16, there are in fact two vestibulospinal tracts on each side. The unqualified term refers to the lateral vestibulospinal tract.)

RAPHESPINAL TRACT

The raphespinal tract originates in and beside the raphe nucleus situated in the midline in the medulla oblongata. It descends on both sides within the posterolateral tract of Lissauer. Its function is to modulate sensory transmission between first- and second-order neurons in the

LOWER MOTOR NEURON DISEASE

Disease of lower motor neurons may be caused by a variety of infectious agents—notably the virus of poliomyelitis. The term *motor neuron disease*, or MND, is used to describe a symptom complex characterized by degeneration of upper and lower motor neurons in late middle age. The etiology is unknown; the variable manifestations of the disease are suggestive of more than one cause. During the first year or two, lower motor neurons alone may be involved, especially in the upper limbs. This phase is called *progressive muscular atrophy*. It has the following manifestations:

1 *Weakness* of the muscles affected, together with
2 *Wasting.* The wasting is not merely a disuse atrophy but results from loss of a trophic (nourishing) factor produced by motoneurons and conveyed to muscle by axonal transport.
3 *Loss of tendon reflexes* (areflexia) in the wasted muscles.
4 *Fasciculations,* which are visible twitchings of small groups of muscle fibers in the early stage of wasting. They arise from spontaneous discharge of motoneurons with activation of motor units. It should be stressed that fasciculations are sometimes observed in healthy muscle, especially after exercise.
5 *Fibrillations,* which are minute contractions detectable only by needle electromyography (a recording electrode in the form of a needle is inserted into the muscle).

Fibrillations are the result of denervation supersensitivity: following denervation, additional ACh receptors develop along the surface of muscle fibers, to the extent that the fibers respond to minute amounts of free acetylcholine in the circulating blood.

Sooner or later, *signs of upper motor neuron disease* appear. The lower limbs become weak, with increased muscle tone and brisk reflexes. This condition is called amyotrophic lateral sclerosis. Motor cranial nerve nuclei in the pons and medulla oblongata may be involved from the start (progressive bulbar palsy, Chapter 15) or only terminally. Death from respiratory complications usually occurs within 5 years of onset.

The absence of significant sensory disturbances is small comfort to these patients. *'Whatever you do, don't get motor neuron disease. It's bloody awful.'*—actor David Niven, who died of it.

The search for etiological clues is intense. Damage to motoneurons by free radicals has long been suspected, and it is of interest that mutation of a free-radical scavenging enzyme has been detected in some of the 10% of patients who inherit MND in an autosomal dominant mode. Other research targets concern the numbers and nature of neurofilaments, the question of autoimmune disorder, and possible benefits of neurotrophic (nerve growth) factors.

posterior gray horn—particularly with respect to pain (see Chapter 19).

AMINERGIC PATHWAYS

Aminergic pathways descend from specialized cell groups in the pons and medulla oblongata (Chapter 19). The principal neurotransmitters involved are *norepinephrine* and *serotonin*, both of which are classed as *biogenic amines*. The aminergic pathways descend in the outer parts of the anterior and lateral funiculi, and are dis-

tributed widely in the spinal gray matter. In general terms, they have inhibitory effects on sensory neurons and facilitatory effects on motor neurons.

CENTRAL AUTONOMIC PATHWAYS

Central sympathetic and parasympathetic fibers descend beside the intermediate gray matter (*Figure 13.6*). They originate in part from autonomic control centers in the hypothalamus and in part from several nuclear groups in the brain-

CLINICAL PANEL 13.4

SPINAL CORD INJURY

In the Western world, automobile accidents are the commonest cause of spinal cord injury. More than half of the victims are in the 15–30 year age group, and the cervical cord is most commonly affected.

Injury at thoracic or lumbar segmental level results in *paraplegia* (paralysis of lower limbs). Injury at cervical level causes *tetraplegia* (*quadriplegia*), in which the extent of upper limb paralysis depends on the number or level of cervical segments involved.

Spinal shock
The following features are found below the segmental level of the injury in the first few days following a complete cord transection:

- Paralysis of movement. The limbs are flaccid and tendon reflexes are absent
- Anesthesia (loss of all forms of sensation)
- Paralysis of the bladder and rectum.

In addition, the patient develops *postural hypotension* when raised from the recumbent position, because of interruption of the baroreceptor reflex. Wearing an abdominal binder may be sufficient to compensate for the lost reflex.

Return of spinal function
Several days or weeks later, reflex functions of the cord become progressively restored, and 'upper motor neuron signs' appear. Muscle tone becomes excessive (spastic). Tendon reflexes become abnormally brisk. A Babinski sign can be elicited on both sides. Ankle clonus is commonly seen when a patient's leg is lifted into contact with the footplate of a wheelchair.

If extensor spasticity in the lower limbs is dominant, the patient develops *paraplegia in extension*; if flexor spasticity is dominant, *paraplegia in flexion*. An extended posture may permit *spinal standing*; it is promoted by appropriate passive placement of the limbs, and it is the rule following cord injury which is either incomplete or low. A flexed posture is promoted by repetitive mass flexor reflexes involving the ankles, knees and hips; mass reflexes can follow any cutaneous stimulation of the legs if the flexor reflex internuncial neurons of the cord are already sensitized by afferent discharges from a bedsore or from an infected bladder.

The condition of the bladder is of great importance because of the twin dangers of infection and formation of bladder stones. For the initial, *atonic* bladder, a sterile catheter is inserted in order to ensure unobstructed drainage. Later, the bladder becomes *automatic*, emptying itself every 4–6 hours through a reflex arc involving the sacral autonomic center in the conus medullaris.

In animals, much of the damage done to the cord by injury has been shown to be secondary to local shifts in electrolyte concentrations, and to vascular changes including arterial spasm and venous thrombosis. Some modest success is being achieved in counteracting these effects. Another line of experimental research is to implant *embryonic* spinal gray matter at the site of injury. These grafts often survive and establish local synaptic connections, but the goal of functional recovery has not been attained.

stem. They terminate in the intermediolateral cell columns that give rise to the preganglionic sympathetic and parasympathetic fibers of the peripheral autonomic system.

The central sympathetic pathway is required for normal *baroreceptor reflex* activity. If the spinal cord is crushed in a neck injury, the patient loses consciousness if raised from the recumbent position within the first week or so because a fall of blood pressure in the carotid sinus on sitting up normally causes a compensatory increase in sympathetic activity in order to maintain blood flow to the brain.

The central parasympathetic pathway is required for normal bladder (and rectal) function. The fibers concerned originate in the reticular formation, mainly at the level of the pons (*Chapter 19*). The pontine center has a tonic inhibitory action on the sacral parasympathetic system. Severe injury to the spinal cord or cauda equina results in reflex voiding when the bladder is only half full (*Panel 13.4*).

Note on the rubrospinal tract

The rubrospinal tract is an important motor pathway in cats and dogs, where it arises in the contralateral red nucleus and descends in front of the corticospinal tract. In monkeys this tract is small and in humans it is quite negligible.

BLOOD SUPPLY OF THE SPINAL CORD

ARTERIES

Close to the foramen magnum, the two vertebral arteries give off **anterior** and **posterior spinal branches**. The anterior branches fuse to form a single **anterior spinal artery** in front of the anterior median fissure (*Figure 13.7*). Branches are given alternately to the left and right sides of the spinal cord. The posterior spinal arteries descend along the line of attachment of the dorsal nerve roots on each side.

The three spinal arteries are boosted by several **radiculospinal branches** from the vertebral arteries and from intercostal arteries. They are distinguishable from the small **radicular arteries** which enter every intervertebral foramen to nourish the nerve roots. The largest radiculospinal artery is the **artery of Adamkiewicz**, which arises from a lower intercostal artery or upper lumbar artery on the left side and supplies the lumbar enlargement and conus medullaris.

Vascular disorders of the spinal cord are quite rare. As part of a generalized atherosclerosis, a branch of the anterior spinal artery may become occluded, causing necrosis of the anterior half of the cord on one side. The clinical picture has some resemblance to a one-sided amyotrophic lateral sclerosis owing to destruction of anterior horn motoneurons and diminished function in the lateral corticospinal tract on the same side. However, arterial disease should be suspected here because of the relatively abrupt onset of symptoms and because concurrent damage to the spinothalamic pathway produces loss of pain and

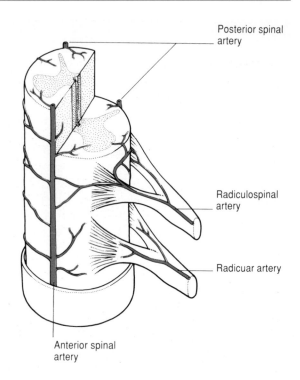

Figure 13.7   Arteries of spinal cord and spinal nerve roots.

of thermal sense on the opposite side, below the level of the lesion.

The artery of Adamkiewicz has to be borne in mind by the vascular surgeon attempting to deal with an abdominal aortic aneurysm. If a clamp is placed across the aorta and the artery happens to arise below that level, the patient is at risk of postoperative paraplegia with incontinence!

VEINS

The venous drainage of the cord is by means of anterior and posterior spinal veins, which drain outward along the nerve roots. Any obstruction to the venous outflow is liable to produce edema of the cord, with progressive loss of function.

CORE INFORMATION

Fibers of the corticospinal tract (CST) governing voluntary movement originate in motor, premotor and supplementary motor areas of the cerebral cortex; fibers governing sensory transmission during movement originate in the parietal lobe. The CST includes corticonuclear fibers innervating motor cranial nerve nuclei. The lateral CST innervates anterior horn cells supplying trunk and limb muscles; 90% of these fibers cross in the pyramidal decussation, 10% are entirely ipsilateral. Lateral CST targets include alpha and gamma motoneurons, Ia inhibitory internuncials, and Renshaw cells.

Clinically, the CST is the upper motoneuron. Damage (e.g. in hemiplegia from stroke) is characterized by initial flaccid paralysis, later by spasticity, brisk reflexes, clonus and Babinski sign. Lower motor neuron (anterior horn cell) disease is characterized by muscle weakness, wasting, fasciculation and loss of related segmental reflexes. Spinal cord transection is characterized by initial flaccid paraplegia/tetraplegia with areflexia, atonic bladder and (permanent) anesthesia below the segmental level involved; later, by spasticity, hyperreflexia, clonus,

Babinski sign, and automatic bladder.

Reticulospinal tracts are activated by premotor cortex. For locomotion, they originate in a midbrain pattern generator and travel to pattern generators in the cord. For postural fixation, they originate in pons and medulla and supply motoneurons via internuncials.

The tectospinal tract descends (crossed) from colliculi to anterior horn; it operates to direct the gaze toward visual/auditory/tactile stimuli. The (lateral) vestibulospinal tract (uncrossed) increases antigravity tone on the side to which the head is tilted. The raphespinal tract descends from the medullary raphe nucleus to the posterior horn via Lissauer's tract; it modulates sensory transmission, especially for pain.

A central sympathetic pathway from hypothalamus/brain stem to the lateral horn belongs to the efferent limb of the baroreflex. A central parasympathetic pathway activates the bladder and rectum.

The cord receives spinal branches from the vertebral arteries, boosted by radiculospinal arteries at segmental levels. Venous drainage is into segmental veins.

SELF TEST

Answer A if the item is associated with A only
B if associated with B only
C if associated with both A and B
D if associated with neither A nor B

A Alpha motoneurons
B Gamma motoneurons
C Both
D Neither

1 Innervated by corticospinal neurons
2 Axons emerge in posterior roots
3 Innervated by reticulospinal neurons
4 Inhibited by Renshaw cells
5 Fusimotor in nature

A Characteristic of upper motor neuron lesion
B Characteristic of lower motor neuron lesion
C Both
D Neither

6 Weakness
7 Rapid wasting
8 Fasciculation
9 Babinski sign
10 Sensory loss

Results of spinal cord transection at T12 level
A Immediate
B Late
C Both
D Neither

11 Motor paralysis of legs
12 Atonic bladder
13 Brisk reflexes
14 Ankle clonus
15 Sensory loss up to nipple level

REFERENCES

Ashby, P. (1993) The neurophysiology of human spinal spasticity. In *Science and Practice in Clinical Neurology* (Gandevia, S.C., Burke, D. and Anthony, M., eds.), p. 106–130. Cambridge: University Press.

Ashe, J. and Ugerbil, K. (1994) Functional imaging of the motor system. *Current Opin. Neurol.* **4:** 832–839.

Crone, C. and Nielson, J. (1994) Central control of disynaptic inhibition in humans. *Acta Physiol. Scand.* **152:** 351–363.

Jeanmonod, D. (1991) Neuroanatomical bases of spasticity. In *Neurosurgery for Spasticity* (Sindou, M., Abbott, R. and Keravel, Y., eds), pp. 3–14. New York: Springer-Verlag.

Levin, M.L. and Feldman, A.G. (1994) The role of stretch reflex threshold regulation in normal and impaired motor control. *Brain Res.* **657:** 23–30.

Massion, J. (1992) Movement, posture and equilibrium: interaction and coordination. *Prog. Neurobiol.* **38:** 35–56.

Meinck, H.M., Benecke, R., Kuster, S. and Konrad, B. (1983) Cutaneomuscular (flexor) reflex organization in normal man and in patients with motor disorders. In *Motor Control Systems in Health and Disease* (Desmedt, J.E., ed), pp. 787–796. New York: Raven Press.

Mitz, A.R. and Winstein, C. (1993) The motor system. 1, lower centers. In *Neuroscience for Rehabilitation* (Cohen, M., ed), pp.141–175. Philadelphia: Lippincott.

Morrison, K.E. (1995) Mechanisms in motor neuron disease - clues from genetic studies. *Molec. Med. Today* **1:** 195–201.

Nathan, P.W. and Smith, M.C. (1982) The rubrospinal and central tegmental tracts in man. *Brain* **105:** 223–269.

Schoenen, J. and Faull, R.L.M. (1990) Spinal cord: cytoarchitectural, dendroarchitectural, and myeloarchitectural organization. In *The Human Nervous System* (Paxinos, G., ed), pp. 19-54. San Diego: Academic Press.

Ugawa, Y., Uesaka, Y., Terao, Y., Hanajima, R. and Kanazawa, I. (1994) Magnetic stimulation of corticospinal pathways at the foramen magnum level in humans. *Ann. Neurol.* **36:** 618–624.

14

BRAINSTEM

Chapter Summary

Spinomedullary junction

Middle of medulla oblongata

Upper part of medulla oblongata

Pons

Isthmus

Midbrain

Orientation of brainstem 'slices' in MR images

Study Guidelines

1 This chapter is largely to do with identification of structures in photographs of brainstem taken at six levels. Try to become familiar enough to be able to name four out of five with the lists of labels covered up. That should suffice because all of the structures come up again later on.
2 Note that in MRI images the brainstem slices appear upside down.
3 Special attention *now*, to the four brainstem decussations will pay handsome returns later on. Their arrangement (*Figure 14.6*) does have an inner logic to it!

The following description of the internal anatomy of the brainstem is centered on six transverse sections stained by the Weigert method for myelin sheaths. The positions of the more important sensory and motor pathways are indicated, as well as the nuclei of cranial nerves. The course of the cranial nerves attached to the brainstem is given in the next four chapters. The reticular formation is described separately in Chapter 19.

SPINOMEDULLARY JUNCTION
(Figure 14.1)

In the ventral region, the chief feature is the **pyramidal decussation,** which gives rise to the **lateral (crossed) corticospinal tract.** On each side of the decussation at this level is the anterior gray horn of the spinal cord.

In the lateral region, the posterior gray horn of the spinal cord has merged with the **nucleus of the spinal tract of the trigeminal nerve.** *This nucleus is clinically significant in receiving nociceptive information from virtually the entire head and neck.* Nociceptive afferents to the 'spinal nucleus' come from the extracranial and intracra-nial territories of the trigeminal, glossopharyngeal, vagus, and upper three spinal nerves. The nucleus mediates such diverse pains as headache, toothache, earache, and pain in the neck.

In the dorsal region, the gracile and cuneate fasciculi can be identified. Next to the midline, the **nucleus gracilis** has made an appearance. In the interval between the two posterior column tracts and the pyramidal decussation is the **central gray matter** surrounding the central canal.

The locations of some smaller ascending and descending pathways are indicated. Most of the small tracts cannot be identified individually on the basis of the Weigert stain alone.

MIDDLE OF MEDULLA OBLONGATA
(Figure 14.2)

In the ventral region, the two **pyramids** are separated by the **anterior median sulcus.** Immediately behind each pyramid is the lower end of the inferior olivary nucleus (see next section).

In the lateral region the **spinal tract** and **nucleus** of the **trigeminal nerve** can be identified. On their lateral side is the **posterior spinocerebellar tract.**

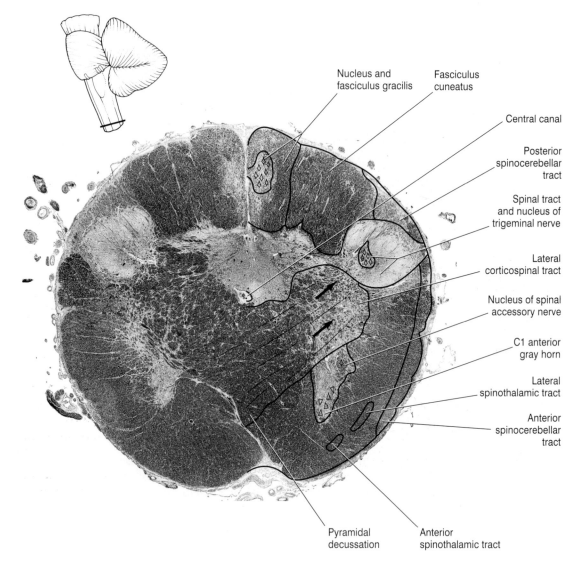

Figure 14.1 Cross–section at level of spinomedullary junction (see inset). Arrows indicate course of fibers crossing from the pyramid to form the lateral corticospinal tract. *(Note:* The photographs in this chapter are reproduced from The Human Brain, by N. Gluhbegovic and T.H. Williams, by kind permission of the authors and of J. B. Lippincott, Inc.)

In the dorsal region are the **gracile** and **cuneate nuclei**. These nuclei receive the first-order afferents serving conscious proprioception and discriminative touch. They give rise to second-order afferents which cross the midline and ascend to the contralateral thalamus. Initially, the second-order afferents comprise **internal arcuate fibers** sweeping ventrally and medially between the spinal trigeminal nucleus and the central gray matter. They intersect with their opposite numbers in the great **sensory decussation**. Having crossed, they turn rostrally as the medial lemniscus (see next section).

Density of staining in Weigert sections reflects thickness of myelin sheaths. As mentioned in Chapter 8, myelin thickness is in proportion to the length of the internodal myelin segments of nerve fibers, and therefore to velocity of conduction. The fastest (darkest) fibers are those of the posterior spinocerebellar tract and fasciculus gracilis. The spinal tract of the trigeminal nerve is light because of the preponderance there of unmyelinated (Group C) fibers.

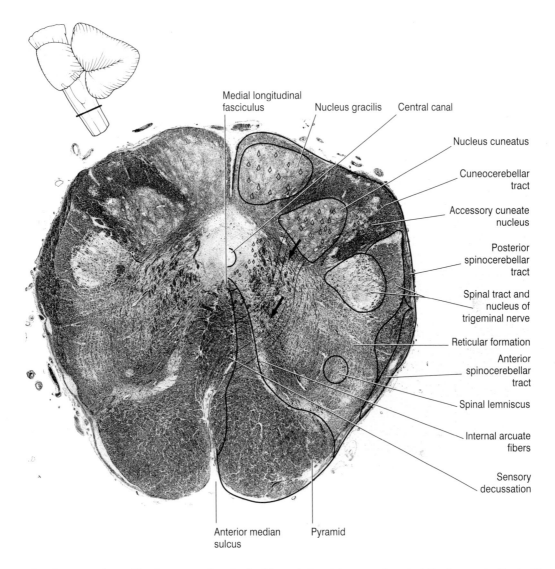

Medial longitudinal fasciculus
Nucleus gracilis
Central canal
Nucleus cuneatus
Cuneocerebellar tract
Accessory cuneate nucleus
Posterior spinocerebellar tract
Spinal tract and nucleus of trigeminal nerve
Reticular formation
Anterior spinocerebellar tract
Spinal lemniscus
Internal arcuate fibers
Sensory decussation
Anterior median sulcus
Pyramid

Figure 14.2 Cross–section of brainstem at level of mid-medulla oblongata (see inset). Arrows indicate fibers entering the sensory decussation from the cuneate nucleus.

UPPER PART OF MEDULLA OBLONGATA
(Figure 14.3)

The most striking feature is the wrinkled **inferior olivary nucleus** (ION), which creates the olive of gross anatomy. The principal cells of the ION give rise to the **olivocerebellar tract,** which intersects with other pathways before entering the opposite inferior cerebellar peduncle. The ION receives afferents from the motor cortex and red nucleus of its own side, and it has a powerful excitatory effect on the principal (Purkinje) cells of the cerebellar cortex. There is reason to believe that the ION is involved in some way when novel motor skills are being acquired (see Chapter 20).

Medial to the main inferior olivary nucleus are two **accessory olivary nuclei,** which are older phylogenetically.

Dorsal to the pyramid is the **medial lemniscus,** which is disposed dorsoventrally. Dorsal to the lemniscus in turn is the **medial longitudinal fasciculus** (MLF). The MLF runs the entire length of the brainstem and links the vestibular nucleus to the ocular motor nuclei (cranial nerves III, IV, and VI).

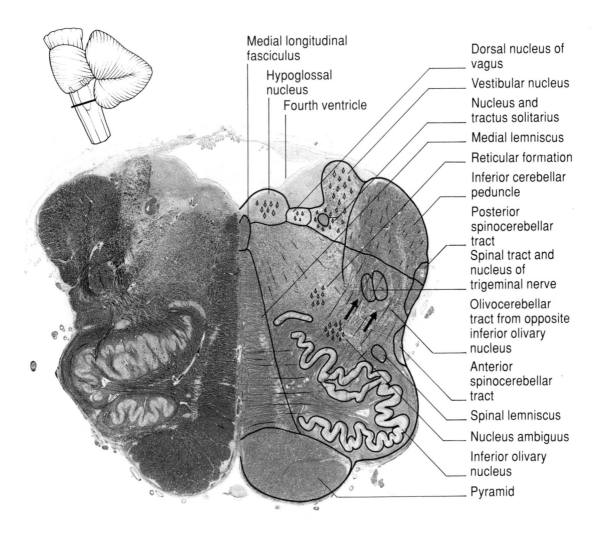

Figure 14.3 Cross-section of brainstem at level of upper part of medulla oblongata (see inset). Arrows indicate course of olivocerebellar fibers derived from the opposite inferior olivary nucleus.

Its chief component in the medulla is the **medial vestibulospinal tract,** which regulates the posture of the head in relation to the trunk (Chapter 16).

The central canal has opened into the caudal part of the **fourth ventricle.** In the central gray matter lining the floor of the ventricle are three cranial nerve nuclei:

1 Near the midline is the **hypoglossal nucleus,** which gives rise to the **hypoglossal nerve** for the supply of the lingual muscles.
2 Lateral to the hypoglossal nucleus is the **dorsal nucleus of the vagus.** This is a parasympathetic motor nucleus supplying preganglionic fibers to autonomic ganglia in the wall of the gastrointestinal tract.

3 The most lateral nucleus at this level is the **vestibular nucleus,** which **receives** special sense afferents from the vestibular labyrinth. As well as the medial vestibulospinal tract, this nucleus gives rise to the larger, **lateral vestibulospinal tract,** which helps to sustain the upright posture by acting upon motoneurons supplying extensor (antigravity) muscles.

Ventral to the vestibular nucleus is the **nucleus solitarius,** which surrounds the **tractus solitarius.** The solitary tract contains several kinds of primary afferent fibers terminating at different levels of the nucleus. The largest number are *visceral afferents* from the territory of the glossopharyngeal and vagus nerves.

The final nucleus to be mentioned here is the **nucleus ambiguus,** located in the tegmentum dorsal to the inferior olivary nucleus. The nucleus ambiguus gives rise to the **cranial accessory nerve,** which is distributed by the vagus. It also contains the *cardioinhibitory center (Chapter 15).*

Figure 14.4 shows the position of the various nuclei in a dorsal view of the brainstem.

PONS

The section shown in *Figure 14.5* is taken through the upper part of the pons, where the **superior cerebellar peduncles** are converging as they run upward on either side of the fourth ventricle.

The ventral two-thirds of the section are taken up by the massive **basilar pons,** in which two sets of myelinated fibers are obvious. One set consists of the **transverse fibers of the pons,** which originate in **nuclei pontis** on one side and cross over to enter the opposite **middle cerebellar peduncle.**

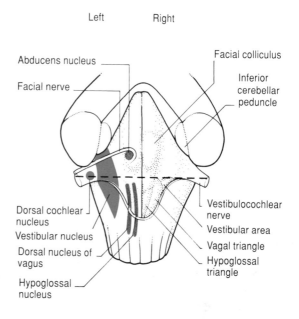

Figure 14.4 Cranial nerve nuclei beneath the floor of the fourth ventricle. Dashed line indicates pontomedullary junction. *Left:* position of the nuclei and of the facial nerve. *Right:* surface appearances, with descriptive anatomical terms.

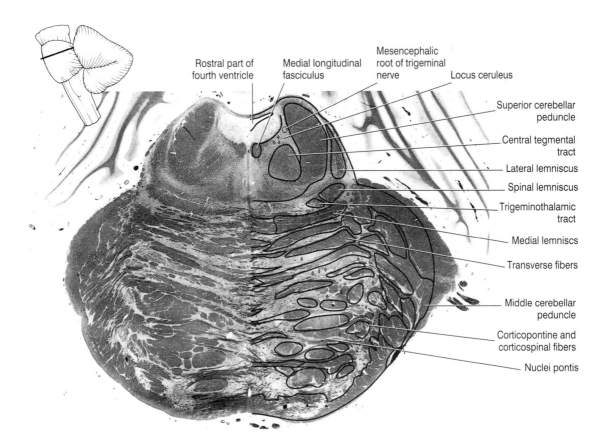

Figure 14.5 Cross-section through the upper part of the pons (see inset).

The other set is seen in cross section and comprises corticopontine and corticospinal fibers.

The **corticopontine fibers** descend from association areas of the cerebral cortex and synapse in the nuclei pontis. Together with the transverse set, they make up the *corticopontocerebellar pathway*, through which the cerebral cortex informs the contralateral cerebellar hemisphere about intended movements (*Figure 14.6*).

The corticospinal fibers constitute the **corticospinal (pyramidal) tract**. The tract is separated into individual fascicles by the transverse fibers. At this level, the corticospinal and corticopontine fascicles look alike.

Dorsal to the basilar region, the profile of the medial lemniscus is horizontal. At its outer border is the **spinal lemniscus** (conjoint anterior and lateral spinothalamic tracts). Alongside these is the **trigeminothalamic tract,** containing second-order sensory neurons from the head and neck. Outside the superior cerebellar peduncle is the **lateral lemniscus,** consisting of auditory fibers ascending to the inferior colliculus of the midbrain.

Medial to the peduncle is the **central tegmental tract,** containing fibers descending from the red nucleus to the inferior olivary nucleus.

ISTHMUS *(Figure 14.7)*

The **isthmus rhombencephali** is the relatively narrow junctional region of the pons with the midbrain. The ventral region shows the same features as the previous section (transverse fibers, corticopontine and corticospinal fibers). The intermediate, tegmental region is massively invaded by the **decussation of the superior cerebellar peduncles**. These consist of heavily myelinated axons that arise in the central cerebellar nuclei of one side and project to the opposite thalamus and red nucleus.

Dorsal to the decussation, the tegmentum contains the medial longitudinal fasciculus and the central tegmental tract. The medial and spinal lemnisci have been displaced to the side, and the lateral lemniscus is approaching the **inferior colliculus** of the midbrain.

The central canal has narrowed to form the caudal end of the **aqueduct**. The **periaqueductal gray matter** is bounded on each side by the **locus ceruleus** and the **mesencephalic trigeminal nucleus**. The locus ceruleus contains much the largest collection of noradrenergic neurons in the CNS.

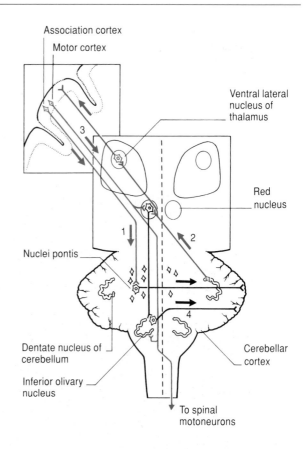

Figure 14.6 The four principal motor decussations of the brainstem. Contributory pathways are numbered in accordance with their usual sequence of activation in voluntary movements. **(1)** Corticopontocerebellar; **(2)** dentato-thalamo-cortical; **(3)** corticospinal; **(4)** olivocerebellar. Also shown is the rubro-olivary connection.

(These and other aminergic neurons are described in Chapter 19.)

MIDBRAIN

The section in *Figure 14.8* is taken from the upper part of the midbrain, where the tegmentum is blending with the thalamus.

Most ventral is the **crus cerebri,** which contains all of the 20 million corticopontine fibers descending to the nuclei pontis, and the one million fibers of the corticospinal tract (including corticonuclear fibers distributed to motor cranial nerve nuclei). The medial part of the crus contains corticopontine fibers from the frontal lobe; the lateral part contains corticopontine fibers

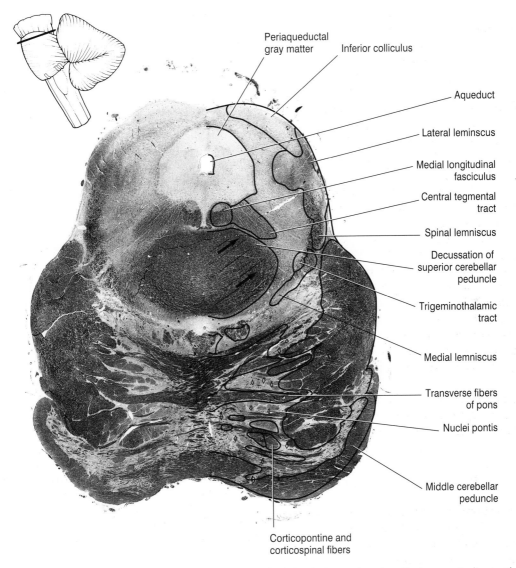

Periaqueductal gray matter

Inferior colliculus

Aqueduct

Lateral lemniscus

Medial longitudinal fasciculus

Central tegmental tract

Spinal lemniscus

Decussation of superior cerebellar peduncle

Trigeminothalamic tract

Medial lemniscus

Transverse fibers of pons

Nuclei pontis

Middle cerebellar peduncle

Corticopontine and corticospinal fibers

Figure 14.7 Cross-section of the brainstem at the level of the isthmus (see inset). Arrows indicate the course of fibers emerging from the decussation of the superior cerebellar peduncles.

from the parietal, occipital, and temporal lobes. The middle of the crus contains the corticospinal tract, mingled to some extent with neighboring corticopontine fibers.

The most ventral part of the tegmentum contains the **substantia nigra** ('black substance'). The pigment is *neuromelanin,* produced during synthesis of dopamine transmitter. The **nigrostriatal pathway** runs from here to the corpus striatum in the base of the cerebral hemisphere. Clinically, the nigrostriatal pathway is highly significant in relation to Parkinson's disease (Chapter 25). A second set of dopaminergic neurons occupies the **ventral tegmental area,** dorsal to the substantia nigra. These neurons project **mesolimbic fibers** to

the limbic lobe of the brain, and **mesocortical fibers** to large areas of the cerebral cortex. *The mesolimbic dopaminergic pathway seems to be significant in relation to psychiatric disorders including schizophrenia* (Chapter 26).

The medial part of the tegmentum contains the **red nucleus,** whose content of iron gives it a pink hue in the fresh state. The red nucleus receives ascending afferents from the contralateral central cerebellar nuclei. It receives descending fibers from the motor cortex, many of these being collaterals of corticospinal and corticobulbar fibers. The human red nucleus is almost entirely *parvocellular* (small-celled), and projects to the ipsilateral inferior olivary nucleus, to the cerebellum

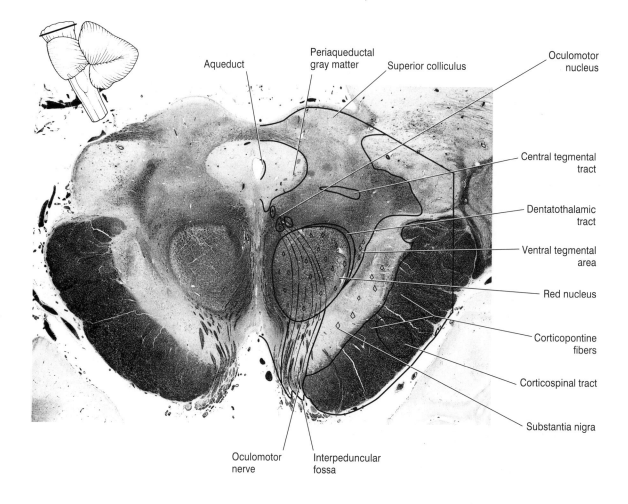

Aqueduct · Periaqueductal gray matter · Superior colliculus · Oculomotor nucleus · Central tegmental tract · Dentatothalamic tract · Ventral tegmental area · Red nucleus · Corticopontine fibers · Corticospinal tract · Substantia nigra · Oculomotor nerve · Interpeduncular fossa

Figure 14.8   Cross-section of the brainstem at the level of the upper part of the midbrain (see inset).

and reticular formation, and to the thalamus. The minute *magnocellular* part projects to the caudal part of the reticular formation. In laboratory mammals such as the cat, the magnocellular part of the nucleus is substantial and projects as the *rubrospinal tract* to motoneurons at all levels of the spinal cord. In humans this tract is, at most, negligible.

The lateral part of the tegmentum contains cerebellothalamic fibers; also the medial and spinal lemnisci and the trigeminothalamic tract. The dorsal part contains the central tegmental tract and the medial longitudinal fasciculus. Ventral to the periaqueductal gray matter is the **oculomotor nucleus,** which gives rise to the **oculomotor nerve.** The nerve passes through the medial part of the tegmentum and emerges from the brain into the interpeduncular fossa.

Dorsal to the periaqueductal gray matter is the **superior colliculus,** the principal subcortical center for visual reflexes. The central tegmental tract no longer contains rubro-olivary fibers but it becomes continuous at higher levels with the medial forebrain bundle (see Chapter 22).

ORIENTATION OF BRAINSTEM 'SLICES' IN MR IMAGES

Figure 14.9 shows the orientation of brainstem 'slices' in MR images (see also *Figure 4.6*). The orientation is the opposite of that in the sections. This is because, in photographs and drawings, the convention is to represent anterior structures below; in CT and MRI scans, on the other hand, anterior structures are represented above.

CORE INFORMATION

In the medulla oblongata, motor cranial nerve nuclei (c.n.n.) are the hypoglossal n., motor n. of vagus and n. ambiguus. Sensory c.n.n. are the spinal n. of trigeminal, vestibular n. and n. solitarius. Pathway nuclei include the gracile and cuneate which are cell stations on the posterior column-medial lemniscal pathway to the contralateral thalamus, and the inferior olivary nucleus receiving ipsilateral inputs from the motor cortex and red nucleus and giving rise to the (crossed) olivocerebellar tract.

In the pons are the motor and the pontine sensory n. of the trigeminal; and the abducens, facial and vestibulocochlear c.n.n. The basilar pons contains the CST but its bulk is composed of corticopontine fibers from ipsilateral association areas and pontocerebellar fibers crossing into the middle peduncle from the nuclei pontis. In the tegmentum are the medial, lateral, spinal and trigeminal lemnisci and the central tegmental tract.

In the isthmus rhombencephali the superior cerebellar peduncles decussate before passing to the contralateral thalamus and red nucleus.

In the midbrain proper are the oculomotor and trochlear c.n.n. The crus cerebri contains corticopontine and corticospinal fibers. The tegmentum contains the red nucleus; also dopaminergic neurons projecting from substantia nigra to striatum, and from ventral tegmental area to limbic lobe and large areas of cerebral cortex. The tectum comprises the superior colliculus (visual) and the inferior colliculus (auditory).

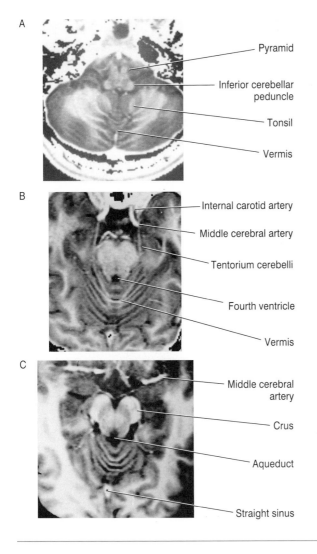

A — Pyramid, Inferior cerebellar peduncle, Tonsil, Vermis

B — Internal carotid artery, Middle cerebral artery, Tentorium cerebelli, Fourth ventricle, Vermis

C — Middle cerebral artery, Crus, Aqueduct, Straight sinus

Figure 14.9 MR images of **(A)** medulla oblongata, **(B)** pons, **(C)** midbrain in the standard radiological orientation. (Kindly provided by Dr Paul Finn, Director, MR Research and Development, Siemens Medical Systems Inc., Iselin, New Jersey.)

SELF TEST

Select the best response:

1 Which of the following nuclei does not occupy the medulla oblongata?

   A Hypoglossal
   B Gracile
   C Dorsal of vagus
   D Inferior olivary
   E Red

2 Which of the following nuclei does not occupy the pons?

   A Nuclei pontis
   B Motor trigeminal
   C Locus ceruleus
   D Nucleus ambiguus
   E Abducens nucleus

3 Which of the following nuclei does not occupy the midbrain?

   A Nucleus solitarius
   B Oculomotor nucleus
   C Substantia nigra
   D Mesencephalic trigeminal
   E Inferior colliculus

4 Which of the following items are not related?

   A Gracile nucleus — internal arcuate fibers
   B Pyramidal decussation — lateral corticospinal tract
   C Medial longitudinal fasciculus — medial vestibulospinal tract
   D Lateral lemniscus — superior colliculus
   E Nuclei pontis — transverse fibers

5 Which of the following is an ascending decussation?

   A Sensory
   B Superior cerebellar peduncles
   C Pyramidal
   D Olicocerebellar
   E Pontocerebellar

6 Example(s) of dopaminergic neurons

   A Nigrostriatal
   B Mesolimbic
   C Mesocortical
   D All of the above
   E A and B only

REFERENCES

Gluhbegovic, N. and Williams, T.H. (1980). *The Human Brain: a Photographic Guide*. New York: Harper & Row.

Nieuwenhuys, R., Voogd, J. and van Huijzen, C. (1988) *The Human Nervous System: a Synopsis and Atlas*, 3rd edn. Berlin: Springer Verlag.

Nathan, P.W. and Smith, M.C. (1982) The rubrospinal and central tegmental tracts in man. *Brain* 105: 223-269.

Toole, J.F. (1990) *Cerebrovascular Disorders*, 4th. edn. New York: Raven Press.

15

THE LAST FOUR CRANIAL NERVES

Chapter Summary

General arrangement of the cranial nerves
Cell columns in the medulla oblongata

Hypoglossal nerve
Motor supply to the hypoglossal nucleus

Spinal accessory nerve

Glossopharyngeal, vagus, and cranial accessory nerves
Nucleus solitarius
Nucleus ambiguus
Glossopharyngeal nerve
Vagus and cranial accessory nerves

CLINICAL PANELS
  Supranuclear lesions of IX, X and XI cranial nerves
  Nuclear lesions of X, XI and XII cranial nerves
  Infranuclear lesions of the last four cranial nerves

Study Guidelines

1 At spinal cord level, we noted two efferent and two afferent cell columns in the gray matter. We must add three more in the brainstem, and adjust the terminology a little to accommodate them.
   Comments on the last four cranial nerves in ascending order:
2 The hypoglossal nerve is straightforward; it is motor to the tongue. The spinal accessory nerve is straightforward; it is motor to the sternomastoid and trapezius.
3 The cranial accessory nerve supplies the intrinsic muscles of larynx and pharynx, and the levator palati. It is *distributed* by the vagus.
4 The vagus nerve proper is the principal preganglionic parasympathetic nerve. It is also the principal visceral afferent nerve.
5 Main features of the glossopharyngeal are: (a) it provides the afferent limb of the gag reflex; (b) it tells us when we have an inflamed throat; (c) it signals bitterness; (d) its carotid branch carries afferents from the carotid sinus monitoring blood pressure and from the carotid body monitoring blood gases; (e) it gives a clinically significant branch to the middle ear.

GENERAL ARRANGEMENT OF THE CRANIAL NERVES

In the thoracic region of the developing spinal cord, four distinct cell columns can be identified in the gray matter on each side (*Figure 15.1A,B*). In the basal plate, the *general somatic efferent column* supplies the striated muscles of the trunk and limbs. The *general visceral efferent column* contains preganglionic neurons of the autonomic system. In the alar plate, the *general visceral afferent column* receives afferents from thoracic and abdominal organs. A general somatic afferent column receives afferents from the body wall.

In the brainstem, these four cell columns can be identified. However, they are fragmented, and

not all of them contribute to each cranial nerve. Their connections are as follows:

■ *General somatic efferent:* supplies the striated musculature of the orbit and of the tongue.
■ *General visceral efferent:* gives rise to the cranial parasympathetic system described in Chapter 10. The target ganglia are the ciliary, pterygopalatine, otic, and submandibular ganglia in the head, and the vagal ganglia in the thorax and abdomen.
■ *General visceral afferent:* receives afferents from the visceral territory of the vagus.
■ *General somatic afferent:* receives afferents from skin and mucous membranes, mainly in the territory of the trigeminal nerve.

Additional cell columns are present for branchial

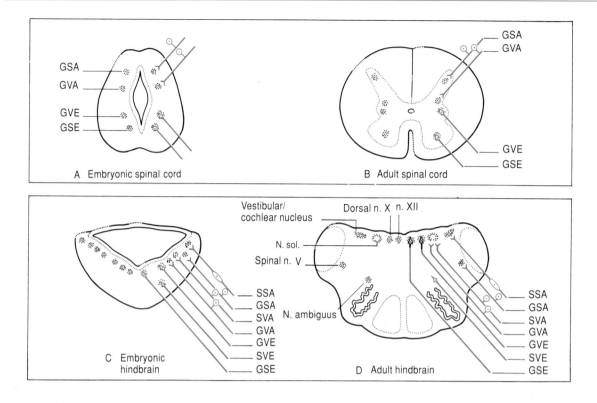

Figure 15.1   Cell columns of the spinal cord and brainstem. **(A)** Embryonic spinal cord; **(B)** adult spinal cord; **(C)** embryonic hindbrain; **(D)** adult hindbrain. Afferent cell columns: GSA, general somatic afferent; GVA, general visceral afferent; SSA, special somatic afferent; SVA, special visceral afferent. Efferent cell columns: GSE, general somatic efferent; GVE, general visceral efferent; SVE, special visceral efferent. N. sol., nucleus solitarius.

arch tissues and for the inner ear (*Figure 15.1C,D*):

■ *Special visceral efferent*: supplies the branchial arch musculature of the face, jaws, larynx and pharynx. These striated muscles have visceral functions in relation to food and air intake (hence the name).
■ *Special visceral afferent*: receives afferents from taste buds located in the endoderm lining the branchial arches.
■ Special sense afferent: receives afferents from the inner ear.

CELL COLUMNS IN THE MEDULLA OBLONGATA *(FIGURE 15.1D)*

■ The somatic efferent cell column is represented by the **hypoglossal nucleus.**
■ The special visceral efferent cell column is represented by the **nucleus ambiguus,** which migrated prenatally to a position dorsal to the inferior olivary nucleus.

■ The general visceral efferent cell column is represented by the **dorsal nucleus of the vagus,** and by the most rostral part of the nucleus ambiguus.
■ The general visceral afferent cell column is represented by the lower end of the **nucleus solitarius.**
■ The special visceral afferent cell column is represented by the upper end of the **nucleus solitarius.**
■ The general somatic afferent cell column is represented by the **spinal trigeminal nucleus,** which migrated prenatally to a lateral position.
■ The special somatic afferent cell column is represented by the **vestibular** and **cochlear nuclei,** located at the pontomedullary junction.

The hypoglossal (XII), accessory (XI), vagus (X), and glossopharyngeal (IX) nerves will now be described. The emphasis will be on functional aspects of the component fibers, at the expense of topographic detail.

HYPOGLOSSAL NERVE

The hypoglossal nerve (cranial nerve XII) contains somatic efferent fibers for the supply of the extrinsic and intrinsic muscles of the tongue. Its nucleus lies close to the midline and extends the full length of the medulla (*Figure 15.2*). The nerve emerges as a series of rootlets in the interval between the pyramid and the olive. It crosses the subarachnoid space and leaves the skull through the hypoglossal canal. Just below the skull it lies close to the vagus and spinal accessory nerves (*Figure 15.3*). It descends on the carotid sheath to the level of the angle of the mandible, then passes forward on the surface of the hyoglossus muscle where it gives off its terminal branches.

In the neck, proprioceptive fibers enter the nerve from the cervical plexus, for distribution to about 100 muscle spindles in the same half of the tongue.

Phylogenetic note

In reptiles, the lingual muscles, the geniohyoid muscle and the infrahyoid muscles develop together from the uppermost mesodermal

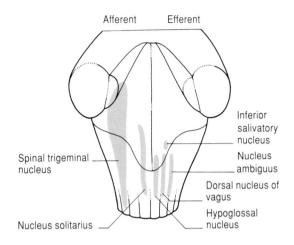

Figure 15.2 Cell columns for the last four cranial nerves.

somites. The somatic efferent neurons supplying this *hypobranchial muscle sheet* form a continuous ribbon of cells extending from lower medulla to spinal segment C3. In mammals, the hypoglossal nucleus is located more rostrally and its rootlets emerge separately from the cervical rootlets. However, the caudal limit of the hypoglossal nucleus remains linked to the cervical

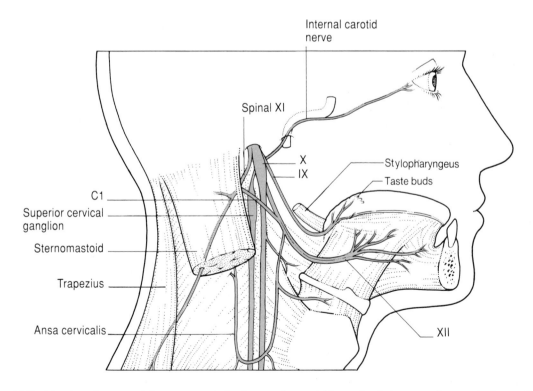

Figure 15.3 The last four cranial nerves and the internal carotid branch of the superior cervical ganglion.

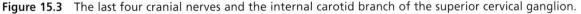

motor cell column by the *supraspinal nucleus*, from which the thyrohyoid muscle is supplied via the first cervical ventral root. In rodents, some of the intrinsic muscle fibers of the tongue receive their motor supply indirectly, from axons which leave the most caudal cells of the hypoglossal nucleus and emerge in the first cervical nerve to join the hypoglossal nerve trunk in the neck. Whether this arrangement holds for primates is not yet known.

MOTOR SUPPLY TO THE HYPOGLOSSAL NUCLEUS

The hypoglossal nucleus receives inputs from the reticular formation, whereby it is recruited for stereotyped motor routines in eating and swallowing. The delicate movements of the tongue during speech require a corticobulbar supply to the nucleus from the large area of the motor cortex involved in this function (*Figure 15.4*). Most of the corticobulbar fibers for the tongue cross over in the upper part of the pyramidal decussation; some remain uncrossed and supply the ipsilateral nucleus.

Supranuclear, nuclear, and infranuclear lesions of the hypoglossal nerve are described together with lesions of the accessory nerve (see *Panels 15.1-15.3*).

Notes on the terms 'corticobulbar' and 'supranuclear'

The *'bulb'* is an archaic term for the medulla oblongata. In clinical usage, it includes the pons as well. *Corticobulbar* (*supranuclear*) fibers are fibers of the pyramidal tract which act upon the motor cranial nerve nuclei of the pons (trigeminal and facial) and medulla (hypoglossal and nucleus ambiguus). The spinal accessory nucleus is also included, although it occupies the spinal cord.

Neither term is used with respect to the ocular motor nuclei (oculomotor, trochlear, abducens) because their cortical supply is separate from the pyramidal tract (see Chapter 18).

SPINAL ACCESSORY NERVE

The spinal accessory (cranial nerve XI) is a purely motor nerve attached to the uppermost five segments of the spinal cord. The nucleus of origin is a column of α and γ motoneurons in the base of the anterior gray horn.

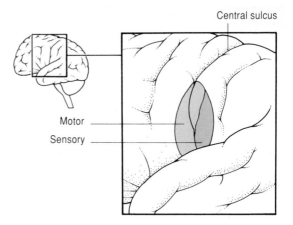

Figure 15.4 Areas of the precentral gyrus and postcentral gyrus containing cortical representations of the tongue. The cells concerned are interspersed among others devoted to the face. (Adapted from Picard, C. and Olivier, A. (1983) *J. Neurosurg.* **59:** 781-789)

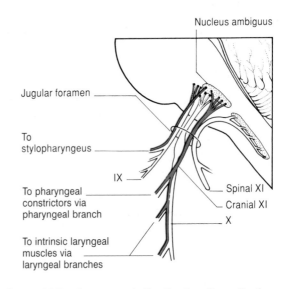

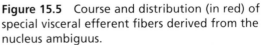

Figure 15.5 Course and distribution (in red) of special visceral efferent fibers derived from the nucleus ambiguus.

The nerve runs upward in the subarachnoid space, behind the denticulate ligament. It enters the cranial cavity through the foramen magnum and leaves it again through the jugular foramen. While in the jugular foramen, it shares a dural sheath with the cranial accessory nerve, but there is no exchange of fibers (*Figure 15.5*).

CLINICAL PANEL 15.1

SUPRANUCLEAR LESIONS OF THE IX, X, AND XI CRANIAL NERVES

The corticonuclear supply to the IX, X, and XI cranial nerves is shown in *Figure CP 15.1.1*. Supranuclear lesions of all three are commonly seen following vascular strokes damaging the pyramidal tract in the cerebrum or brainstem.

Effects of unilateral supranuclear lesions
1 The supranuclear supply to the hypoglossal nucleus is mainly crossed. The usual picture following a hemiplegic stroke is as follows: during the first few hours or days the tongue, when protruded, deviates toward the paralyzed side because of the stronger pull of the healthy genioglossus. Later, the tongue does not deviate on protrusion.
2 The supranuclear supply to the nucleus ambiguus is bilateral. Phonation and swallowing will therefore not be affected.
3 The supranuclear supply to the spinal XI nucleus is uncrossed for sternomastoid motoneurons and crossed for trapezius motoneurons. The explanation for this arrangement is as follows. When an object in the (say) left hand is held up for inspection, the left trapezius is used to support the weight of the object and the right sternomastoid is used to turn the head. Both actions are effected by the right pyramidal tract.

Effects of bilateral supranuclear lesions
The supranuclear supply to the hypoglossal

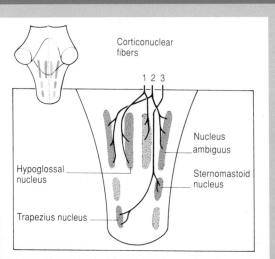

Figure CP 15.1.1 Corticonuclear inputs to XI and XII motoneurons. For numbers see text.

nucleus and nucleus ambiguus may be compromised *bilaterally* by thrombotic episodes in the brainstem in patients suffering from arteriosclerosis of the vertebrobasilar arterial system. The motor nuclei of the trigeminal nerve (to the masticatory muscles) and of the facial nerve (to the facial muscles) may be affected as well. The characteristic picture, known as *pseudobulbar palsy*, is that of an elderly patient who has spastic (tightened) oral and pharyngeal musculature, with consequent difficulty with speech articulation, chewing, and swallowing. The gait is slow and shuffling because of involvement of corticospinal fibers descending to the spinal cord.

CLINICAL PANEL 15.2

NUCLEAR LESIONS OF THE X, XI, AND XII CRANIAL NERVES

Lesions of the hypoglossal nucleus and nucleus ambiguus occur together in *progressive bulbar palsy*, a variant of progressive muscular atrophy (Chapter 13) in which the cranial motor nuclei of the pons and medulla are attacked at the outset. The patient quickly becomes distressed by a multitude of problems: difficulty in chewing and articulation

(mandibular and facial nuclei, Chapter 17) and difficulty in swallowing and phonation (hypoglossal and cranial accessory nuclei).

Unilateral lesions at nuclear level may be caused by thrombosis of the vertebral artery or of one of its branches (see Lateral Medullary Syndrome in Chapter 16). The distribution of motor weakness is the same as for infranuclear lesions (see *Panel 15.3*).

INFRANUCLEAR LESIONS OF THE LAST FOUR CRANIAL NERVES

Jugular foramen syndrome

The last four cranial nerves, and the internal carotid (sympathetic) nerve nearby, are at risk of entrapment by a tumor spreading along the base of the skull. The tumor may be a primary one in the nasopharynx, or a metastatic one within lymph nodes of the upper cervical chain. In the second case the primary tumor may be in an air sinus or in the tongue, larynx, or pharynx. In either case a mass can usually be felt behind the ramus of the mandible. The symptomatology varies with the number of nerves caught up in the tumor, and the degree to which the nerves are compromised.

Symptoms

■ Pain in or behind the ear, attributable to irritation of the tympanic/auricular branches of the IX and X nerves. *Whenever an adult complains of constant pain in one ear, without evidence of middle ear disease, a cancer of the pharynx must be suspected.*

■ Headache, from irritation of the meningeal branch of the vagus.

■ Hoarseness, due to paralysis of laryngomotor fibers.

■ Dysphagia (difficulty in swallowing) due to paralysis of pharyngomotor fibers.

Signs (see *Figure CP 15.3.1*)

■ Horner's syndrome (ptosis of the upper eyelid, with some pupillary constriction) from interruption of the internal carotid nerve.

■ Infranuclear paralysis of the hypoglossal nerve, with wasting of the affected side of the tongue and deviation of the tongue to the affected side on protrusion.

■ When the patient is asked to say 'Aahh' the uvula is pulled away from the affected side by the unopposed healthy levator palati.

■ Sensory loss in the oropharynx on the affected side.

■ On laryngoscopic examination, inability to adduct the vocal cord to the midline.

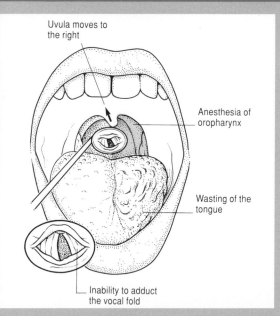

Figure CP 15.3.1 Left-sided jugular foramen syndrome. A laryngeal mirror is being used to inspect the vocal folds during an attempt to cough.

■ Interruption of the spinal accessory nerve produces weakness and wasting of the sternomastoid and trapezius.

A jugular foramen syndrome may also be caused by invasion of the jugular foramen from above, for instance by a tumor extending from the cerebellopontine angle (Chapter 17). In this case the sympathetic and spinal accessory nerves will be out of reach, and unaffected.

Isolated lesion of the spinal accessory nerve

The surface marking for the spinal accessory nerve in the posterior triangle of the neck is a line drawn from the posterior border of the sternomastoid one-third of the way down to the anterior border of the trapezius two-thirds of the way down. It may be injured in this part of its course by a stab wound, or during a surgical procedure for removal of cancerous lymph nodes. The trapezius is selectively paralyzed, whereupon the scapula and clavicle sag noticeably because trapezius normally helps to

CLINICAL PANEL 15.3 (continued)

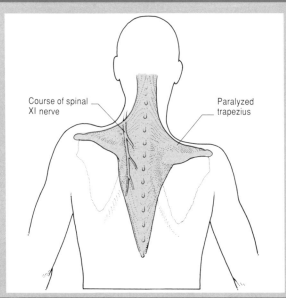

Course of spinal XI nerve

Paralyzed trapezius

carry the upper limb. Shrugging of the shoulder is weakened because the levator scapulae must work alone. Progressive atrophy of the muscle leads to characteristic scalloping of the contour of the neck (see *Figure CP 15.3.2*).

Figure CP 15.3.2   Visible effects of right-sided spinal XI paralysis: scalloping of the neck and drooping of the shoulder.

Upon leaving the cranium it crosses the transverse process of the atlas and enters the sternomastoid in company with twigs from roots C2 and C3 of the cervical plexus. It emerges from the posterior border of the sternomastoid and crosses the posterior triangle of the neck to reach the trapezius. It pierces the trapezius in company with twigs from roots C3 and C4 of the cervical plexus. In the posterior triangle the nerve is vulnerable, being embedded in prevertebral fascia and covered only by investing cervical fascia and skin.

The spinal accessory nerve provides the extrafusal and intrafusal motor supply to the sternomastoid and trapezius. The branches from the cervical plexus are proprioceptive in function to the sternomastoid and to the craniocervical part of the trapezius. The thoracic part of the trapezius, which arises from the spines of all the thoracic vertebrae, receives its proprioceptive innervation from the posterior rami of the thoracic spinal nerves. Some of the afferents supplying muscle spindles in the thoracic trapezius do not meet up with the fusimotor supply before reaching the spindles. This is the only instance, *in any muscle,* where the fusimotor and afferent fibers to some spindles travel by completely independent routes.

GLOSSOPHARYNGEAL, VAGUS, AND CRANIAL ACCESSORY NERVES

Especially relevant to nerves IX, X, and cranial XI are the nucleus solitarius and the nucleus ambiguus. These two nuclei will be described before the three individual nerves are considered.

NUCLEUS SOLITARIUS

In the center of this nucleus is the **tractus solitarius,** so named because it is made 'solitary' by the sleeve of neurons surrounding it. The original and meaningful name of the neuronal sleeve was *nucleus of the tractus solitarius.*

The nucleus solitarius extends from the lower border of the pons to the level of the nucleus gracilis. Its lower end reaches the midline and forms the **commissural nucleus.** Neuronal packing density in the nucleus solitarius is high and there is neurochemical diversity.

Anatomically, the nucleus is divisible into eight parts. Functionally, four *regions* have been clarified (*Figure 15.6*):

1   The uppermost region is the **gustatory nucleus,** which receives primary afferents supplying taste buds in the tongue and palate.

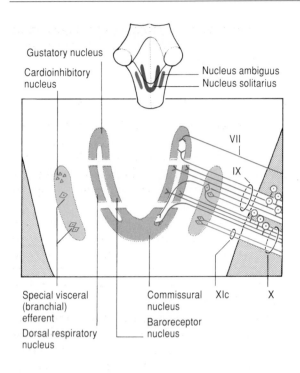

Gustatory nucleus

Cardioinhibitory
nucleus

Nucleus ambiguus
Nucleus solitarius

VII

IX

Special visceral
(branchial)
efferent

Dorsal respiratory
nucleus

Commissural
nucleus

XIc   X

Baroreceptor
nucleus

Figure 15.6 Composition of nucleus ambiguus and nucleus solitarius.

2 The lateral midregion is the **dorsal respiratory nucleus** (see Chapter 19).
3 The medial midregion is the **baroreceptor nucleus,** which receives the primary afferents supplying the blood pressure detectors in the carotid sinus and aortic arch (see later).
4 The most caudal region, including the commissural nucleus, is the major **visceral afferent nucleus** of the brainstem. It receives primary afferents supplying the alimentary tract and respiratory tract.

NUCLEUS AMBIGUUS

Originally of uncertain function (hence the name), the nucleus ambiguus lies immediately behind the inferior olive. Functionally, two regions have been clarified (*Figure 15.6*):

1 The most rostral cells are *parasympathetic*. They give rise to the preganglionic nerve supply to the heart.
2 The remaining cells of the nucleus *are special visceral efferent*. They supply the branchial muscles of the pharynx (stylopharyngeus and the three pharyngeal constrictors) and of the larynx (the intrinsic muscles); also the levator palati.

GLOSSOPHARYNGEAL NERVE

The glossopharyngeal nerve is almost exclusively sensory. It carries no less than five different kinds of afferent fibers traveling to five separate afferent nuclei in the brainstem. The largest of its peripheral territories is the oropharynx, which is bounded in front by the back of the tongue; hence the name for the nerve.

The glossopharyngeal rootlets are attached behind the upper part of the olive. The nerve accompanies the vagus through the anterior compartment of the jugular foramen (the posterior compartment contains the bulb of the internal jugular vein). Within the foramen, the nerve shows small superior and inferior ganglia; these contain unipolar sensory neurons.

Immediately below the skull, the glossopharyngeal nerve finds itself in the company of three other nerves (*Figure 15.3*): the vagus, the spinal accessory, and the internal carotid (sympathetic) branch of the superior cervical ganglion. Together with the stylopharyngeus, it slips between the superior and middle constrictor muscles to reach the mucous membrane of the oropharynx.

Functional divisions and branches

■ Before emerging from the jugular foramen the IX nerve gives off a **tympanic branch** which ramifies on the tympanic membrane and is a potential source of referred pain (Panel 15.3). The central processes of the tympanic branch synapse in the spinal nucleus of the trigeminal nerve, which receives nociceptive and thermal information from almost the entire head and neck (Chapter 17).
■ Some fibers of the tympanic branch are parasympathetic. They pierce the roof (tegmen tympani) of the middle ear as the **lesser petrosal nerve,** leave the skull through the foramen, and synapse in the **otic ganglion.** Postganglionic fibers supply secretomotor fibers to the parotid gland. The preganglionic fibers originate in the **inferior salivary nucleus,** which is adjacent to the nucleus ambiguus.
■ The branch to the stylopharyngeus comes from the nucleus ambiguus.
■ Branches serving 'common sensation' (touch) supply the mucous membranes bounding the oropharynx (throat), including the posterior one-third of the tongue. The neurons synapse centrally in the commissural nucleus. The

glossopharyngeal branches provide the afferent limb of the *gag reflex*—contraction of the pharyngeal constrictors in response to stroking the wall of the oropharynx. (The gag reflex is unpleasant because of accompanying nausea. To test the integrity of the IX nerve, it is usually sufficient to test sensation on the pharyngeal wall.) Generalized stimulation of the oropharynx elicits a complete swallowing reflex, through a linkage between the commissural nucleus and a specific swallowing center nearby (Chapter 19).

■ Gustatory neurons supply the taste buds contained in the circumvallate papillae; they terminate centrally in the gustatory nucleus.

■ An important *carotid branch* descends to the bifurcation of the common carotid artery. This branch contains two different sets of afferent fibers. One set ramifies in the wall of the carotid sinus (at the commencement of the internal carotid artery), terminating in *stretch receptors* responsive to systolic blood pressure; these **baroreceptor neurons** terminate centrally in the medial part of the nucleus solitarius.

■ The second set of afferents in the carotid branch supplies glomus cells in the carotid body. These nerve endings are *chemoreceptors* monitoring the carbon dioxide and oxygen levels in the blood. The central terminals enter the dorsal respiratory nucleus.

VAGUS AND CRANIAL ACCESSORY NERVES

The vagus is *the* parasympathetic nerve. Its preganglionic component has a huge territory which includes the heart, the lungs, and the alimentary tract from esophagus through transverse colon (Chapter 10). At the same time the vagus is the largest visceral afferent nerve; afferents outnumber parasympathetic fibers by four to one. Overall, the vagus contains the same seven fiber classes as the glossopharyngeal, and they will be listed in the same order.

The rootlets of the vagus and cranial accessory nerves are in series with the glossopharyngeal, and the three nerves travel together into the jugular foramen. At this point the cranial accessory shares a dural sheath with the spinal accessory, but there is no exchange of fibers (*Figure 15.5*). Just below the foramen, the cranial accessory is incorporated into the vagus. The vagus itself shows a small, jugular, and a large, nodose ganglion; both are sensory.

Functional divisions and branches

■ An **auricular branch** supplies skin lining the outer ear canal, and a **meningeal branch** ramifies in the posterior cranial fossa. Both branches have their cell bodies in the **jugular ganglion;** the central processes enter the spinal trigeminal nucleus.

■ **Cardioinhibitory neurons** of the nucleus ambiguus synapse in cardiac ganglia close to the great veins and coronary sinus. The parasympathetic neurons for the respiratory and alimentary tracts originate from the dorsal nucleus of the vagus.

■ Special visceral efferent neurons of the nucleus ambiguus make up the *entire* cranial accessory nerve. The fibers constitute the motor elements in the pharyngeal and laryngeal branches of the vagus. They supply the following striated muscles of branchial origin: levator palati; pharyngeal constrictors; intrinsic muscles of the larynx; upper third of esophagus.

■ General visceral afferent fibers from the heart, and from the respiratory and alimentary tracts have their cell bodies in the nodose ganglion and synapse centrally in the commissural nucleus. They serve important reflexes including the *Bainbridge reflex* (cardiac acceleration brought about by distension of the right atrium); the *cough reflex* (stimulation of a coughing center (Chapter 19) by irritation of the tracheobronchial tree); and the *Hering-Breuer reflex* (inhibition of the dorsal respiratory center by pulmonary stretch receptors). In addition, afferent information from the stomach (in particular) is forwarded to the hypothalamus and influences feeding behavior (Chapter 21).

■ A few taste buds on the epiglottis report to the gustatory center.

■ Some *baroreceptors* in the aortic arch, and

■ *Chemoreceptors* in the tiny aortic bodies, supplement the corresponding receptors at the carotid bifurcation.

Supranuclear, nuclear, and infranuclear lesions of the IX, X, and XI nerves are described in the Clinical Panels.

CORE INFORMATION

Hypoglossal nerve

XII contains somatic efferent neurons supplying extrinsic and intrinsic muscles of the tongue. Its nucleus is close to midline and is innervated by reticular neurons for automatic/reflex movements and by (mainly crossed) corticonuclear neurons for speech articulation. XII emerges beside the pyramid, exits the hypoglossal canal and descends on the carotid sheath where it collects cervical proprioceptive fibers for the supply of lingual muscle spindles. Supranuclear paralysis of XII is characterized by temporary deviation to the paralyzed side on protrusion. Nuclear/infranuclear paralysis is characterized by wasting and fasciculation as well as deviation.

Spinal accessory nerve

Spinal XI is purely motor. From motoneurons of spinal segments 1–5, the axons enter the foramen magnum and exit the jugular foramen; they pierce and supply sternomastoid, then pass deep to trapezius and supply it. Proprioceptive connections are received from cervical and thoracic spinal nerves. Supranuclear lesions are characterized by weakness of ipsilateral sternomastoid and contralateral trapezius; nuclear/infranuclear lesions by ipsilateral wasting of the two muscles and drooping of the scapula.

Glossopharyngeal nerve

IX emerges behind the olive and exits the jugular foramen where it shows two unipolar-cell ganglia and gives off a tympanic branch which is partly sensory to the middle ear, partly parasympathetic to the parotid gland via the otic ganglion. IX then passes between superior and middle constrictors to gain the oropharynx, where it supplies sensation to that mucous membrane including the posterior third of tongue (hence the name), and taste fibers to the circumvallate papillae. A carotid branch supplies the carotid sinus and carotid body.

Vagus and cranial accessory nerves

X and c.XI rootlets emerge behind the olive and unite in the jugular foramen. c. XI fibers arise in n. ambiguus and utilize laryngeal and pharyngeal branches of X to supply the intrinsic muscles of larynx and pharynx, and levator palati.

Preganglionic fibers from neurons in the upper end of nucleus ambiguus run in X to innervate parasympathetic ganglia in the wall of the heart. Others from the dorsal nucleus of X travel to intramural ganglia in the walls of bronchi and alimentary tract. Visceral afferents from these three regions, and from larynx and pharynx, have unipolar cell bodies in the nodose ganglion and project to the commissural nucleus.

SELF TEST

Match the cell columns on the left with the nuclei on the right:

1 Somatic efferent	A Hypoglossal
2 General visceral efferent	B Spinal trigeminal
3 General somatic afferent	C Cochlear
4 Special visceral efferent	D Nucleus ambiguus
5 Special somatic afferent	E Dorsal of vagus

Match the nerves on the left with the functions on the right:

6 Hypoglossal	A Protruding the tongue
7 Spinal accessory	B Slowing the heart
8 Vagus	C Turning the head
9 Glossopharyngeal	D Throat sensation
10 Cranial accessory	E Phonation

11 Which of the following items are not related:
A Nucleus ambiguus — trapezius
B Inferior salivatory nucleus — gustatory nucleus
C Commissural nucleus — visceral afferents
D Nucleus ambiguus — heart
E Supranuclear — corticobulbar

REFERENCES

Andresen, M.C. (1994) Nucleus tractus solitarii - gateway to neural circulatory control. *Ann. Rev. Physiol.* **56**: 93-116.5.

Saxina, P.R. (1995) Serotonin receptors: subtypes, functional responses and therapeutic relevance. *Pharmacol. Therap.* **66**: 339-368

Dampney, R.A.L. (1994) Functional organization of the central pathways regulating the cardiovascular system. *Physiol. Rev.* **74**: 323-364.

FitzGerald, M.J.T. and Sachithanandan, S.R. (1979) The structure and source of lingual proprioceptors in the monkey. *J. Anat.* **128**: 523-552.

FitzGerald, M.J.T., Comerford, P.T. and Tuffery, A.R. (1982) Sources of innervation of the neuromuscular spindles in sternomastoid and trapezius. *J. Anat.* **134**: 174-190.

Mtui, E.P., Anwar, M., Reis, D.J. and Ruggiero, D.A. (1995) Medullary visceral reflex circuits: local afferents to nucleus tractus solitarii synthesize catecholamines and project to thoracic spinal cord. *J. Comp. Neur.* **351**: 5-26.

Patten, J.P. (1980) **Neurological Differential Diagnosis**. London: Harold Stark.

Sawchenko, P.E. (1983) Central connections of the sensory and motor nuclei of the vagus nerve. *J. Auton. Nerv. Syst.* **9**: 13-26.

16
VESTIBULOCOCHLEAR NERVE

Chapter Summary

Introduction

Vestibular system
Static labyrinth: anatomy and
  actions
Kinetic labyrinth: anatomy
  and actions

Auditory system
The cochlea
Cochlear nerve
Central auditory pathways
Descending auditory pathways
Deafness

CLINICAL PANELS
Vestibular disorders
Lateral medullary syndrome
Two kinds of deafness

Study Guidelines

Vestibular nerve
1 The static labyrinth is primarily concerned with maintenance of balance when the head is off center.
2 The dynamic labyrinth enables us to maintain our gaze on a particular object while the head is moving.
3 Clinically, the lateral semicircular is the canal of choice for testing labyrinthine function.

Cochlear nerve
1 Vibrations created by sound waves cross the vestibular membrane to reach the organ of Corti, where cochlear nerve fibers terminate.
2 The central auditory pathway is partly ipsilateral, to the extent that damage on one side does not compromise hearing unduly.
3 Nuclei strung along the brainstem part of the pathway serve to magnify tiny differences in the intensity of sounds entering the two ears.

INTRODUCTION

The vestibulocochlear nerve is primarily composed of the centrally directed axons of bipolar neurons housed in the petrous temporal bone (*Figure 16.1*). The peripheral processes are applied to neuroepithelial cells in the cochlea and vestibular labyrinth. The nerve enters the brainstem at the junctional region of the pons and medulla oblongata. The functional anatomy of the two component nerves and end organs will be considered separately.

VESTIBULAR SYSTEM

The **bony labyrinth** of the inner ear is a very dense shell containing **perilymph,** which resembles extracellular fluid in general. The perilymph provides a water jacket for the **membranous labyrinth,** which encloses the sense organs of bal-

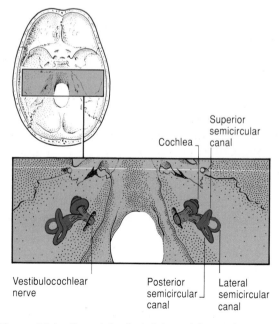

Figure 16.1 Bony labyrinth, viewed from above.

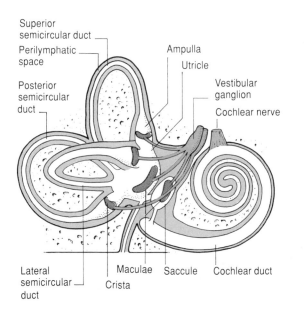

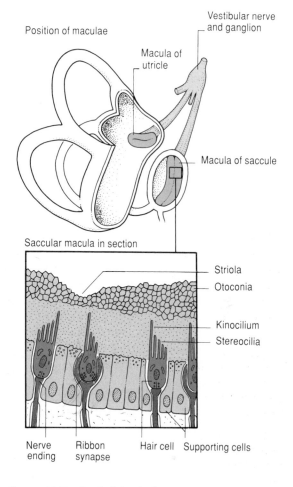

Figure 16.2 Locations of the five vestibular sense organs.

Figure 16.3 Static labyrinth.

ance and of hearing. The sense organs are bathed in **endolymph**. The endolymph resembles intracellular fluid, being potassium-rich and sodium-poor.

The vestibular labyrinth comprises the **utricle,** the **saccule,** and three **semicircular ducts** (*Figure 16.2*). The utricle and saccule each contain a 3 × 2 mm³ **macula**. Each semicircular duct contains an **ampulla** at one end, and the ampulla houses a **crista**.

The two maculae are the sensory end organs of the *static labyrinth,* which signals head position. The three cristae are the end organs of the *kinetic* or *dynamic labyrinth,* which signals head movement.

The bipolar cells of the **vestibular ganglion** occupy the internal acoustic meatus. Their peripheral processes are applied to the five sensory end organs. Their central processes, which constitute the **vestibular nerve,** cross the subarachnoid space and synapse in the vestibular nucleus.

The vestibular nucleus is made up of four individual nuclei, **lateral, medial, inferior,** and **superior.**

STATIC LABYRINTH: ANATOMY AND ACTIONS

The position and structure of the maculae are shown in *Figure 16.3*. The **utricular macula** is rela-

tively horizontal, the **saccular macula** is relatively vertical. The cuboidal cells lining the membranous labyrinth become columnar **supporting cells** in the maculae. Among the supporting cells are so-called **hair cells,** to which vestibular nerve endings are applied. Some hair cells are almost completely enclosed by large nerve endings whereas others (phylogenetically older) receive only small contacts. At the cell bases are **ribbon synapses,** the synaptic vesicles being lined up along synaptic bars. Projecting from the free surface of each hair cell are about 100 **stereocilia** and, close to the cell margin, a single, long **kinocilium**. The hair cells discharge continuously, the resting rate being about 100 Hz.

The cilia are embedded in a gelatinous matrix containing protein-bound calcium carbonate crystals called **otoconia** ('ear sand'). (The term 'otolith', when used, refers to the larger, 'ear stones' of reptiles.) The otoconia exert gravitational drag on the hair cells. Whenever kinocilia are dragged away from stereocilia, depolarization is facilitated. As indicated in *Figure 16.3*, the macula has a central groove (**striola**) and the hair cell orientations have a mirror arrangement in relation to the groove. Electrical activity of hair cells is facilitated on one side of the groove by a given gravitational vector, and disfacilitated on the other side.

The maculae also respond to linear acceleration of the head in the horizontal plane (e.g. during walking) or in the vertical (gravitational) plane. Also, when the tilted head is stationary in a flexed or extended position, the facilitated half of the utricular macula discharges intensely in both ears; the saccular ones are more responsive when the head is held to the side. Both receptors are linked by the vestibular nerve to the lateral, medial, and inferior vestibular nuclei.

The primary function of the static labyrinth is to signal the position of the head relative to the trunk. In response to this signal, the vestibular nucleus initiates compensatory movements, with the effect of maintaining the center of gravity between the feet (in standing) or just in front of the feet (during locomotion), and of keeping the head horizontal. These effects are mediated by the vestibulospinal tracts.

The **lateral vestibulospinal tract** (Deiterospinal tract) arises from large neurons in the **lateral vestibular nucleus of Deiters**. The fibers descend in the anterior funiculus on the same side and synapse upon extensor (antigravity) motoneurons in the spinal cord. Both α and γ motoneurons are excited, and a significant part of the increased muscle tone is exerted by way of the gamma loop (Chapter 13). During standing, the tract is tonically active on both sides of the spinal cord. During walking, activity is selective for the quadriceps motoneurons of the leading leg; this commences at the moment of heel strike and continues during the stance phase (when the other leg is off the ground). Deiters' nucleus is somatotopically organized, and the functionally appropriate neurons are selected by the flocculonodular lobe of the cerebellum. The flocculonodular lobe (Chapter 20) has two-way connections with all four vestibular nuclei.

Antigravity action is triggered mainly from the horizontal macula of the utricle. The vertical macula of the saccule, on the other hand, is maximally activated by a *free fall*. The shearing effect produces powerful extensor thrust in anticipation of a hard landing.

A small, **medial vestibulospinal tract** arises in the medial and inferior vestibular nuclei. It descends in the medial longitudinal fasciculus and terminates ipsilaterally upon *inhibitory* internuncials in the cervical part of the cord. It operates *head-righting reflexes,* which serve to keep the head—and the gaze—horizontal when the body is craned forward or to one side. Good examples of head-righting reflexes are to be seen around pool tables and in bowling alleys. An added twist can be provided, if required, by torsion of the eyeballs (up to 10°) within the orbital sockets. This eye-righting reflex is mediated by axons *ascending* the medial longitudinal fasciculus from the *lateral* vestibular nucleus to reach nuclei controlling the extraocular muscles. Evidence derived from unilateral vestibular destruction (*Panel 16.1*) indicates that the horizontal position of the eyes when the head is upright is the result of a canceling effect of bilateral tonic activity in these Deitero-ocular pathways.

The medial vestibulospinal tract is also activated by the kinetic labyrinth.

The static labyrinth contributes to the sense of position. The sense of position of the body in space is normally provided by three sensory systems: the visual system, the conscious proprioceptive system, and the vestibular system. Deprived of one of the three, the individual can stand and walk by using information provided by the other two. Following loss of vision, for example, the subject can get about, although the constraints imposed by blindness are known to all. Following loss of conscious proprioception instead, the subject uses vision as a substitute for proprioceptive sense, and is disabled by closure of the eyes (sensory ataxia, Chapter 12). If the static labyrinths alone are inactive, closure of the eyes may lead to a heavy fall.

KINETIC LABYRINTH: ANATOMY AND ACTIONS

Basic features of macular epithelium are repeated in the three cristae. Again there are supporting cells, and hair cells to which vestibular nerve endings are applied. The kinocilia of the hair cells are long, penetrating deeply into a gelatinous projection called the **cupula** (*Figure 16.4*). The cupula is bonded to the opposite wall of the ampulla. The cristae are sensitive to angular acceleration of the labyrinths. Angular acceleration occurs during rotary 'yes' and 'no' movements of the head. The endolymph tends to lag behind

---

CLINICAL PANEL 16.1

VESTIBULAR DISORDERS

Unilateral vestibular disease

Acute failure of one vestibular labyrinth may follow spread of disease from the middle ear or thrombosis of the labyrinthine artery. A common cause of unilateral vestibular symptoms in the elderly is a *transient ischemic attack* involving the vertebrobasilar arterial system. Transient ischemic attacks last 15 minutes or less and leave no residual neurological deficit. However, they are commonly followed by a vascular thrombosis somewhere in the brain within 6 months.

The effects of unilateral vestibular disease are well demonstrated when the vestibular system is inactivated surgically, either during removal of an acoustic neuroma (Chapter 17) or as a last resort in treating paroxysmal attacks of vertigo. During the immediate postoperative period, the patient shows triple effects of loss of tonic input from the static labyrinth:

■ Loss of function in the Deitero-ocular pathway on one side leads to about 10° of torsion of both eyeballs toward that side. The

patient's perception of the horizontal shows a corresponding tilt, so that reaching movements become inaccurate.

■ The head tilts to the same side, being no longer controlled on that side by the head-righting reflex.

■ The patient tends to fall to the same side, because the Deiterospinal tract no longer compensates for tilting of the head.

Because function continues in the normal lateral semicircular canal, there is a nystagmus to the normal side.

Bilateral vestibular disease

Following total loss of static labyrinthine function, visual guidance becomes important, and the patient dare not walk out-of-doors after twilight. By day, any distraction causing the patient to look overhead may result in a heavy fall. Loss of kinetic labyrinthine function makes it impossible to fix the gaze on an object while the head is moving. During walking, the scene bobs up and down as if it were being viewed through a hand-held camera.

---

because of its inertia, and the cupula balloons like a sail when thrust against it. The disposition of the kinocilia is uniform across each crista, and is such that the *lateral* ampullary crista is facilitated by cupular displacement *toward* the utricle; the *superior* and *posterior* cristae are facilitated by cupular displacement *away from* the utricle. In practical terms, the left lateral ampulla is activated by turning the head to the left; both superior ampullae are activated by flexion of the head; and both posterior ampullae by extension of the head.

Afferents from the cristae terminate in the medial and superior vestibular nuclei. As with the macular afferents, there are two-way connections with the flocculonodular lobe of the cerebellum.

The function of the kinetic labyrinth is to provide information for compensatory movements of the eyes in response to movement of the head. *Vestibulo-ocular reflexes* operate to maintain the gaze on a selcted target. A simple example is our ability to gaze at the period (full stop) at the end

of a sentence, while moving the head about. The two eyes move *conjugately,* i.e. in parallel.

The basic pathway for the horizontal vestibulo-ocular reflex is shown in *Figure 16.5*. In the example shown in *Figure 16.4*, the right lateral ampullary crista was activated by a head turn to the right. Under cerebellar guidance, the medial vestibular nucleus projects to the contralateral abducens nucleus where it selects two kinds of neurons: (a) motoneurons to abduct the left eye, and (b) internuclear neurons which send large axons along the medial longitudinal bundle to the right oculomotor nucleus, where they seek out motoneurons which adduct the right eye.

The superior vestibular nucleus simultaneously *inhibits* the motoneurons serving the antagonist muscles (left medial and right lateral rectus).

Appropriate point-to-point connections also exist between the vestibular nuclei and motoneurons of the oculomotor and trochlear nerves for similar reflexes in the vertical plane.

In order to control the vestibulo-ocular reflexes, the cerebellum needs to be informed about the

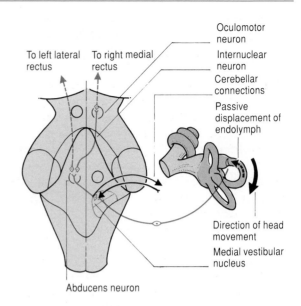

Figure 16.5 Minimal pathway for a horizontal vestibulo-ocular reflex originating in the right semicircular canal.

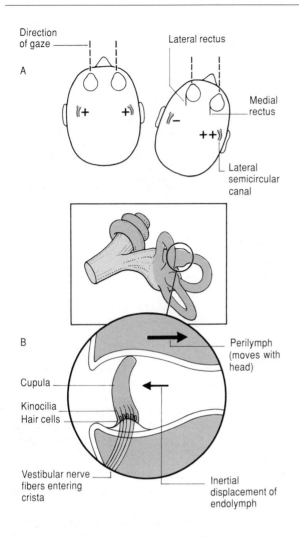

Figure 16.4 Kinetic labyrinth, showing the response of the lateral semicircular duct and crista to a rightward turn of the head.

initial position of the head in relation to the trunk. This information is provided by a great wealth of muscle spindles in the deep muscles surrounding the cervical vertebral column. The spindle afferents enter the rostral spinocerebellar tract and relay in the accessory cuneate nucleus.

Nystagmus

A horizontal vestibulo-ocular reflex can be elicited by warming or cooling the endolymph in the semicircular canals. In routine tests of vestibular function, advantage is taken of the proximity of the lateral semicircular canal to the middle ear. The canal is angled at 30° to the horizontal plane. Tilting the head back by 60° brings the canal into the vertical plane, with the ampulla uppermost.

In the *warm caloric test*, water at 44°C is then instilled into the ear. The air in the middle ear is heated, and heat transfer to the lateral canal produces convection currents within the endolymph. Whether through displacement of the cupula or by some other mechanism, the crista of the warmer lateral ampulla becomes more active than its opposite number. The result is a slow drift of the eyes away from the stimulated side. It is as if the head had been turned to the side being tested. The drift is followed by a recovery phase in which the eyes snap back to the resting position. Slow and fast phases are repeated several times per second. This is *vestibular nystagmus*. The direction of the nystagmus is named in accordance with the fast phase because of the obvious 'beat'. A warm caloric test applied to the right ear should produce a right-beating nystagmus ('nystagmus to the right'). Subjectively, nystagmus is accompanied by vertigo—a sense of rotation of self in relation to the external world, or vice versa.

Unilateral and bilateral vestibular syndromes are considered in *Panel 16.1*. A vascular syndrome involving the vestibular system in the medulla oblongata is described in *Panel 16.2*.

Vestibulocortical connections

Second-order sensory neurons project from the vestibular nucleus to the contralateral thalamus.

CLINICAL PANEL 16.2

LATERAL MEDULLARY SYNDROME

Thrombosis of the vertebral or posterior inferior cerebellar artery may produce an infarct (area of necrosis) in the lateral part of the medulla. The clinical picture depends on the extent to which the various nuclei and pathways are damaged. Brainstem pathology must always be suspected when a cranial nerve lesion on one side is accompanied by 'upper motor neuron signs' on the other side—so-called *alternating* or *crossed hemiplegia*.

Lateral medullary syndrome (see Figure CP 16.2.1)

1 Damage to the vestibular nucleus leads to vertigo (often with initial vomiting), together with the symptoms of unilateral disconnection of the labyrinth described in *Panel 16.1*.

2 Interruption of posterior and rostral spinocerebellar fibers may produce signs of cerebellar ataxia in the ipsilateral limbs. Cerebellar ataxia is a prominent feature if blood flow is interrupted in the posterior inferior cerebellar artery.

3 Damage to the spinal tract of the trigeminal nerve interrupts fine primary afferent fibers descending the brainstem from the trigeminal ganglion (Chapter 17). These fibers are functionally equivalent to those of Lissauer's tract in the spinal cord (Chapter 12). The result of interruption is loss of pain and thermal senses from the face on the same side.

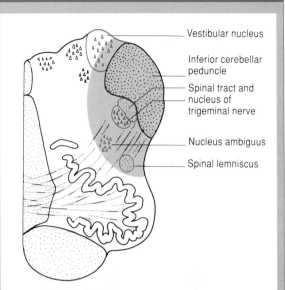

Figure CP 16.2.1 Lateral medullary infarct (shaded).

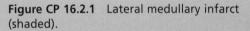

4 Interruption of the central sympathetic pathway to the spinal cord produces a complete Horner's syndrome (ptosis, miosis, anhidrosis).

5 Damage to the nucleus ambiguus causes hoarseness, and sometimes difficulty in swallowing.

6 The only *contralateral* sign is loss of pain and temperature sense in the trunk and limbs, resulting from damage to the lateral spinothalamic tract. There is no motor weakness because the corticospinal tract is spared.

The fibers terminate in company with trigeminothalamic fibers in the ventral posterior nucleus. The main cortical area in receipt of third-order vestibular fibers seems to be a patch immediately behind the face representation on the somatic sensory cortex. In conscious patients with the cortex exposed at operation, a mild electrical stimulus to this patch may elicit a sensation of vertigo.

AUDITORY SYSTEM

The auditory system comprises the cochlea, the cochlear nerve, and the central auditory pathway from the cochlear nucleus in the brainstem to the cortex of the temporal lobe. The central auditory pathway is more elaborate than the somatosensory or visual pathway. This is because the same sounds are detected by both ears. In order to signal the location of a sound, a very complex neuronal network is in place, with numerous connections (mainly inhibitory) between the two central pathways in order to magnify minute differences in intensity and timing of sounds that exist during normal, binaural hearing.

THE COCHLEA

The main features of cochlear structure are seen

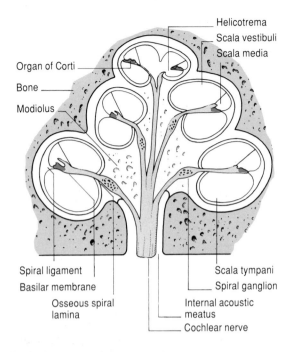

Figure 16.6   The cochlea in section.

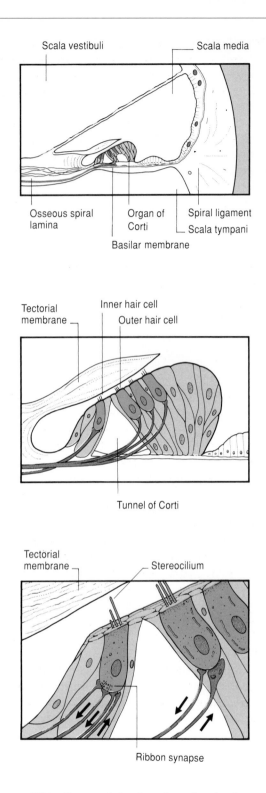

Figure 16.7   Organ of Corti at three levels of magnification. Arrows indicate directions of impulse traffic.

in *Figures 16.6* and *16.7*. The cochlea is pictured as though it were upright, but in life it lies on its side, as shown in *Figure 16.1*. The central bony pillar of the cochlea (the **modiolus**) is in the axis of the internal acoustic meatus. Projecting from the modiolus, like the flange of a screw, is the **osseous spiral lamina**. The **basilar membrane** is attached to the tip of this lamina; it reaches across the cavity of the bony cochlea to become attached to the **spiral ligament** on the outer wall. The osseous spiral lamina and spiral ligament become progressively smaller as one ascends the two and one half turns of the cochlea, and the fibers of the basal lamina become progressively longer.

The basal lamina and its attachments divide the cochlear chamber into upper and lower compartments. These are the **scala vestibuli** and the **scala tympani,** respectively, and they are filled with perilymph. They communicate at the apex of the cochlea, through the **helicotrema**. A third compartment, the **scala media (cochlear duct)**, lies above the basilar membrane and is filled with endolymph. It is separated from the scala vestibuli by the delicate **vestibular membrane**.

Sitting on the basilar membrane is the **spiral organ (organ of Corti)**. The principal sensory receptor epithelium consists of a single row of **inner hair cells,** each one having up to 20 large

afferent nerve endings applied to it. The hair cells rest upon **supporting cells,** and there are ancillary cells as well. The organ of Corti contains a central tunnel, filled with perilymph diffusing through the basilar membrane. On the outer side of the tunnel are several rows of **outer hair cells,** attended by supporting and ancillary cells.

All of the hair cells are surmounted by **stereocilia.** Unlike the vestibular hair cells, they have no kinocilium in the adult state. The stereocilia of the outer hair cells are embedded in the overlying tectorial membrane. Those of the inner hair cells lie immediately below the membrane.

The outer hair cells are contractile (at least in tissue culture), and they have substantial efferent nerve endings (*Figure 16.7*). In theory at least, oscillatory movements of outer hair cells could influence the sensitivity of the inner hair cells through effects on the tectorial or basilar membrane.

Sound transduction

The vibrations of the tympanic membrane in response to sound waves are transmitted along the ossicular chain. The footplate of the stapes fits snugly into the oval window, and vibrations of the stapes are converted to pressure waves in the scala vestibuli. The pressure waves are transmitted through the vestibular membrane to reach the basilar membrane. High frequency pressure waves, created by high–pitched sounds, cause the short fibers of the basilar membrane in the basal turn of the cochlea to resonate and absorb their energy. Low–frequency waves produce resonance in the apical turn where the fibers are longest. The basilar membrane is therefore *tonotopic* in its fiber sequence. Not surprisingly, the inner hair cells have a similar tonotopic sequence. In response to local resonance, the cells become depolarized and liberate excitatory transmitter substance from synaptic ribbons (*Figure 16.7*).

The nerve fibers supplying the hair cells are the peripheral processes of the bipolar spiral ganglion cells lodged in the base of the osseous spiral lamina.

COCHLEAR NERVE

The bulk of the cochlear nerve consists of the myelinated central processes of some 30 000 large bipolar neurons of the spiral ganglion. Unmyelinated fibers come from small ganglion cells supplying dendrites to the outer hair cells. (Motor fibers do not travel in the cochlear nerve trunk.) The nerve traverses the subarachnoid

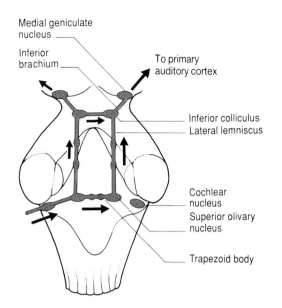

Figure 16.8 Dorsal view of brainstem showing basic plan of central auditory pathways. The upper horizontal arrow denotes the collicular commissure.

space in company with the vestibular and facial nerves, and it enters the brainstem at the pontomedullary junction.

CENTRAL AUDITORY PATHWAYS

The general plan of the central auditory pathway from the left cochlear nerve to the cerebral cortex is shown in *Figure 16.8*. The first cell station is the **cochlear nucleus,** where all cochlear nerve fibers terminate upon entry to the brainstem. From here, some second-order fibers project all the way to the opposite **inferior colliculus** by way of the **trapezoid body** and **lateral lemniscus.** The **inferior brachium** links the inferior colliculus to the **medial geniculate body,** which projects to the **primary auditory cortex** in the temporal lobe.

A small but important purely ipsilateral relay passes from the superior olivary nucleus to the higher auditory centers.

Functional anatomy (Figure 16.9)

Cochlear nucleus

The cochlear nucleus comprises dorsal and ventral nuclei, on the corresponding surfaces of the inferior cerebellar peduncle. Many incoming fibers of the cochlear nerve bifurcate and enter both nuclei. The cells in both are tonotopically arranged.

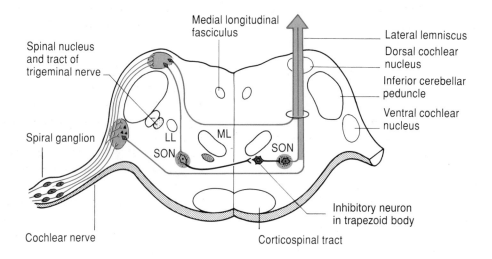

Figure 16.9 Transverse section of lower end of the pons showing central connections of the cochlear nerve. LL, lateral lemniscus; ML, medial lemniscus; SON, superior olivary nucleus.

Responses of many cells in the ventral nucleus are called primary-like, because their frequency (firing rate) resembles that of primary afferents. Most of the output neurons project to the nearby superior olivary nucleus.

The cells of the dorsal nucleus are heterogeneous. At least six different cell types have been characterized by their morphology and electrical behavior. Most of the output neurons project to the contralateral inferior colliculus. Individually, they exhibit an extremely narrow range of tonal responses, being 'focused' by collateral inhibition.

Superior olivary nucleus
The superior olivary complex of nuclei is relatively small in the human brain. It contains *binaural neurons* affected by inputs from both ears. Ipsilateral inputs are excitatory to the binaural neurons whereas contralateral inputs are inhibitory. The inhibitory effect is mediated by internuncial neurons in the **nucleus of the trapezoid body.**

The superior olivary nucleus is responsive to differences in intensity and timing between sounds entering both ears simultaneously. On the side ipsilateral to a sound, stimulation of the cochlea, and of the nucleus, is earlier and more intense than on the contralateral side. By exaggerating these differences through crossed inhibition, the superior olivary nucleus helps to indicate the spatial direction of incoming sounds. At the same time, the excited nucleus projects to the inferior colliculus of both sides, giving rise to binaural responses in the neurons of the inferior colliculus and beyond.

Lateral lemniscus
Fibers of the lateral lemniscus arise from the dorsal and ventral cochlear nuclei and from the superior olivary nuclei—in each case, mainly contralaterally. The tract terminates in the **central nucleus of the inferior colliculus.** Nuclei within the lateral lemniscus participate in reflex arcs (see later).

Inferior colliculus
Spatial information from the superior olivary nucleus, intensity information from the ventral cochlear nucleus, and pitch information from the dorsal cochlear nucleus are integrated in the inferior colliculus. The main (central) part of the nucleus is laminated in a tonotopic manner. Within each tonal lamina, cells differ in their responses: some have a characteristic 'tuning curve' (they respond only to a particular tone); some fire spontaneously but are inhibited by sound; and some respond only to a moving source of sound.

As well as projecting to the medial geniculate nucleus, the inferior colliculus exerts inhibitory effects on its opposite number through the **inferior collicular commissure** (*Figure 16.8*). It also contributes to the tectospinal tract.

Medial geniculate nucleus

The medial geniculate nucleus is the specific thalamic nucleus for hearing. The main (ventral) nucleus is laminated and tonotopic, and the large (magnocellular) principal neurons project as the **auditory radiation** to the primary auditory cortex.

Primary auditory cortex

The upper surface of the temporal lobe shows one or two **transverse temporal gyri**. The anterior one (the **gyrus of Heschl**) contains the **primary auditory cortex** (see Chapter 24). Tonotopic arrangement is preserved in Heschl's gyrus, its posterior part being responsive to high tones and its anterior part to low tones. The cortex responds to auditory stimuli within the *contralateral sound field*. In cats, destruction of a patch of primary cortex on one side produces a *sigoma* or 'deaf spot' in the contralateral sound field. In humans, ablation of the superior temporal gyrus (in the course of tumor removal) does not cause deafness, but it significantly reduces ability to judge the direction and distance of a source of sound.

Brainstem acoustic reflexes

Fibers emerge from the lateral lemniscus and form the internuncial linkage for certain reflex arcs:

- Fibers entering the motor nuclei of the trigeminal and facial nerves link up with motoneurons supplying the tensor tympani and stapedius, respectively. These muscles exert a damping action on the ossicles of the middle ear. The tensor tympani is activated by the subject's own voice, the stapedius by external sounds.
- Fibers entering the reticular formation have an important arousal effect on the state of consciousness, as exemplified by the alarm clock. Sudden loud sounds cause the subject to flinch; this is the 'startle response', mediated by outputs from the reticular formation to the spinal cord and to the motor nucleus of the facial nerve.

DESCENDING AUDITORY PATHWAYS

A cascade of descending fibers runs from the

CLINICAL PANEL 16.3

TWO KINDS OF DEAFNESS

All forms of deafness can be grouped into two categories. *Conductive deafness* is caused by disease in the outer ear canal or in the middle ear. *Sensorineural deafness* is caused by disease in the cochlea or in the neural pathway from cochlea to brain.

Common causes of conductive deafness include accumulation of cerumen (wax) in the outer ear, and *otitis media* (inflammation in the middle ear). *Otosclerosis* is a disorder of the oval window in which the capsule of the synovial joint between the footplate of the stapes and the vestibule of the bony labyrinth is progressively replaced by bone. The stapes becomes immobilized, with severe impairment of hearing throughout the full tonal range. Replacement of the stapes by a prosthesis (artificial substitute) often restores normal hearing.

Sensorineural deafness usually originates within the cochlea. The commonest form is the high-frequency hearing loss of the elderly, resulting from deterioration of the organ of Corti in the basal turn. As a result, the elderly have difficulty in distinguishing among high-frequency consonants (d, s, t); vowels, which are low frequency, are quite audible. The elderly should be addressed distinctly rather than loudly.

Occupational deafness arises from a noisy environment at work. A persistent noise, especially indoors, may eventually lead to degeneration of the organ of Corti in the region corresponding to the particular frequency.

Ototoxic deafness may follow administration of drugs, including streptomycin, neomycin, and quinine.

Infectious deafness may follow more or less complete destruction of the cochlea by the virus of mumps or congenital rubella (German measles).

An important cause of sensorineural deafness in adults is an *acoustic neuroma*. Because the trigeminal and facial nerves may be affected as well as the cochlear and vestibular, this tumor is described in Chapter 17.

primary auditory cortex to the medial geniculate nucleus and inferior colliculus, and from the inferior colliculus to the superior olivary nucleus. The **olivocochlear bundle** emerges in the vestibular nerve and carries efferent, cholinergic fibers to the cochlea, with some for the vestibular labyrinth. The cochlear fibers apply large synaptic boutons to outer hair cells, and small boutons to the afferent nerve endings on inner hair cells.

The function of the olivocochlear bundle is uncertain. Experimental evidence indicates an involvement in enhancing detection of faint sounds.

DEAFNESS

Deafness is a widespread problem in the community. About 10% of adults suffer from it in some degree. The cause may lie in the outer, middle, or inner ear, or in the cochlear neural pathway. The two fundamental types of deafness are described in *Panel 16.3*.

CORE INFORMATION

Vestibular nerve

The static labyrinth comprises the maculae in utricle and saccule. The dynamic labyrinth comprises the semicircular ducts and their cristae. Vestibular bipolar neurons supply all five and synapse in the vestibular nucleus, which is controlled by the flocculonodular lobe of cerebellum. The static labyrinth functions to control balance, via the lateral vestibulospinal tract, by increasing antigravity tone on the side to which the head is tilted. This system is in partnership with proprioceptors and retina in maintaining upright posture. In the absence of good vision, a fall is likely if the system has been compromised.

The dynamic labyrinth operates vestibuloocular reflexes so as to keep the gaze on target during rotatory movements of the head. For sideways rotation the main projection is from medial vestibular nucleus to ipsilateral abducens nucleus where the lateral rectus muscle is activated and where internuclear neurons project to the contralateral medial rectus.

Clinically, this pathway can be activated by the caloric test, which normally elicits nystagmus.

Cochlear nerve

The bipolar neurons occupy the osseous spiral lamina of the modiolus. Their peripheral processes supply hair cells in the organ of Corti. Their central processes end in the cochlear nucleus; from here, a polyneuronal pathway leads mainly through the trapezoid body and via the lateral lemniscus to the inferior colliculus, but there is a significant ipsilateral pathway too. From the inferior colliculus fibers run to the medial geniculate nucleus, and from there to the primary auditory cortex on the upper surface of the temporal lobe of the brain.

Clinically, deafness is of two kinds: conductive, involving disease in the outer or middle ear; and sensorineural, involving disease of the cochlea (usually) or of central auditory pathways. Hearing is seldom significantly compromised by central pathway lesions because of the bilateral projections to the inferior colliculus.

SELF TEST

Select the best response:

1 Which of the following are vestibular sense organs?

   A Maculae
   B Cristae
   C Organ of Corti
   D All of the above
   E A and B only

2 Which of the following are unique to the static labyrinth?

   A Otoconia
   B Gelatinous matrix
   C Kinocilia
   D All of the above
   E A and B only

3 Which cristae are facilitated by flexion of the head?

   A Both superior
   B Both inferior
   C Both lateral
   D Right lateral
   E Left lateral

4 Which of the following are involved in antigravity extensor thrust reflex?

   A Utricular macula
   B Lateral vestibular nucleus
   C Inferior ampullary cristae
   D All of the above
   E A and B only

5 Which of the following sits on the basilar membrane?

   A Spiral ganglion
   B Osseous spiral lamina
   C Spiral organ
   D Spiral ligament
   E Spiral membrane

6 The lateral lemniscus contains:

   A Axons from the ipsilateral superior olivary nucleus
   B Axons from the contralateral nucleus
   C Nuclei serving reflex arcs
   D All of the above
   E A and B only

REFERENCES

VESTIBULAR SYSTEM

Anniko, M. (1988) Functional morphology of the vestibular system. In *Physiology of the Ear* (Jahn, A.F. and Santos-Sacchi, J., eds), pp. 457–475. New York: Raven Press.

Elliott, L.L. (1994) Functional brain imaging and hearing. *J. Acoust. Soc. Am.* 96: 1397–1408.

Fitzpatrick, R. and McCloskey, D. I. (1994) Proprioceptive, visual and vestibular thresholds for the perception of sway during standing in humans. *J. Physiol.* 478: 173–186.

Hart, C.W., McKinley, P.A. and Peterson, B.W. (1987) Compensation following acute unilateral total loss of peripheral vestibular function. In *The Vestibular System: Neurologic and Clinical Research* (Graham, M.D. and Kemink, J.L., eds), pp. 187–192. New York: Raven Press.

Markham, C.H. (1987) Vestibular control of muscular tone and posture. *Can. J. Neurol. Sci.* 14: 493–496.

Spoendlin, H. (1988) Neural anatomy of the inner ear. In *Physiology of the Ear* (Jahn, A.F. and Santos-Sacchi, J., eds), pp. 201–219. New York: Raven Press.

Adams, J.C. (1986) Neuronal morphology in the human cochlear nucleus. *Arch. Otolaryngol. Head Neck Surg.* 112: 1253–1261.

Aitkin, L.M. (1989) The auditory system. In *Handbook of Chemical Neuroanatomy*, Vol. 7: Integrated Systems of the CNS, Part II (Bjorklund, A., Hokfeld, T. and Swanson, L.W., eds), pp. 165–218. New York: Elsevier.

Corwin J.T. and Warchol, M.E. (1991) Auditory hair cells: structure, function, development, and regeneration. *Ann. Rev. Neurosci.* 14: 301–333.

Phillips, D.P. (1988) Introduction to anatomy and physiology of the central auditory nervous system. In *Physiology of the Ear* (Jahn, A.F. and Santos-Sacchi, J., eds), pp. 407–427. New York: Raven Press.

17

TRIGEMINAL AND FACIAL NERVES

Chapter Summary

Trigeminal nerve
Motor nucleus of the V nerve
Sensory nuclei of the V nerve
Innervation of the teeth
Innervation of the cerebral
　arteries
　Trigeminothalamic tract
Mastication

Facial nerve
Facial nerve proper
Nervus intermedius

CLINICAL PANELS
Trigeminal neuralgia
Referred pain in diseases of
　the head and neck
Lesions of the facial nerve
Syndromes of the
　cerebellopontine angle

Study Guidelines

Trigeminal nerve
1 The motor nucleus of V supplies the muscles of mastication.
2 The unipolar sensory neurons of the V provide sensory innervation to the face and related mucous membranes.
3 The 'spinal' nucleus is of special clinical importance because of its huge nociceptive territory.

Facial nerve
1 VII is the most commonly paralyzed of all peripheral nerves, owing to the great length (approx. 7 cm) of its canal in the temporal bone. Because VII supplies the muscles of facial expression, the effects of facial paralysis are obvious to all.
2 Learn the distinctions between upper and lower motor neuron lesions of VII.
3 Note that VII participates in several important reflex arcs.

TRIGEMINAL NERVE

The trigeminal nerve has a very large sensory territory which includes the skin of the face, the oronasal mucous membranes and the teeth, the dura mater and major intracranial blood vessels. The nerve is also both motor and sensory to the muscles of mastication. The **motor root** lies medial to the large **sensory root** at the site of attachment to the pons. The **trigeminal (Gasserian) ganglion,** near the apex of the petrous temporal bone, gives rise to the sensory root and consists of unipolar neurons.

Details of the distribution of the ophthalmic, maxillary, and mandibular divisions are available in gross anatomy textbooks. Accurate appreciation of their respective territories on the face is essential if trigeminal neuralgia is to be distinguished from other sources of facial pain (*Panel 17.1*).

MOTOR NUCLEUS OF THE V NERVE
(FIGURE 17.1)

The motor nucleus is the special visceral nucleus supplying the muscles derived from the embryonic mandibular arch. These comprise the masticatory muscles attached to each half of the mandible (*Figure 17.2*), along with the tensor tympani and tensor palati. The nucleus occupies the lateral pontine tegmentum. Embedded in its upper pole is a node of the reticular formation, the **supratrigeminal nucleus,** which acts as a pattern generator for masticatory rhythm.

Voluntary control is provided by corticonuclear projections from each motor cortex to both motor nuclei.

SENSORY NUCLEI OF THE V NERVE

Three sensory nuclei are associated with the trigeminal nerve: **mesencephalic, pontine,** and **spinal.**

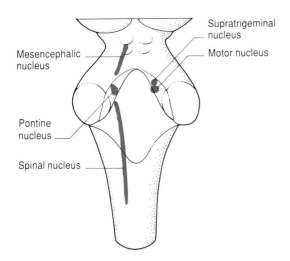

Figure 17.1 Trigeminal nuclei. *Left:* sensory nuclei; *right:* motor nucleus, supratrigeminal nucleus.

Mesencephalic nucleus

The mesencephalic nucleus is unique in being the only nucleus in the CNS that is composed of unipolar neurons. In humans their peripheral processes enter the sensory root via the **mesencephalic tract** of the trigeminal. Some travel in the mandibular division to supply stretch receptors (neuromuscular spindles) in the masticatory muscles. Others travel in the maxillary and mandibular divisions to supply stretch receptors (Ruffini endings) in the periodontal ligaments of the teeth.

The central processes of the mesencephalic afferent neurons descend through the pontine tegmentum in the small *tract of Probst*. Most fibers of this tract terminate in the supratrigeminal nucleus; others end in the motor nucleus or in the pontine sensory nucleus; a few travel as far as the dorsal nucleus of the vagus.

Pontine nucleus

The pontine (chief, principal) nucleus is homologous with the posterior column nuclei (gracilis and cuneatus). It processes discriminative tactile information from the skin of the face.

CLINICAL PANEL 17.1

TRIGEMINAL NEURALGIA

Trigeminal neuralgia is an important condition, characterized by attacks of excruciating pain in the territory of one or more divisions of the trigeminal nerve. The patient (who is usually more than 60 years old) is able to map out the affected division(s) accurately. Because the condition has to be distinguished from many other causes of facial pain, the clinician should be able to mark out a trigeminal sensory map (see *Figure CP 17.1.1*). Sometimes there is an underlying osteitis of the petrous temporal bone, or compression of the sensory root by an arterial loop, but usually no explanation is found.

Most patients respond well to drug therapy. For those who do not, the usual practice is to carry out electrocoagulation of the affected division, through a needle electrode inserted through the foramen ovale from below. The intention is to heat the nerve sufficiently to destroy only the finest fibers, in which case analgesia is produced but touch (including the corneal reflex) is preserved. An alternative

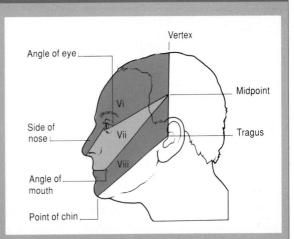

Figure CP 17.1.1 Five lines used to delineate the divisions of the trigeminal nerve on the face.

procedure is *medullary tractotomy*: the spinal root is sectioned through the dorsolateral surface of the medulla. In successful cases, pain and temperature sensitivity is lost from the face but touch (mediated by the pontine nucleus) is preserved.

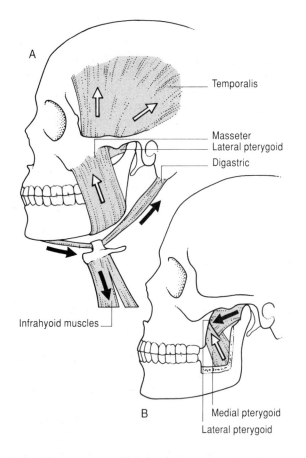

Figure 17.2 (A) Masticatory and infrahyoid muscles viewed from the left side; (B) medial view of the pterygoid muscles of the right side. Clear arrows indicate directions of pull of jaw-closing muscles. Black arrows indicate directions of pull of jaw openers.

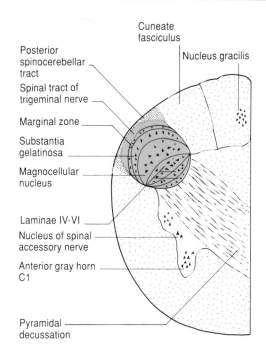

Figure 17.3 Spinal tract and nucleus of trigeminal nerve, at level of spinomedullary junction.

Spinal nucleus

The spinal nucleus extends from the lower part of the pons to the third cervical segment of the spinal cord (hence the term 'spinal').Two minor nuclei in its upper part (called pars oralis and pars interpolaris) receive afferents from the mouth. The main spinal nucleus (called pars caudalis) receives tactile, nociceptive, and thermal information from the entire trigeminal area, and even beyond.

In section, the main spinal nucleus is seen to be an expanded continuation of the outer laminae (I–III) of the posterior horn of the cord (*Figure 17.3*). The inner three laminae (IV–VI) are relatively compressed. Laminae III and IV are referred to as the magnocellular part of the nucleus. In animals, nociceptive-specific neurons are

found in lamina I. 'Polymodal' neurons are in the magnocellular nucleus and correspond to lamina V neurons lower down; they respond to tactile stimuli applied to the trigeminal skin area as well as to noxious mechanical stimuli (pinching the skin with a forceps). Whereas the nociceptive-specific neurons have small receptive fields confined to one territory (a patch of skin or mucous membrane), many of the polymodal neurons show the phenomenon of *convergence* to a marked degree. In anesthetized animals, a single neuron may be responsive to noxious stimuli applied to a tooth, and to facial skin, and to the temporomandibular joint. This finding provides a plausible basis of explanation for erroneous localization of pain by patients. Examples are given in *Panel 17.2*.

Arrangements for pain modulation appear to be the same as for the spinal cord (see Chapter 19). They include the presence of enkephalinergic and GABAergic internuncials in the substantia gelatinosa, and aminergic projections from the nucleus raphe magnus (partly serotonergic) and the locus ceruleus (noradrenergic).

Afferents to the spinal nucleus come from three sources (*Figure 17.4*):

CLINICAL PANEL 17.2

REFERRED PAIN IN DISEASES OF THE HEAD AND NECK

Cervical headache

Experiments in healthy volunteers have demonstrated that noxious stimulation of tissues supplied by the upper cervical nerves may induce pain referred to the head. Tissues tested include the ligaments of the upper cervical joints, the suboccipital muscles, and the sternomastoid and trapezius. The pain is primarily occipital, as would be expected from the cutaneous distribution of nerves C2 and C3, but it may radiate to the forehead. A common source of cervical headache in the elderly is spondylosis, a degenerative arthritis in which bony excrescences compress the emerging spinal nerves (Chapter 11). Another source appears to be myofascial disease of the sternomastoid-trapezius continuum close to the base of the skull. Trigger points—tender nodules within the muscles which give rise to occipital pain when compressed—are often detected by physical therapists during palpation of these muscles.

Earache

Earache is most often due to an acute infection of the outer ear canal or middle ear. However, pain may be referred to a perfectly healthy ear from a variety of sources. The outer ear skin receives small sensory branches from the mandibular, facial, vagus, and upper cervical nerves; the middle ear epithelium is supplied by the glossopharyngeal and vagus. Earache may be a leading symptom of disease in the territory of one of these nerves. Important examples include:

- Cancer of the pharynx—perhaps concealed in the piriform fossa beside the larynx, or near the tonsil.
- An impacted wisdom tooth in the mandible.
- Temporomandibular joint disease.
- Spondylosis of the upper cervical spine.

Pain in the face

- Important causes of pain referred to the face below the eye include:
- Dental caries or an impacted wisdom tooth in the upper jaw.
- Cancer in a mucous membrane supplied by the maxillary nerve: maxillary air sinus, nasal cavity, nasopharynx.
- Acute maxillary sinusitis.
- Trigeminal neuralgia affecting the maxillary nerve.

---

1 *Trigeminal afferents* are the central processes of Gasserian ganglion cells. The peripheral processes terminate in tactile and nociceptive endings in the territory of the three divisions of the nerve. Most often involved clinically are the nociceptive terminals in: (a) the teeth; (b) the cornea; (c) the temporomandibular joint; and (d) the dura mater of the anterior and middle cranial fossae. Topographic representation of the trigeminal territory is onion-like (*Figure 17.5*); the mandibular fibers terminate in the rostral part of the nucleus, the maxillary fibers in the midregion, and the ophthalmic fibers caudally.

2 *Cervical afferents* come from the territory of the first three cervical posterior nerve roots. (The first posterior nerve root is either small or absent.) Most often involved clinically are nociceptive fibers supplying (a) the intervertebral joints and spinal dura mater, and (b) the dura mater of the posterior cranial fossa, reached by cervical fibers ascending through the hypoglossal canal.

3 *Nociceptive afferents* from the mucous membranes of the pharyngotympanic tube, middle ear, pharynx and larynx. These afferents are often involved in acute inflammatory processes during wintertime. Their cell bodies occupy the sensory ganglia of the glossopharyngeal and vagus nerves.

INNERVATION OF THE TEETH

From the superior and inferior alveolar nerves, Aδ and C fibers enter the root canals of the teeth and form a dense plexus within the pulp. Individual fibers terminate in the pulp, in the predentin, and in dentinal tubules. Most dentinal tubules underlying the occlusal surfaces of the teeth contain single nerve fibers; however, the

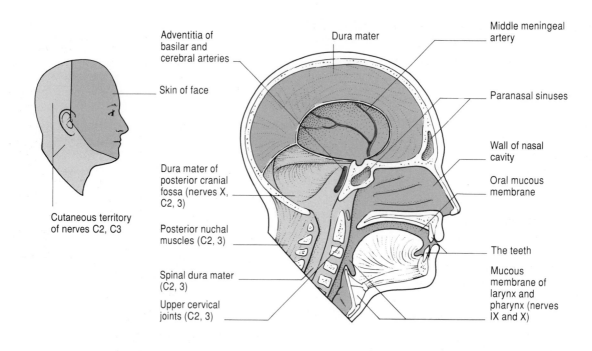

Figure 17.4 Illustration to indicate the extensive nociceptive territory of the spinal trigeminal nucleus. Structures labeled without qualification are supplied directly by the trigeminal nerve. The remainder are supplied by other nerves having central nociceptive projections to the spinal trigeminal nucleus.

fibers are restricted to the inner ends of the tubules whereas pain can be elicited from the outer surface of dentin after removal of the enamel. Hydrodynamic and chemical factors have been invoked to fill the gap, as well as possible participation of odontoblasts as intermediaries.

The periodontal ligaments are richly innervated by the nerves supplying the oral epithelium including the gums. Some of the nerve endings are a potential source of pain during dental extraction or periodontal disease. Others function as tension receptors comparable to Ruffini endings found in joint capsules; tension receptors would be anticipated because the periodontal ligaments are arranged like hammocks around the roots of the teeth.

INNERVATION OF CEREBRAL ARTERIES

The ophthalmic divison of the trigeminal comes close to the internal carotid artery in the cavernous sinus. Here it gives off afferent fibers which accompany the artery to its point of bifurcation into anterior and middle cerebral branches. The nerve fibers accompany these, and also reach the posterior cerebral artery. Several peptide substances have been detected in these

axons; they include substance P, the peptide particularly associated with nociceptive transmission.

The function of the *trigeminovascular neurons* (as they are called) is the subject of speculation.

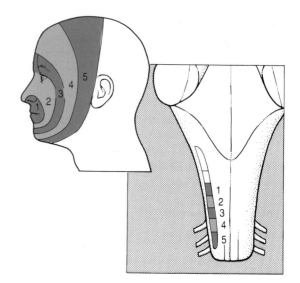

Figure 17.5 Representation of the face in the spinal trigeminal nucleus. (Adapted from Sears and Franklin (1980).)

Their presence accounts well for the *frontal headache* associated with distortion of the cerebral arteries by space-occupying lesions.

TRIGEMINOTHALAMIC TRACT
(FIGURE 17.6)

The trigeminothalamic tract originates in the supratrigeminal, pontine, and spinal trigeminal nuclei. Nearly all of its fibers cross the midline before ascending to the ventral posterior nucleus of the thalamus. The tract has features in common with the medial lemniscus (it mediates conscious proprioception and discriminative touch) and the spinal lemniscus (it mediates tactile, nociceptive, and thermal sense). At the level of the midbrain, it is also called the trigeminal lemniscus.

From the thalamus, third-order afferents project to the large area of facial representation in the lower half of the somatic sensory cortex.

Trigeminoreticular fibers synapse in the parvocellular reticular formation on both sides of the brainstem. They are counterparts of the spinoreticular tract, and they mediate the arousal effect of stroking or slapping the face, and of the old-fashioned 'smelling salts' (the ammonia irritates trigeminal afferents in the nose).

MASTICATION

Mastication is a complex activity requiring orchestration of the nuclear groups supplying the muscles that move the mandible, tongue, cheeks, and hyoid bone. The chief controlling center seems to be an area of the premotor cortex directly in front of the face representation on the motor cortex. Stimulation of this area produces masticatory cycles.

Brainstem control of mandibular activity resides in the **supratrigeminal nucleus,** which functions as a pattern generator. The supratrigeminal nucleus receives proprioceptive information from the spindle-rich jaw-closing muscles (masseter, temporalis, medial pterygoid) and from the periodontal ligaments. The supratrigeminal nucleus also receives tactile information (food in the mouth) from the pontine nucleus, and nociceptive information from the spinal nucleus. It gives rise to an ipsilateral trigeminocerebellar projection and a contralateral trigeminothalamic projection, both of which contain proprioceptive information. It controls mastication directly by means of excitatory and inhibitory inputs to the trigeminal motor nucleus.

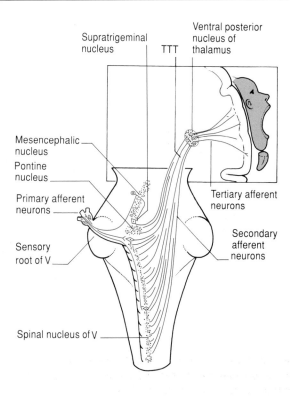

Figure 17.6 Primary, secondary, and tertiary trigeminal afferents.

The *jaw-closing reflex* is initiated by contact of food with the oral mucous membrane. The response of the pattern generator is to activate the jaw-closing motoneurons so that the teeth are brought into occlusion.

The *jaw-opening reflex* is initiated by periodontal stretch afferents activated by dental occlusion. The pattern generator responds by inhibiting the closure motoneurons and activating the jaw openers. Muscle spindles are especially numerous in the anterior part of the masseter, and when stretch reaches a critical level the pattern generator is switched to a jaw-closing mode.

The jaw jerk

The jaw jerk is a tendon reflex elicited by tapping the chin with a downward stroke. The normal response is a twitch of the jaw-closing muscles, because muscle spindle afferents make some direct synaptic contacts upon trigeminal motoneurons. Supranuclear lesions of the motor nucleus (e.g. pseudobulbar palsy, Chapter 15) may be accompanied by an 'exaggerated' (abnormally brisk) jaw jerk.

The supratrigeminal nucleus is seldom dormant. In the erect posture, it activates the jaw closers to keep the mandible elevated. During sleep, it activates the lateral pterygoid so that the pharynx is not occluded by the tongue. (The root of the tongue is anchored to the mandible.) However, the nucleus is *inactivated by general anesthesia*, in which circumstance the ramus of the mandible must be held forward constantly in order to prevent choking.

FACIAL NERVE

The facial (VII cranial) is the nerve of supply to the second branchial arch. The facial **nerve proper** supplies the muscles of facial expression, as well as the stapedius, stylohyoid, and posterior digastric. Accompanying the facial nerve proper for part of its course is the **nervus intermedius** which supplies secretomotor fibers to glands in the eye, nose and mouth, and taste fibers to the tongue and palate.

The facial nerve is of clinical importance in being the most frequently paralyzed of all the peripheral nerves.

FACIAL NERVE PROPER

The facial nerve proper arises from the branchial (special visceral) efferent cell column caudal to the motor nucleus of the trigeminal. The **facial motor nucleus** occupies the lateral region of the tegmentum in the caudal part of the pons (*Figure 17.7*). Before emerging from the brainstem, the nerve loops around the abducens nucleus, creating the **facial colliculus** in the floor of the fourth ventricle (Chapter 14).

The facial nerve emerges at the lower border of the pons together with the nervus intermedius. The two nerves cross the subarachnoid space in company with the vestibulocochlear nerve to reach the internal acoustic meatus. The facial nerve enters a narrow bony canal above the vestibule of the labyrinth, bends backward at the genu, and descends to the stylomastoid foramen in the interval between the middle ear and the mastoid process. In this interval, it supplies the stapedius muscle. Upon leaving the skull, the facial nerve supplies the posterior belly of the occipitofrontalis, the stylohyoid, and the posterior belly of the digastric. It then turns forward within the substance of the parotid gland and breaks up into the five named branches which

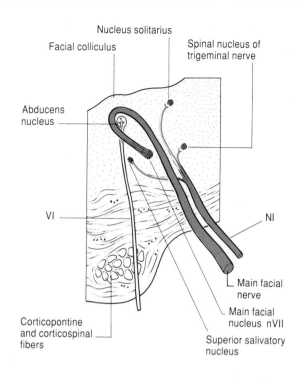

Figure 17.7 Transverse section of the pons showing components of the facial nerve and of the nervus intermedius. NI, nervus intermedius.

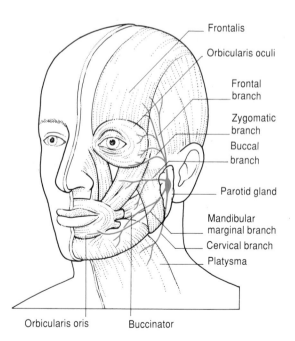

Figure 17.8 Principal extracranial branches of the facial nerve.

supply the muscles of facial expression (*Figure 17.8*).

Supranuclear connections

All of the cells of the main motor nucleus receive a corticonuclear supply from the 'face' area of the contralateral motor cortex. In addition, the cells supplying the muscles of the upper face (occipitofrontalis and orbicularis oculi) receive an equal supply from the *ipsilateral* motor cortex. The bilateral supply for the upper facial muscles is reflected in their normally paired activities in wrinkling the forehead, or blinking, or squeezing the eyes shut. The muscles around the mouth, in contrast, can be activated discretely. The partial bilateral supply helps to distinguish a supranuclear from a nuclear or infranuclear lesion of the facial nerve (*Panel 17.3*).

More than any other muscle group, the muscles of facial expression are responsive to emotional states. A limbic contribution to the supranuclear supply is to be expected, and its most likely source is the **nucleus accumbens** at the base of the forebrain. The nucleus accumbens is a ventral part of the basal ganglia, which in turn influence the motor cortex (Chapter 25). That circuit is compromised in Parkinson's disease, which is characterized by a mask-like, emotionless demeanor.

Nuclear connections

Five reflex arcs involving the facial nucleus are listed in *Table 17.1*. Most important clinically is the corneal reflex.

Corneal reflex

The usual test is to touch the cornea with a cotton wisp. This should elicit a bilateral blink response. The afferent limb of the reflex is the ophthalmic division of the trigeminal nerve (nasociliary branch). The efferent limb is the facial nerve (branch to palpebral element of orbicularis oculi). Since the reflex can still be elicited following section of the spinal tract of the trigeminal nerve (tractotomy operation), internuncials projecting from the pontine nucleus to both facial nuclei must be sufficient to complete the reflex arc.

The corneal reflex may be lost following a lesion of either the ophthalmic or facial nerves. A gradual compression of ophthalmic fibers in the sensory root of the trigeminal nerve may damage corneal neurons selectively. For this reason, the corneal reflex must be tested in patients under suspicion of an acoustic neuroma (*Panel 17.4*).

NERVUS INTERMEDIUS

The nervus intermedius enters the facial nerve proximal to the genu. It contains two sets of parasympathetic fibers and two sets of special sense fibers (*Figure 17.9*).

The *parasympathetic root* of the nerve arises from the **superior salivatory nucleus** in the pons. It forms the motor component of the greater petrosal and chorda tympani nerves. The greater petrosal nerve synapses in the **pterygopalatine ganglion** whose postganglionic fibers supply the lacrimal and nasal glands. The motor component of chorda tympani synapses in the **submandibular ganglion** whose postganglionic fibers supply the submandibular and sublingual glands.

Table 17.1 Brainstem reflexes involving the facial nerve

	Corneal reflex	Sucking reflex	Blinking to light	Blinking to noise	Sound attenuation
Receptor	Cornea	Lips	Retina	Cochlea	Cochlea
Afferent	Ophthalmic nerve	Mandibular nerve	Optic nerve	Cochlear nucleus	Cochlear nucleus
First synapse	Spinal nucleus of trigeminal	Pontine nucleus of trigeminal	Superior colliculus	Inferior colliculus	Superior olivary nucleus
Second synapse	Facial nucleus	Facial nucleus	Facial nucleus	Facial nucleus	Facial nucleus
Muscle	Orbicularis oculi	Orbicularis oris	Orbicularis oculi	Orbicularis oculi	Stapedius

CLINICAL PANEL 17.3

LESIONS OF THE FACIAL NERVE

Supranuclear lesions
Much the commonest cause of a supranuclear lesion of the seventh nerve is a vascular stroke, in which corticonuclear and corticospinal fibers are interrupted at the level of the internal capsule or cerebral cortex. The usual effect of a stroke is to produce a contralateral motor weakness of the lower part of the face and of the limbs. The upper face escapes because of the bilateral supranuclear supply to the upper part of the facial nucleus.

Nuclear lesions
The main motor nucleus may be involved in thrombosis of one of the pontine branches of the basilar artery. As might be anticipated from the relationships depicted in *Figure 17.7*, the usual result of such a lesion is an *alternating (crossed) hemiplegia*: complete paralysis of the facial and/or abducens nerve on one side combined with motor weakness of the limbs on the opposite side.

Infranuclear lesions
Bell's palsy is a common disorder caused by a neuritis (possibly viral in origin) of the facial nerve. The inflammation causes the nerve to swell, and conduction is compromised by the tight fit of the nerve in the bony canal between the geniculate ganglion and the stylomastoid foramen. There may be some initial pain in the ear, but the condition is otherwise painless.

Facial paralysis is usually complete. On the affected side the patient is unable to raise the eyebrow, close the eye, or retract the lip. Tears may spill from the lax lower eyelid, and saliva may drool from the corner of the mouth. The patient may experience *hyperacusis:* ordinary sounds may be unpleasantly loud due to loss of the damping action of the stapedius muscle.

The segment of nerve between geniculate ganglion and stylomastoid foramen is usually compromised. Tests may reveal blockage of nervus intermedius fibers on the affected side, in the form of reduced lacrimal salivary secretions and loss of taste from the anterior part of the tongue.

Four out of five cases recover completely within a few weeks because the nerve has only

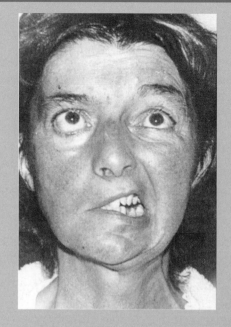

Figure CP 17.3.1 Complete facial nerve paralysis, patient's right side. The patient has been asked to show her teeth and to look upward. To compare the two sides, cover the left and right halves of the photograph alternately with a card. On the paralyzed side, note (paralyzed muscles in parentheses): inability to raise the eyebrow (frontalis muscle); drooping of the lower eyelid (orbicularis oculi); inability to retract the mouth (buccinator); no webbing of the neck (platysma). The patient was also unable to abduct the right eye (abducens nerve paralysis, Chapter 18). Together with a history of other disturbances, the clinical picture was suggestive of multiple sclerosis with a current patch of demyelination deep to the facial colliculus, affecting the emerging fibers of the facial and abducens nerves (cf. *Figure 17.6*). (Photograph reproduced from Parsons, M. (1987) *Diagnostic Picture Test in Clinical Neurology.* London: Wolfe Medical Publications, with the kind permission of the author and publisher.)

suffered a conduction block or neuropraxia. In the remainder, the nerve undergoes Wallerian degeneration (Chapter 7); recovery takes about 3 months and is often incomplete. During regeneration, some preganglionic fibers of the nervus intermedius may enter the greater petrosal nerve instead of the chorda tympani, with the result that the lacrimal gland becomes active at mealtimes (so-called 'crocodile tears').

CLINICAL PANEL 17.3 *Continued*

Other causes of infranuclear palsy include a patch of demyelination in the course of multiple sclerosis (*Figure CP 17.3.1*), tumors in the cerebellopontine angle (*Panel 17.4*), middle ear disease, and tumors of the parotid gland. *Herpes zoster oticus* is a rare but well recog-

nized viral infection of the geniculate ganglion. Severe pain in one ear precedes the appearance of a vesicular rash in and around the external acoustic meatus. Swelling of the geniculate ganglion may be sufficient to cause a complete facial palsy (Ramsay Hunt syndrome).

CLINICAL PANEL 17.4

SYNDROMES OF THE CEREBELLOPONTINE ANGLE

The *cerebellopontine angle* is the recess between the hemisphere of the cerebellum and the lower border of the pons. The petrous temporal bone, laterally, completes a triangle having the V nerve at its upper corner and the IX and X at its lower corner; the triangle is bisected by the VII and VIII nerves (*Figure CP 17.4.1*).

Several kinds of space-occupying lesions may compromise one or more nerves in the angle. The most frequent is an *acoustic neuroma,* which is a slow-growing benign tumor of Schwann cells (a neurolemmoma). The tumor originates in the vestibular nerve within the internal acoustic meatus, but the initial symptoms are more often cochlear than vestibular. *An acoustic neuroma must be suspected in every middle-aged or elderly patient presenting*

with auditory or vestibular symptoms. Early diagnosis is important because of the difficulty of removing a large neuroma extending into the posterior cranial fossa; also because the cumulative motor and sensory disturbances may not show significant improvement after surgery.

The following is a fairly typical sequence of symptoms and signs in a case escaping early detection:

- *Tinnitus* is experienced on the affected side, in the form of a high-pitched ringing or fizzing sound.
- *Deafness* on the affected side is slowly progressive over a period of months or years.
- *Vertigo* occurs episodically. Severe vertigo with nystagmus signifies compression of the brainstem.
- *Loss of the corneal reflex* is an early sign of distortion of the V nerve by a tumor emerging from the internal acoustic meatus into the posterior cranial fossa.
- *Weakness of the masticatory muscles* is a later sign of V nerve involvement. The jaw deviates toward the affected side when the mouth is opened, because the normal lateral pterygoid is unopposed. Wasting of the masseter may be obvious on palpation of the cheek.
- *Weakness of the facial musculature* develops as the VII nerve becomes stretched.
- *Anesthesia of the oropharynx* signifies involvement of the IX nerve.
- *Ipsilateral 'cerebellar signs'* in the arm and leg appear when the cerebellum is compressed.
- *'Upper motor neuron signs'* in the limbs signify compression of the brainstem.
- *Signs of raised intracranial pressure* (headache, drowsiness, papilledema) signify obstruction of cerebrospinal fluid circulation either inside or around the brainstem.

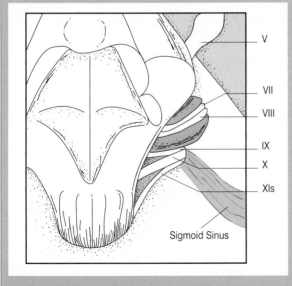

Figure CP 17.4.1 An acoustic neuroma invading the right posterior cranial fossa. XIs, spinal XI nerve.

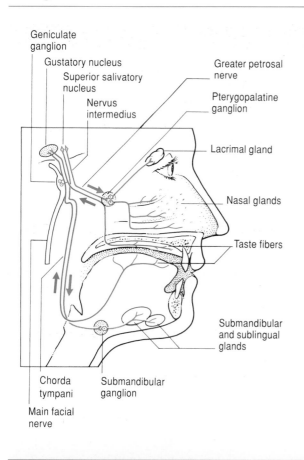

Geniculate ganglion
Gustatory nucleus
Superior salivatory nucleus
Nervus intermedius
Greater petrosal nerve
Pterygopalatine ganglion
Lacrimal gland
Nasal glands
Taste fibers
Submandibular and sublingual glands
Chorda tympani
Submandibular ganglion
Main facial nerve

Figure 17.9 The nervus intermedius and its branches. Arrows indicate direction of impulse traffic.

The *special sense root* of the nerve has unipolar cell bodies in the **geniculate ganglion** of the facial nerve. The peripheral processes of the ganglion cells supply taste buds in the palate via the great petrosal nerve, and taste buds in the anterior two-thirds of the tongue via the chorda tympani. The central processes enter the gustatory nucleus, which also receives fibers from the glossopharyngeal nerve (Chapter 15). From here, second-order neurons project to the thalamus on the *same* side, for relay to the anterior parts of insula and cingulate cortex.

A few cells of the geniculate ganglion supply skin in and around the external acoustic meatus.

CORE INFORMATION

Trigeminal nerve

The motor root of V enters the mandibular division to supply the six muscles of mastication, the tensor tympani and the tensor palati. Automatic control is from the supratrigeminal nucleus, voluntary control bilaterally from the motor cortex.

The V ganglion (unipolar cells) sends peripheral processes into all three divisions, providing sensory endings in the face and oronasal mucous membranes and teeth. The central processes synapse in the pontine and spinal nuclei of V. Peripheral processes proprioceptive to teeth and masticatory muscles come from the (unipolar) mesencephalic nucleus.

The pontine nucleus processes tactile information from the face and oronasal mucous membranes. The spinal nucleus receives nociceptive signals from the entire trigeminal sensory field, also from the territory of the IX, X and upper cervical nerves.

The pontine and spinal nuclei project fibers into the reticular formation (for arousal) and to the somatic sensory cortex via the thalamus.

Facial nerve

From the facial motor nucleus, VII winds around VI creating the facial colliculus, emerges at lower border of pons, enters the int. auditory meatus to reach a long bony canal that takes it to the stylomastoid foramen. It supplies the muscles of facial expression, stapedius and posterior digastric. The motor nucleus receives a bilateral supranuclear supply from the motor cortex to its upper half, a contralateral supply to its lower half.

The nervus intermedius travels in part with VII. The superior salivatory nucleus forms the motor components of greater petrosal (for lacrimal and nasal glands via pterygopalatine ganglion) and chorda tympani (for submandibular and sublingual glands via submandibular ganglion). The geniculate ganglion of VII has unipolar neurons that supply taste sensation to the palate via great petrosal and tongue via chorda tympani. A few of the unipolar neurons supply skin in and around the external acoustic meatus.

SELF TEST

Answer **A** if 1, 2, and 3 only are correct
       B if 1 and 3 only are correct
       C if 2 and 4 only are correct
       D if 4 only is correct
       E if all four are correct

1 Which of the following nerves convey nociceptive information to the spinal trigeminal nucleus:
1 Glossopharyngeal
2 Inferior alveolar
3 Ophthalmic
4 Lower three cervical

2 The motor nucleus of the trigeminal nerve contains neurons that:
1 Emerge lateral to the sensory root
2 Enter the maxillary nerve
3 Innervate lingual muscles
4 Receive bilateral corticonuclear projections

3 Disease here may produce pain referred to the ear:
1 Nasopharynx
2 Temporomandibular joint
3 Molar tooth
4 Piriform fossa

4 The facial nerve supplies the following muscle(s):
1 Masticatory
2 Facial expression
3 Tensor tympani
4 Stapedius

5 Which of the following nuclei are connected to the facial nerve?
1 Superior salivatory
2 Abducens
3 Nucleus solitarius
4 Vestibular

6 Which of the following reflexes involve(s) the facial nerve?
1 Startle
2 Sound attenuation
3 Blink to light
4 Jaw jerk

REFERENCES

Trigeminal nerve

Bogduk, N., Corrigan, B., Kelly, P., Schneider, G., and Farr, R. (1985) Cervical headache. *Aust. J.Med.* **143**: 202–207.

Bovim, G., Berg, R. and Dale, L.G. (1992) Cervicogenic headache. *Pain* **49**: 315–320.

Lambert, G.A. (1993) Pathways for headache. In *Science and Practice in Clinical Neurology* (Gandevia, S.C., Burke, D., and Anthony, M., eds), pp. 284–302. Cambridge: University Press.

Ogawa, H. (1994). Gustatory cortex of primates: anatomy and physiology. *Neurosci. Res.* **20**: 1–13.

Rappaport, Z.H. (1994) Trigeminal neuralgia: the role of self-sustaining discharge in the trigeminal ganglion. *Pain* **56**: 127–138.

Sears, E.S. and Franklin, G.M. (1980) Diseases of the cranial nerves. In *Neurology* (Rosenberg, R.N., ed), pp. 471–494. New York: Grune & Stratton.

Sessle, B.J. (1990) Anatomy, physiology and pathophysiology of orofacial pain. In *Headache and Facial Pain* (Jacobson, A.L. and Donlon, W.C., eds), pp. 1–24. New York: Raven Press.

Yokota, T. (1988) Anatomy and physiology of intra- and extracranial nociceptive afferents and their central projections. In *Basic Mechanisms of Headache* (Olesen, J. and Edvinsson, L., eds), pp. 117–128. Amsterdam: Elsevier.

Facial nerve

Lang, J. (1984) Clinical anatomy of the cerebellopontine angle and internal acoustic meatus. *Adv. Oto-Rhino-Laryng.* **34**: 8–24.

Manni, J.J. and Stennert, E. (1984) Diagnostic methods in facial nerve pathology. *Adv. Oto-Rhino-Laryng.* **34**: 202–213.

Parnes, S. M. (1988) The facial nerve. In *Physiology of the Ear* (Jahn, A.F. and Santos-Sacchi, J., eds), pp. 125–142. New York: Raven Press.

18

OCULAR MOTOR NERVES

<table>
<tr><td>

Chapter Summary

The nerves
Oculomotor nerve
Trochlear nerve
Abducens nerve

Nerve endings
Motor endings
Sensory endings

Pupillary light reflex

Accommodation
The near response
The far response

Occular palsies

Notes on the sympathetic pathway to the eye

Control of eye movements
Scanning
Tracking

CLINICAL PANEL
Ocular palsies

</td><td>

Study Guidelines

General
Because of the immense diagnostic and therapeutic importance of ocular innervation, and because of its inherent complexity, neuro-ophthalmology has become a branch of medicine in its own right.

It is especially important to appreciate the way in which premotor centers are able to operate bilaterally in order to keep the gaze on target, even when the head is moving.

Particular
1 In addition to nerves III, IV, and VI, the sympathetic supply to the eye is reviewed here because it counterbalances the parasympathetic innervation contained in III.
2 The nerve supply to the six muscles that move the eyeball is straightforward. However, III also supplies the elevator of the upper eyelid.
3 The autonomic supply to the eye is straightforward. For the sympathetic, think of someone being startled awake at night. For the parasympathetic, think of someone eyeing food on a fork.

</td></tr>
</table>

THE NERVES

The ocular motor nerves comprise the **oculomotor** (III cranial), **trochlear** (IV cranial) and **abducens** (VI cranial) **nerves**. They provide the motor nerve supply to the four recti and two oblique muscles controlling movements of the eyeball on each side (*Figure 18.1*). The oculomotor nerve contains two additional sets of neurons: one to supply the levator of the upper eyelid, the other to control the sphincter of the pupil and the ciliary muscle.

The nuclei serving the extraocular muscles (extrinsic muscles of the eye) belong to the somatic efferent cell column of the brainstem, in line with the nucleus of the hypoglossal nerve. The oculomotor nucleus has an additional,

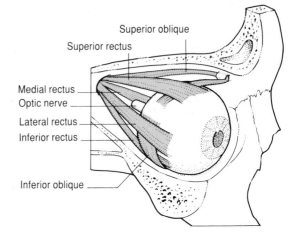

Superior oblique
Superior rectus
Medial rectus
Optic nerve
Lateral rectus
Inferior rectus
Inferior oblique

Figure 18.1 Extrinsic ocular muscles.

parasympathetic nucleus which belongs to the general visceral efferent cell column.

OCULOMOTOR NERVE

The nucleus of the third nerve is at the level of the superior colliculi. It is partly embedded in the periaqueductal gray matter (*Figure 18.2A*). It is composed of five individual nuclei for the supply of striated muscles, and one parasympathetic nucleus.

The nerve pases through the tegmentum of the midbrain and emerges into the interpeduncular arachnoid cistern. It crosses the apex of the petrous temporal bone, pierces the dural roof of the cavernous sinus, runs in the lateral wall of the sinus and breaks into upper and lower divisions within the superior orbital fissure. The upper division supplies the superior rectus and the levator palpebrae superioris; the lower division supplies the inferior and medial recti and the inferior oblique.

The parasympathetic fibers originate in the **Edinger-Westphal nucleus**. They accompany the main nerve as far as the orbit, then leave the branch to the inferior oblique and synapse in the **ciliary ganglion**. Postganglionic fibers emerge from the ganglion in the **short ciliary nerves,** which pierce the *lamina cribrosa* ('sieve-like layer') of the sclera and supply the *ciliaris* and *sphincter pupillae.*

TROCHLEAR NERVE

The nucleus of the fourth nerve is at the level of the inferior colliculus. The nerve itself is unique in two respects (*Figure 18.2B*): it is the only nerve to emerge from the back of the brainstem; and it crosses the midline.

The IV nerve winds around the crus of the midbrain and travels through the cavernous sinus in company with the III nerve (*Figure 18.3*). It passes through the superior orbital fissure and supplies the *superior oblique* muscle.

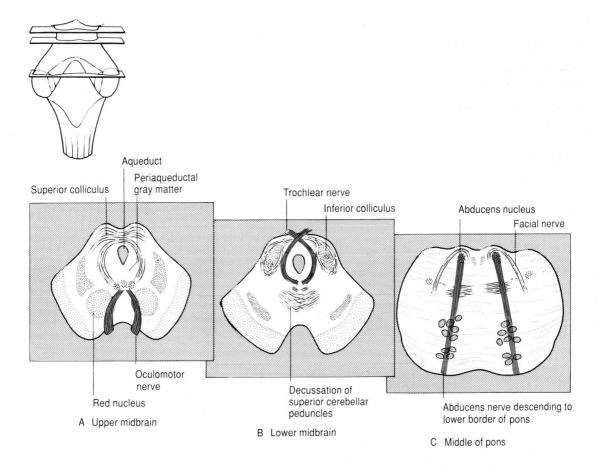

Figure 18.2A-C Transverse sections of the brainstem showing the origins of the ocular motor nerves.

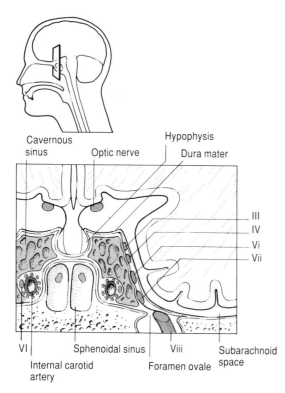

Figure 18.3 Coronal section of the cavernous sinus and related structures.
III, oculomotor nerve
IV, trochlear nerve
VI, abducens nerve
Vi, Vii, Viii ophthalmic, maxillary, mandibular divisions of trigeminal nerve.

ABDUCENS NERVE

The nucleus of the sixth nerve is at the level of the facial colliculus, in the middle of the pons (*Figure 18.2C*). The nerve emerges at the lower border of the pons and runs up the pontine subarachnoid cistern, beside the basilar artery. It angles over the apex of the petrous temporal bone and passes through the cavernous sinus beside the internal carotid artery (*Figure 18.3*). It enters the orbit through the superior orbital fissure and supplies the *lateral rectus* muscle, which abducts the eye.

NERVE ENDINGS

MOTOR ENDINGS

All of the ocular motor units are small, containing 5–10 muscles fibers apiece (compared with 1000 or more in the tibialis anterior).

Type A fibers produce the fast twitches required for saccadic movements. *Type B* are slow-twitch and may be used for smooth pursuit. *Type C* show only local contractions beneath the individual plates. Type C fibers may be involved in keeping the visual axes of the two eyes parallel with one another. Since the visual axes diverge following administration of muscle relaxants, keeping them parallel must require continuous muscle action, even during sleep.

SENSORY ENDINGS

In addition to neuromuscular spindles of standard type, numerous *palisade endings* exist in the form of nerve spirals around individual muscle fibers.

The extraocular muscle proprioceptors are the peripheral terminals of neurons in the mesencephalic nucleus of the trigeminal nerve. In monkeys, some of the central processess of these neurons reach as far caudally as the accessory cuneate nucleus in the medulla oblongata. This nucleus also receives proprioceptive terminals from the neck muscles, and it projects both to the ipsilateral cerebellum and to the contralateral superior colliculus. The conjunction of ocular and cervical proprioceptive information presumably assists in the coordination of simultaneous movements of the eyes and head.

PUPILLARY LIGHT REFLEX *(FIGURE 18.4)*

Constriction of the pupils in response to light involves four sets of neurons, as follows:

1 The afferent limb commences in the ganglionic layer of the retina, which gives rise to the optic nerve. It enters both optic tracts and terminates in the **pretectal nucleus,** situated just rostral to the superior colliculus on each side.
2 The pretectal nucleus is linked by internuncial neurons to both Edinger-Westphal (parasympathetic) nuclei; the contralateral nucleus is reached by way of the **posterior commissure.**
3 Preganglionic parasympathetic fibers enter the oculomotor nerve, leave the branch to the inferior oblique and synapse in the ciliary ganglion.
4 Postganglionic fibers run in the short ciliary nerves and enter the iris to supply the sphincter pupillae.

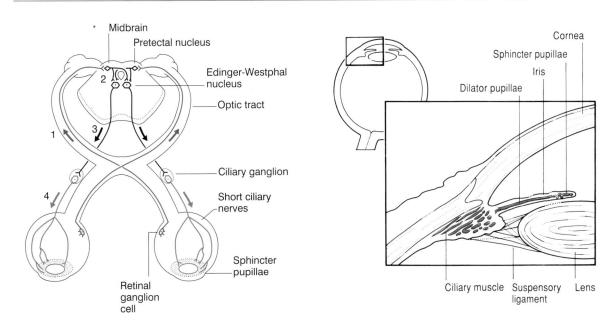

Figure 18.4 Pupillary light reflex. For numbers, see text.

Figure 18.5 Intrinsic muscles of the eye.

ACCOMMODATION

THE NEAR RESPONSE

When the eyes view an object close up, the ciliary muscle contracts reflexly, thereby relaxing the suspensory ligament of the lens (*Figure 18.5*). Since the lens at rest is somewhat compressed (flattened) by tension exerted on the lens capsule by the suspensory ligament, the lens bulges passively when the ciliary muscle contracts. The thicker lens has the greater refractive power required to bring close-up objects into focus on the retina. The response of the lens is one of *accommodation*.

The *accommodation reflex,* as understood clinically, involves two other features. The sphincter pupillae contracts in order to eliminate passage of light through the peripheral, thinner part of the lens. At the same time, the visual axes of the two eyes converge, as a result of increased tone in the medial rectus muscles.

The three features described are also known as the *near response.*

Pathway for the accommodation reflex

In order to execute the near response, a stereoscopic analysis of the object is carried out at the level of the visual association cortex. The afferent limb of the reflex passes from the retina to the occipital lobe via the lateral geniculate nucleus. The efferent limb passes from the occipital lobe to the midbrain, where some fibers activate the Edinger-Westphal nucleus and others activate vergence cells in the reticular formation. The vergence cells activate the nuclear groups serving the medial recti, with the effect of *fixating* the object on to the fovea centralis of each eye. The (con)vergence response is called the *fixation reflex.*

THE FAR RESPONSE

Just as the state of the pupil depends upon the balance of sympathetic and parasympathetic activity, so does the state of the lens. At rest, both are in midposition. The resting focal length of the lens averages 1 meter (with considerable variation between individuals). This is because the ciliary muscle is tonically active. In order to bring a distant object into focus, the ciliary muscle must be inhibited, so that the suspensory ligament becomes taut and the lens flat. The sphincter of the pupil is inhibited as well.

The sympathetic system innervates all of the intrinsic muscles. It has a dual mode of action. It causes contraction of the dilator pupillae by way of *alpha receptors* on the muscle fibers; and it causes *relaxation* of the ciliary muscle and pupillary sphincter, by way of *beta receptors*. This dual effect constitutes the *far response*, and it is used to focus the eyes upon objects at a distance.

In stressed individuals, heightened sympathetic activity may interfere with the normal process of accommodation. For example, students taking an important written test may have difficulty in bringing the questions into proper focus.

NOTES ON THE SYMPATHETIC PATHWAY TO THE EYE

The great length of the sympathetic pathway is indicated in *Figure 18.6*.

1 *Central fibers* descending from the hypothalamus cross to the other side in the midbrain. In the pons and medulla they are joined by ipsilateral fibers descending from the reticular formation.
2 *Preganglionic fibers* emerge in the first thoracic ventral nerve root, and run up in the sympathetic chain to the superior cervical ganglion.
3 *Postganglionic fibers* run along the external and internal carotid arteries and their branches.

The *external* carotid sympathetic fibers accompany all of the branches of the external carotid artery. Those accompanying the facial artery supply the arterioles of the cheek and lips and are particularly responsive to emotional states. Those accompanying the maxillary artery supply the cavernous tissue covering the nasal conchae (turbinate bones).

Two sets of sympathetic fibers accompany the *internal* carotid artery. One set joins the ophthalmic division of the V nerve in the cavernous sinus, leaves it in the long and short ciliary nerves, and supplies the vessels and smooth muscles of the eyeball. The second set forms a plexus around the internal carotid artery and its branches including the ophthalmic artery. The ophthalmic artery gives off supratrochlear and supraorbital branches which carry sympathetic fibers to the skin of the forehead and scalp.

Interruption of the postganglionic fibers at the

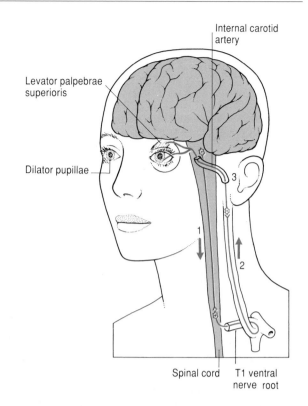

Figure 18.6 Three neuron pathway from the hypothalamus to the eye. Arrows indicate directions of impulse conduction. For numbers, see text.

CLINICAL PANEL 18.1

OCULAR PALSIES

One or more of the three ocular motor nerves may be paralyzed by disease within the brainstem (e.g. multiple sclerosis, vascular thrombosis), in the subarachnoid space (e.g. meningitis, aneurysm in the circle of Willis, or distortion by an expanding intracranial lesion), or in the cavernous sinus (e.g. thrombosis of the sinus, aneurysm of the internal carotid artery).

Oculomotor nerve
Complete III nerve palsy
The three characteristic signs of complete third nerve paralysis are shown in *Figure CP 18-1.1*. They are:

1 Complete ptosis of the eyelid (unopposed orbicularis oculi)
2 A fully dilated, non-reactive pupil (unopposed dilator pupillae)

CLINICAL PANEL 18.1 *Continued*

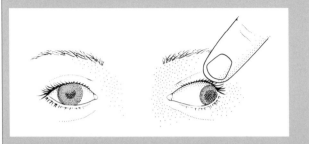

Figure CP 18.1.1 Complete III nerve paralysis. The closed eyelid has been raised by the examiner's finger.

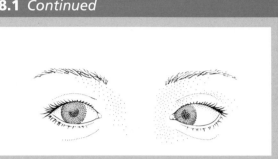

Figure CP 18.1.2 Complete left VI nerve paralysis.

3   A fully abducted eye (unopposed lateral rectus), which is also depressed (unopposed superior oblique)

Partial III nerve palsy
The pupils are *always* monitored when cases of head injury come to medical attention. Rapidly increasing intracranial pressure, resulting from an acute extradural or subdural hematoma (Chapter 4), often compresses the third nerve on the crest of the petrous temporal bone. The autonomic fibers are superficially placed and are the first to suffer, and the pupil dilates progressively on the affected side. *Pupillary dilatation is an urgent indication for surgical decompression of the brain.*

Trochlear nerve
The IV nerve is rarely paralyzed alone. The cardinal symptom is diplopia (double vision) on looking down, for example when going down stairs. This happens because the inferior rectus normally assists the inferior rectus in pulling the eye downward, especially when the eye is in a medial position.

Abducens nerve
The effect of a *complete* VI nerve paralysis is shown in *Figure CP 18-1.2*. The eye is fully adducted by the unopposed pull of the medial rectus.
  The abducens has the longest course in the subarachnoid space of any cranial nerve. It also bends sharply over the crest of the petrous temporal bone. A space-occupying lesion affecting either cerebral hemisphere may cause compression and paralysis of the nerve.

'Spontaneous' paralysis of the VI nerve may be caused by an arterial aneurysm at the base of the brain or by hardening (atherosclerosis) of the internal carotid artery in the cavernous sinus.

Ocular sympathetic supply
Any one of the three sequential sets of neurons depicted in *Figure 18.6* may be interrupted by local pathology.

1   The *central* set may be interrupted by a vascular lesion of the pons or medulla oblongata. The usual picture is one of Horner's syndrome (ptosis and miosis, as described in Chapter 10) and cranial nerve involvement one one side, together with motor weakness and/or sensory loss in the limbs on the contralateral side. The Horner's syndrome is associated with *anhidrosis*—absence of sweating—in the face and scalp on the same side, together with congestion of the nose (engorged turbinates).
2   The *preganglionic* set is most often interrupted by stony, cancerous deep cervical lymph nodes in the lower part of the neck. A Horner's syndrome is associated with anhydrosis of the face and scalp (and nasal congestion) on the same side.
3   The *postganglionic* set accompanying the *external* carotid artery is rarely damaged directly. The set accompanying the internal carotid artery may be interrupted as part of a jugular foramen syndrome (Chapter 15), or by pathology in the cavernous sinus. Horner's syndrome is accompanied by anhydrosis of the forehead and anterior scalp (territory of the supraorbital and supratrochlear arteries).

jugular foramen (see *jugular foramen syndrome,* Chapter 15) or in the cavernous sinus produces anhidrosis (loss of sweating) on the forehead and scalp.

OCULAR PALSIES

The effects of paralysis of the motor nerves to the eye are described in *Panel 18.1.*

CONTROL OF EYE MOVEMENTS

The eyes normally move as a pair. This *conjugate* movement is of three fundamentally different kinds, as follows:

1 *Scanning.* The eyes flick from one visual target to another, in high-speed movements called *saccades.*
2 *Tracking.* In tracking, or *smooth pursuit,* the eyes follow an object of interest across the visual field.
3 *Compensation.* The gaze can be held on an object of interest during movements of the head. This is the *vestibulo-ocular* or *fixation reflex,* which depends upon displacement of endolymph in the kinetic labyrinth.

SCANNING

Four separate *gaze centers* in the brainstem pick out motoneurons appropriate to the direction of movement: leftward, rightward, upward, or downward. The centers are small nodes in the reticular formation. They contain *burst cells,* which discharge at 1000 Hz (impulses/sec) and entrain the appropriate motoneurons momentarily at this rate.

The paired centers (left and right) for horizontal saccades are in the paramedian pontine reticular formation; hence the designation, PPRF. Each pulls the eyes to its own side (*Figure 18.7*). The midbrain contains a bilateral center for upward saccades located in the rostral end of the medial longitudinal fasciculus (MLF), at the level of the pretectal nucleus. It is called the **rostral interstitial nucleus** (riMLF). At the same level but a little ventral to this is a bilateral center for downward gaze.

Automatic scanning movements are activated by the superior colliculus, on receipt of visual information from the retina through the medial

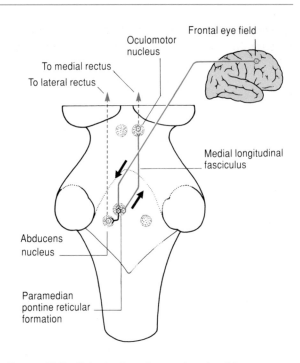

Figure 18.7 Principal pathways involved in a voluntary ocular saccade to the left.

root of the optic tract. Examples of automatic scanning include the sideward glance toward an object attracting attention in the peripheral visual field, and the saccadic movements used in reading. The projections cross the midline before proceeding to the gaze centers. Saccadic accuracy is controlled by the midregion (vermis) of the cerebellum, which receives afferents from the superior colliculi and projects to the gaze control centers.

Voluntary scanning movements are initiated in the frontal eye fields, directly in front of the premotor cortex. From each frontal eye field, a projection descends in the anterior limb of the internal capsule. Most of the fibers cross over before terminating in the gaze centers.

As explained in Chapter 25, the ipsilateral superior colliculus is activated at the same time, to reinforce the excitation of the appropriate gaze center.

The projection from the frontal eye field is interrupted in about one–third of patients who suffer a stroke involving the internal capsule. The result is *paralysis of contraversive horizontal gaze.* 'Contraversive' refers to an inability to make a voluntary saccade away from the side of the lesion. The gaze paralysis vanishes within a week, even if the hemiplegia remains profound—presumably because of takeover by uncrossed fibers.

The best known afferents to the frontal eye field come from the parietal cortex, from cells concerned with *visual attention*. In monkeys, some cells in the posterior parietal cortex become active when an object of interest is seen. These cells project to the frontal eye field and are thought to facilitate eye movement in the direction of the object. In humans, neglect of the contralateral visual field is a well-known feature of damage to the posterior parietal lobe, especially on the right side (Chapter 24).

TRACKING

The neural mechanisms for tracking must be complex because of the following basic requirements: (a) intact visual pathways to monitor the position of the object throughout the movement; (b) neurons to signal the rate of movement of the object (velocity detectors); (c) neurons to coordinate movements of the eyes and head (neural integrator); and (d) a system to monitor smooth execution of the tracking movement. Monkey and cat experiments indicate the following:

■ Object position information is forwarded from the visual cortex to the posterior parietal cortex, and from there to the reticular formation of the pons.

■ Velocity detectors are present in the upper part of the pons, apparently receiving information direct from the retina via the medial root of the optic tract.

■ Head movement is signaled by the dynamic labyrinth, and is integrated with spatial and velocity information in the **nucleus prepositus hypoglossi**—a node of the reticular formation which is in fact closer to the abducens nucleus than to the hypoglossal nucleus. The nucleus prepositus projects to the paramedian pontine reticular formation (PPRF), which controls conjugate eye movements. The pathway to the neck muscles (for turning the head) may involve the superior colliculus.

■ Smooth execution of tracking movements is monitored by the flocculus of the cerebellum, which has two-way connections to the vestibular nucleus and pontine reticular formation.

The dynamic labyrinth and cerebellum cooperate to keep the eyes on target during movement of the head, as described in Chapter 16.

CORE INFORMATION

Oculomotor nerve

Somatic efferent fibers of III arise from the main nucleus at superior collicular level. The nerve passes intact through the cavernous sinus and in two divisions through the superior orbital fissure. The upper division supplies superior rectus and levator palpebrae superioris, the lower division supplies inferior and medial recti and inferior oblique.

Parasympathetic fibers arise from the Edinger–Westphal nucleus, travel with the main nerve and synapse in the ciliary ganglion for supply of sphincter pupillae and ciliaris.

Paralysis of III is shown first by a dilated pupil with ptosis, later by a divergent squint as well.

Trochlear nerve

The nucleus of IV is at inferior collicular level. The fibers cross the midline before emerging below the inferior colliculi. IV passes through the cavernous sinus to supply superior oblique.

Paralysis of IV is characterized by diplopia on looking down.

Abducens nerve

The nucleus of VI is at the level of the facial colliculus in pons. The nerve runs in the subarachnoid space from lower border of pons to apex of petrous temporal bone, passes through cavernous sinus and superior orbital fissure and supplies lateral rectus.

Paralysis of VI is characterized by convergent squint with inability to abduct the affected eye.

Sympathetic

Muscles stimulated are dilator pupillae and levator palpebrae superioris. Paralysis is characterized by ptosis with a constricted pupil (Horner's syndrome).

Reflex pathways

For the pupillary light reflex: optic nerve and tract pretectal nucleus → both E–W nuclei → ciliary ganglion → sphincter pupillae.

For the accommodation reflex: optic nerve and tract → lateral geniculate n. → occipital cortex → E–W ciliary ganglion ciliaris

Oculomotor controls

Scanning (saccading) is locally activated by six gaze centers. Cinically most important is the paramedian pontine reticular formation (PPRF) which operates to pull ipsilateral lateral rectus and contralateral medial rectus conjugately to its own side. Automatic scanning is controlled by superior colliculi, voluntary scanning by the contralateral frontal eye field.

Tracking is complex and involves occipital cortex, dynamic labyrinth, cerebellum, superior colliculus and reticular formation.

SELF TEST

For questions 1-9, answer
A if the item is associated with A only
B if associated with B only
C if associated with both A and B
D if associated with neither A nor B

- A Light reflex
- B Accommodation reflex
- C Both
- D Neither

1 Ganglionic cells of retina are excited
2 Lateral geniculate nucleus is excited
3 Pretectal nucleus is excited
4 Visual cortex is excited

- A Oculomotor nerve
- B Sympathetic system
- C Both
- D Neither

5 Some neurons originate in the pretectal nucleus
6 Orbital neurons originate in the superior cervical ganglion
7 Traverse(s) superior orbital fissure
8 Some neurons supply levator palpebrae superioris
9 Some neurons supply superior rectus

Match the items A–D with the numbers 10–11

- A Convergent squint
- B Divergent squint
- C Ptosis with constricted pupil
- D Paralysis of contraversive gaze

10 Paralysis of oculomotor nerve
11 Paralysis of abducens nerve
12 Paralysis of sympathetic system
13 Damage to frontal eye field

REFERENCES

American Academy of Ophthalmology (1995) *Principles of Ophthalmology*. San Francisco.

Anderson *et al.* (1994) Cortical control of saccades and fixation in man. *Brain* 117: 1073–1084.

Dean, P., Mayhew, J.E.W., and Langdon, P. (1994) Learning and maintaining saccadic accuracy: a model of brain stem-cerebellar interactions. *J. Cog. Neurosci.* 6: 117–38.

Keller, E.L. and Heinen, S.J. (1991) Generation of smooth pursuit eye movements: neuronal mechanisms and pathways. *Neurosci. Res.* 11: 79–07.

Kommerell, G. (1984). Supranuclear and nuclear disorders of eye movement. In *Neuro-ophthalmology*, Vol. 3 (Lessell, S. and van Dalen, J.T.W., eds), pp. 277–289. Amsterdam: Elsevier.

Miyazaki, S. (1985) Location of motoneurons in the oculomotor nucleus and the course of their axons in the oculomotor nerve. *Brain Res.* 348: 57–63.

Oda, K. (1986) Motor innervation and acetylcholine receptor distribution of human extraocular muscle fibers. *J. Neurol. Sci.* 74: 125–133.

Parkinson, D. (1988) Further observations on the sympathetic pathways to the pupil. *Anat. Rec.* 220: 108–109.

Wilhelm, H. (1994) Pupil examination and evaluation of pupillary disorders. *Neuro-ophthalmology* 14: 283–295.

19

RETICULAR FORMATION

Chapter Summary

Organization
Aminergic neurons of the
  brainstem

Functional anatomy
Pattern generators
Bladder control
Respiratory control
Cardiovascular control
Sleeping and wakefulness
Sensory modulation

Study Guidelines

1 The reticular formation has very diverse functions. Some of its
   nuclear groups have direct access to motoneurons in the brainstem and spinal cord. Others have direct access to autonomic
   effector nuclei including cardiovascular controls. Some may act
   simultaneously upon somatic and autonomic nuclei.
2 All of the sensory systems contribute afferents to the reticular
   formation.
3 Ascending projections of the reticular formation to the forebrain are essential for the conscious state.
4 Sets of aminergic neurons embedded in the reticular formation
   have a bearing on psychiatric states including endogenous
   depression and schizophrenia.

INTRODUCTION

The reticular formation is phylogenetically a very
old neural network, being a prominent feature of
the reptilian brainstem. It originated as a slowly
conducting, polysynaptic pathway intimately
connected with olfactory and limbic regions. The
progressive dominance of vision and hearing over
olfaction led to lateralization of sensory and
motor functions within the tectum of the midbrain. Direct spinotectal and tectospinal tracts
bypassed the reticular formation, which was
largely relegated to automatic functions in relation to posture and to the autonomic system. In
mammals, the tectum in turn has been relegated
to minor status with the emergence of very fast
pathways linking the cerebral cortex with the
peripheral sensory and motor apparatus.

In the human brain, the reticular formation
continues to be of importance in relation to automatic and reflex activities, and it has retained its
linkages to the limbic system.

ORGANIZATION

The term *reticular formation* refers only to the
polysynaptic network in the brainstem,
although the network continues rostrally into
the thalamus and hypothalamus, and caudally
into the propriospinal network of the spinal
cord.

The characteristic neuron is *isodendritic*. The
dendrites are long and branch at regular intervals. They have a predominantly transverse orientation and their interstices are penetrated by
long pathways running to and from the thalamus
and cerebral cortex.

The ground plan is shown in *Figure 19.1A*. In
the midline is a series of **raphe nuclei** (pron. 'raf-
fay' and derived from the Greek word for seam).
Next to this is the **magnocellular reticular formation** which, in the lower pons and upper medulla, becomes **gigantocellular** before blending with
the **central reticular nucleus** of the medulla
oblongata. Lateralmost is the **parvocellular reticular formation**, which extends into the midbrain.
Finally, **paramedian** and lateral reticular nuclei in
the medulla have two-way connections with the
cerebellum; the latter also has connections with
the spinal cord.

The parvocellular RF is a predominantly *afferent* system. It receives fibers from all of the sensory pathways, including the special senses:

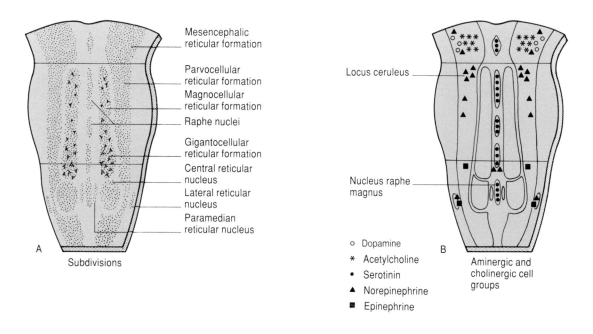

Figure 19.1 Reticular formation. The pons is marked off by the horizontal lines.

- Olfactory fibers are received through the median forebrain bundle, which passes alongside the hypothalamus.
- Visual pathway fibers are received from the superior colliculus.
- Auditory pathway fibers are received from the superior olivary nucleus.
- Vestibular fibers are received from the medial vestibular nucleus.
- Somatic sensory fibers are received from the spinoreticular tracts.

Most parvocellular axons ramify extensively among the dendrites of the magnocellar reticular formation. However, some synapse within the nuclei of cranial nerves and act as pattern generators (see later).

The magnocellular reticular formation is a predominantly *efferent* system. The axons are relatively long. Some ascend to synapse in the midbrain reticular formation or in the thalamus. Others have both ascending and descending branches contributing to the polysynaptic network. The magnocellular component receives corticoreticular fibers from the premotor cortex and gives rise to the pontine and medullary reticulospinal tracts.

AMINERGIC NEURONS OF THE BRAINSTEM

Embedded in the reticular formation are sets of aminergic neurons (*Figure 19.1B*). They include one set producing *serotonin* (5-hydroxytryptamine) and three sets producing *catecholamines*, as listed below.

- The serotoninergic neurons have the largest territorial distribution of any set of CNS neurons. In general, those of the midbrain project rostrally into the cerebral hemispheres; those of the pons ramify in the brainstem and cerebellum; and those of the medulla supply the spinal cord (*Figure 19.2A*). All parts of the CNS gray matter are permeated by serotonin-secreting axonal varicosities. Clinically, enhancement of serotonin activity is part of the treatment for a prevalent condition known as major depression (Chapter 21).
- The *dopaminergic neurons* of the midbrain fall into two groups. Those of the substantia nigra are categorized with the basal ganglia. Dorsal to these are mesolimbic neurons

Table 19.1 Aminergic neurons of the reticular formation

Transmitter	Location
Serotonin	Raphe nuclei of midbrain, pons, medulla
Dopamine	Tegmentum of midbrain
Norepinephrine	Mainly pons (locus ceruleus)
Epinephrine	Medulla oblongata

187

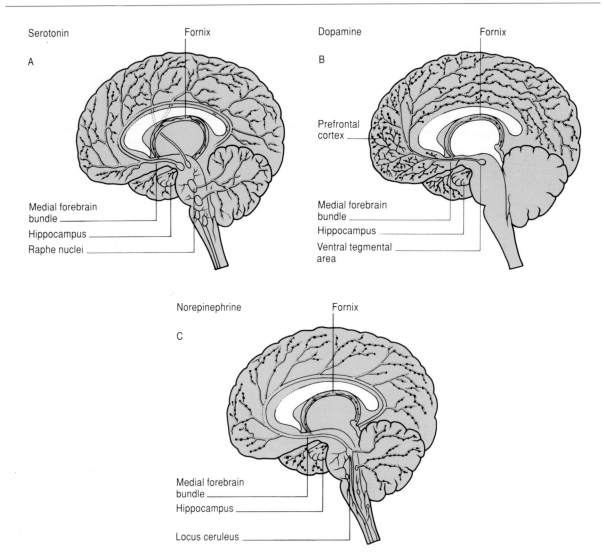

Figure 19.2 **(A)** Serotonergic neurons of the brainstem midline (raphe). **(B)** Dopaminergic projections from the ventral tegmental area of the midbrain. **(C)** Noradrenergic neurons of the pons and medulla oblongata. The medial forebrain bundle is a continuation of the central tegmental tract into the forebrain, passing along the lateral side of the hypothalamus.

categorized with the RF. Their somas occupy the *ventral tegmental area* (of Tsai). They project mainly to frontal and temporal areas of the cerebral cortex which are associated with the limbic system (*Figure 19.2B*).

■ The *noradrenergic neurons* are only marginally less prodigious than the serotoninergic ones. About 90% of the somas are pooled in the locus ceruleus, a 'violet spot' in the floor and side wall of the fourth ventricle at the upper end of the pons (*Figure 19.3*). Neurons of the locus ceruleus project in *all* directions, as indicated in *Figure 19.2C*.

■ Epinephrine-secreting neurons are relatively scarce and are confined to the medulla oblongata. Some project rostrally to the hypothalamus, others project caudally to synapse upon preganglionic sympathetic neurons.

In the cerebral cortex, the ionic and electrical effects of aminergic neuronal activity are quite variable. Firstly, more than one kind of postsynaptic receptor exists for each of the amines. Secondly, some aminergic neurons liberate a peptide substance as well, capable of modulating the transmitter action—usually by prolonging it.

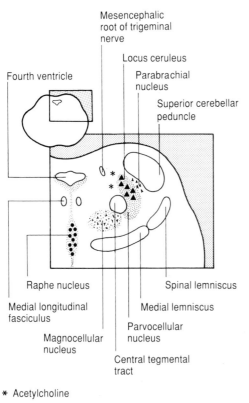

- * Acetylcholine
- • Serotonin
- ▲ Norepinephrine

Figure 19.3 Part of a transverse section through the upper part of the pons, showing elements of the reticular formation.

Table 19.2 Elements of the reticular formation and their functions

RF element	Function
N. gigantocellularis	Posture, locomotion
Premotor cranial nerve nuclei	Patterned cranial nerve activities
Salivatory nuclei	Salivary secretion, lacrimation
Lateral pontine tegmentum	Bladder control
Parabrachial nucleus	Respiratory rhythm
Central nucleus of medulla oblongata	Vital centers (circulation, respiration)
Paramedian and lateral medullary nuclei	Convey somatic and visceral information to the cerebellum
Aminergic neurons	Sleeping and waking, attention and mood, sensory modulation

Thirdly, the larger cortical neurons receive many thousands of excitatory and inhibitory synapses from local circuit neurons and they have numerous different receptors. Activation of a single kind of aminergic receptor may have a large or small effect depending on the current excitatory state.

Although our understanding of the physiology and pharmacology of the monoamines is far from complete, no one disputes their relevance to a wide range of behavioral functions. Monoamine transmitters/receptors are of particular interest to psychiatrists: for example, serotonin and norepinephrine have been implicated in endogenous depression and dopamine in schizophrenia (*Chapter 26*).

FUNCTIONAL ANATOMY

The wide variety of functions served by different parts of the RF is indicated in **Table 19.2.**

PATTERN GENERATORS

The contribution of N. gigantocellularis to posture and locomotion is described in Chapter 13.

Patterned activities involving cranial nerves include:

- Conjugate movements of the eyes controlled by nodal points (gaze centers) in the midbrain and pons feeding into the oculomotor, trochlear, and abducent nerves.
- Rhythmical chewing movements controlled by the supratrigeminal nucleus in the pons.
- Swallowing, vomiting, coughing, and sneezing, controlled by separate nodal points in the medulla feeding into the appropriate cranial nerves and into the respiratory centers.

The salivatory nuclei belong to the parvocellular RF of the pons and medulla oblongata. They contribute preganglionic fibers to the facial and glossopharyngeal nerves.

BLADDER CONTROL

The bladder control center is on the medial side of the locus ceruleus, with interconnections across the midline. The center exerts a tonic inhibitory action on the parasympathetic neurons in sacral segments 2, 3, and 4 of the spinal cord. The pontine center is inhibited in turn from a cortical zone within the precentral gyrus.

When the bladder is half full, vesical afferents in the pelvic splanchnic nerves relay the information through the spinoreticular tract to the pontine center, which responds by suppressing the parasympathetic activity that would otherwise occur through the sacrovesical reflex arc. At the same time, sympathetic activity in the lumbar splanchnic nerves (presumably influenced by the bladder center) assists in two distinct ways: bladder compliance is increased by β_2-receptor inhibition of the trabeculated detrusor musculature; and the tone of the smooth muscle at the bladder neck is increased by way of α receptors.

When the bladder is full and the time is opportune, the pontine center releases the sacral cord from inhibition. If the time is not opportune, the premotor cortex can defer voiding by reinforcing the inhibitory function of the pontine center.

RESPIRATORY CONTROL *(FIGURE 19.4)*

The respiratory cycle is regulated by *dorsal* and *ventral respiratory centers* located at the upper end of the medulla oblongata on each side. The dorsal respiratory center occupies the lateral side of the nucleus solitarius. The ventral center lies behind the nucleus ambiguus. The dorsal respiratory center has an inspiratory function. It

projects to the nuclei on the opposite side of the spinal cord supplying the diaphragm, intercostals, and accessory muscles of inspiration. It receives two major excitatory projections from chemoreceptors in the medullary chemosensitive area and in the carotid body.

Medullary chemosensitive area

Close to the site of attachment of the glossopharyngeal nerve, the choroid plexus of the fourth ventricle pouts through the lateral aperture of the fourth ventricle to lie beside the medulla oblongata. Specifically at this location, RF cells at the medullary surface are exquisitely sensitive to the H^+ ion concentration in the neighboring cerebrospinal fluid. In effect, the *chemosensitive area* samples the CO_2 level in the blood supplying the brain. Any increase in H^+ ions stimulates the dorsal respiratory center through a direct synaptic linkage.

Carotid chemoreceptors

The pin-head **carotid body** is situated beside the stem of the internal carotid artery. A twig from

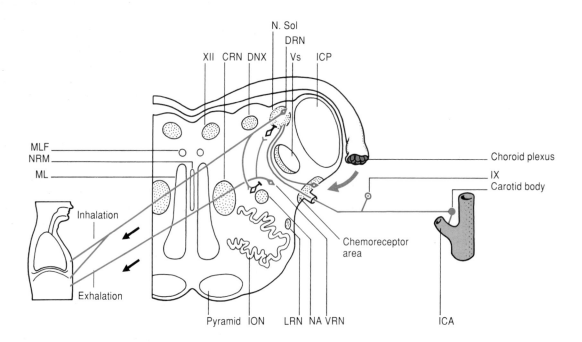

Figure 19.4 Upper part of medulla oblongata showing relationships of the respiratory nuclei. CRN, central reticular nucleus; DNX, dorsal nucleus of vagus; ICP, inferior cerebellar peduncle; ION, inferior olivary nucleus; IX, glossopharyngeal nerve; LRN, lateral reticular nucleus; ML, medial lemniscus; MLF, medial longitudinal fasciculus; NA, nucleus ambiguus; NRM, nucleus raphe magnus; N.sol., nucleus solitarius; VRN, ventral respiratory nucleus; Vs, spinal tract of trigeminal nerve; XII, hypoglossal nerve; ICA, internal carotid artery.

the internal carotid ramifies within it, and the blood flow is so intense that the arteriovenous PO_2 changes by less than 1% during passage. The chemoreceptors are glomus cells to which branches of the sinus nerve (IX) are applied. The carotid chemoreceptors respond to either a fall in PO_2 or a rise in PCO_2. (The chemoreceptors of the aortic bodies seem to be relatively insignificant in humans.)

The ventral respiratory center is expiratory (in the main). During quiet breathing it functions as an oscillator, being engaged in reciprocal inhibition with the inspiratory center. During forced breathing it activates the abdominal and other muscles required to empty the lungs.

The connections shown *Figure 19.4* are a simplification. Animal experiments indicate that excitation of the neurons projecting to the spinal cord is mainly by way of internuncials contacted by the primary afferents. Some of these internuncials discharge to the dorsal respiratory center to initiate inspiration, others project to the ventral respiratory center to initiate expiration.

A third respiratory center, the *medial parabrachial nucleus,* is adjacent to the locus ceruleus. It seems to have a pacemaker function governing respiratory rate (cycles per minute).

CARDIOVASCULAR CONTROL

Because of the prevalence of essential hypertension in late middle age, the neural and endocrine systems controlling cardiac output and peripheral arterial resistance are subjects of major research effort. Particular attention is being given to the medially placed cells of the nucleus solitarius, which receive *baroreceptor afferents* from the carotid sinus and aortic arch. The baroreceptors are stretch receptors (a multitude of free nerve endings) in the adventitial coat of these vessels. Afferents from the carotid sinus travel in the glossopharyngeal nerve; afferents from the aortic arch travel in the vagus. The baroreceptor afferents are known as 'buffer nerves' because they act to correct any deviation of the arterial blood pressure from the norm.

The nucleus solitarius (N. sol.) responds to a rise in arterial pressure by slowing the heart (increased vagal activity) and by lowering peripheral arterial resistance (reduced sympathetic activity). The heart is slowed by an excitatory projection from N. sol. to the cardioinhibitory center in the nucleus ambiguus (Chapter 14). The *barovagal reflex* involves a sequence of four neu-

rons, the final one (on the wall of the heart) being inhibitory.

Animal experiments indicate that the *barosympathetic reflex* uses a sequence of six neurons. It involves a *pressor center* and a *depressor center,* both of these being located in the ventral region of the medulla oblongata. The pressor center has a tonic excitatory effect on the thoracolumbar sympathetic outflow through descending fibers, some of which secrete norepinephrine and others serotonin. The depressor center exerts a GABAergic braking action on the pressor center, and N. sol. reduces sympathetic activity by means of an excitatory (glutamate) projection to the depressor center.

SLEEPING AND WAKEFULNESS

The onset of sleep is accompanied by a change in the electrical group activity of neurons in the cerebral cortex, as revealed by electroencephalography (EEG). The rapid, low voltage pattern of the waking state is replaced by slow waves which have higher voltage because group activity is more synchronized. After about 90 minutes, S (synchronized) sleep is replaced by a D (desynchronized) sleep in which the EEG pattern resembles the waking state. During D sleep dreams take place and there are rapid eye movements (hence the term 'REM sleep'). Several S and D phases occur during a normal night's sleep.

Details of brainstem involvement in sleep phenomena are available in psychology texts. Some salient experimental evidence may be summarized:

- In animal experiments, destruction of the raphe neurons in the midbrain, or pharmacological prevention of serotonin synthesis, results in insomnia lasting for several days.
- Serotonin and norepinephrine neuronal activities fluctuate in parallel. Both are most active during attentive wakefulness, sluggish during S sleep, and virtually silent during REM sleep.
- Brainstem serotonin neurons form numerous surface varicosities on the walls of the third ventricle. Serotonin liberated into the cerebrospinal fluid seems to be metabolized by hypothalamic neurons to form a sleep-inducing substance.
- Cholinergic neurons close to the locus ceruleus are active during REM sleep, and they appear to cause the rapid eye movements by playing upon the ocular motor nuclei.

Ascending reticular activating system (ARAS)

This term refers to the participation of RF neurons in activation of the cerebral cortex, as shown by a change in EEG records from high-amplitude, slow waves to low-amplitude, fast waves during spontaneous arousal from sleep. The strongest candidates for such a role seem to be the sets of cholinergic neurons close to the locus ceruleus (*Figure 19.3*). As well as supplying the above-mentioned fibers to the ocular motor nuclei, these cholinergic neurons project to nearly all of the nuclei of the thalamus, and they have an excitatory effect upon thalamic neurons projecting to the cerebral cortex.

The **hypothalamus** is an important controling center for various body rhythms, including sleep and wakefulness. A second candidate for cortical activation has been found here, namely the **tuberomamillary nucleus**. This nucleus contains histaminergic neurons having widespread projections to the cerebral cortex and brainstem (Chapter 22).

Following arousal, the waking-state EEG pattern seems to be sustained by the continued discharge of the brainstem and hypothalamic neurons mentioned; also by a third set of neurons, embedded in the basal forebrain immediately above the optic chiasma. The third set occupies the **basal nucleus of Meynert** (see Chapter 26) and projects fine, cholinergic axons to most parts of the cerebral cortex.

SENSORY MODULATION: GATE CONTROL

Sensory transmission from primary to secondary afferent neurons (at the levels of the posterior gray horn and posterior column nuclei) and from secondary to tertiary (at the level of the thalamus) is subject to *gating*. The term *gating* refers to the degree of freedom of synaptic transmission from one set of neurons to the next.

Tactile sensory transmission is gated at the level of the posterior column nuclei. Pyramidal tract neurons in the postcentral gyrus may facilitate or inhibit sensory transmission at this level, as described in Chapter 13.

Nociceptive transmission from the trunk and limbs is gated in the posterior gray horn of the spinal cord. From the head and upper part of the neck, it is gated in the spinal trigeminal nucleus. A key structure in both areas of gray matter is the substantia gelatinosa, which is packed with small excitatory and inhibitory internuncial neurons. The excitatory internuncial transmitter is glutamate; the inhibitory one is GABA for some internuncials, enkephalin (an opiate pentapeptide) for others.

Finely myelinated (Aδ) polymodal nociceptive fibers synapse directly upon dendrites of lamina I and lamina V relay neurons of the lateral spinothalamic tract and of its trigeminal equivalent. The Aδ fibers signal sharp, well-localized pain. Unmyelinated, C fiber nociceptive afferents have mainly indirect access to relay cells, via excitatory gelatinosa internuncials. The C fibers signal dull, poorly localized pain. Most of them contain substance P, which may be liberated as a cotransmitter with glutamate.

Segmental antinociception

Large (A) mechanoreceptive afferents from hair follicles synapse upon *anterior* spinothalamic relay cells (and their trigeminal equivalents). They give off collaterals to inhibitory (mainly GABA) gelatinosa cells which synapse in turn upon *lateral* spinothalamic relay cells (*Figure 19.5*). Some of the internuncials exert presynaptic inhibition as well, upon C fiber terminals, either by axo-axonic contacts (which are very difficult to find in experimental material), or by dendro-axonic contacts.

Gating of the spinothalamic response to C fiber activity can be induced by stimulating the mechanoreceptive afferents, thereby recruiting inhibitory gelatinosa cells. This simple circuit accounts for the relief afforded by 'rubbing the sore spot'. It also provides a rationale for the use of *transcutaneous electrical nerve stimulation* (TENS) by physical therapists for pain relief in arthritis and other chronically painful conditions. The standard procedure in TENS is to apply a stimulating electrode to the skin at the same segmental level as the source of noxious C fiber activity, and to deliver a current sufficient to produce a pronounced buzzing sensation.

Supraspinal antinociception

Three supraspinal pathways having antinociceptive functions descend from the reticular formation to the spinal cord and spinal trigeminal nucleus, one from the **nucleus raphe magnus** (NRM), one from the **locus ceruleus,** and one from the **lateral reticular nucleus** of the medulla oblongata (*Figure 19.5*).

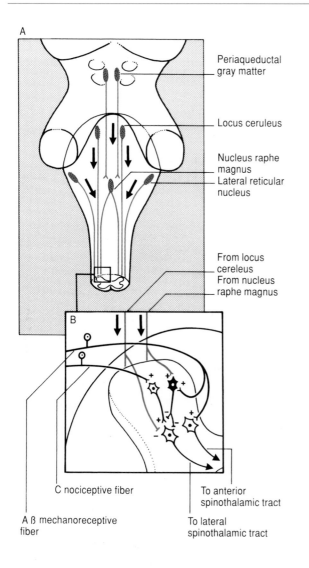

Figure 19.5 **(A)** Three antinociceptive pathways descending (arrows) from brainstem to spinal cord. **(B)** Enlargement from (A) showing excitatory (+) and inhibitory (-) inputs to spinothalamic transmission cells. Solid black = inhibitory internuncial.

Nucleus raphe magnus

From the nucleus raphe magnus (NRM) and adjacent gigantocellular RF, *raphespinal fibers* descend within Lissauer's tract, terminating in the substantia gelatinosa. In animals, electrical stimulation of NRM may produce total analgesia throughout the body, with little effect on tactile sensation. Many fibers of the raphespinal tract liberate *serotonin*, which excites inhibitory internuncials in the posterior gray horn and spinal trigeminal nucleus. The internuncials induce both pre- and postsynaptic inhibition on the relevant relay cells.

■ *Diffuse noxious inhibitory controls.* NRM is not somatotopically arranged, but it does receive inputs from spinoreticular and trigemi-noreticular neurons responding to peripheral noxious stimulation. This anatomical connection accounts for what are called diffuse noxious inhibitory controls. Painful stimulation of one part of the body may produce pain relief in all other parts. The arrangement accounts well for the heterotopic relief of pain in acupuncture, where needles are used to excite nociceptive afferents in the most superficial musculature.

■ *Stimulus-induced analgesia.* NRM is intensely responsive to stimulation of the periaqueductal gray matter (PAG) of the midbrain. This connection has been used to advantage for patients suffering intractable pain: a fine stimulating electrode can be inserted into PAG and wired so that the patient can control the level of self-stimulation.

■ *Stress-induced analgesia.* At rest, the PAG projection to NRM is under tonic inhibition by inhibitory internuncials present within PAG. The internuncials are themselves inhibited by opiate peptides—notably by β-endorphin released from a small set of hypothalamic neurons projecting to PAG. In life-threatening situations, where injury may be the price to be paid for escape, PAG may be released (disinhibited) by the hypothalamus. This seems to be the mechanism whereby a bullet wound may be scarcely noticed in the heat of battle.

Locus ceruleus

The locus ceruleus (*Figure 19.5*) has an antinociceptive action when stimulated. Some ceruleospinal axons descend in the lateral funiculus and exert direct postsynaptic inhibition on spinothalamic relay cells.

Lateral reticular nucleus

Some cells in the lateral reticular nucleus of the medulla oblongata can exert a powerful antinociceptive effect upon the posterior gray horn. Their mode of action is not well understood.

In addition to the segmental and supraspinal controls of nociceptive transmission from primary to secondary afferents, gating occurs within the thalamus (see Chapter 22). Furthermore, perception of the aversive (unpleasant) quality of pain seems to require participation of the anterior cingulate cortex, which is rich in opiate receptors (see Chapter 26).

CORE INFORMATION

Ground plan

The RF extends the entire length of the brain stem. The characteristic neuron is isodendritic, with regularly branched dendrites and a horizontal arrrangement. Obvious collections of RF neurons are the midline raphe nuclei, the magnocellular RF, and laterally the parvocellular RF. Parvo receives afferents from all sensory systems and feeds into magno; magno projects cranially, also caudally as reticulospinal tracts (RST).

Serotonergic neurons of the raphe nuclei project to all parts of the gray matter of the CNS. Dopaminergic neurons project from substantia nigra to striatum and from midbrain ventral tegmental area to cerebral cortex. Noradrenergic neurons of locus ceruleus project to all parts of the CNS gray matter. Epinephrine-secreting neurons of the medulla project to hypothalamus and spinal cord.

Pattern generators include gaze centers for conjugate eye movement; the supratrigeminal nucleus for rhythmical chewing; a pontine bladder center; and in the medulla, respiratory, vomiting, coughing and sneezing centers, and pressor and depressor centers for cardiovascular control.

The medullary chemosensitive area contains RF neurons sensitive to H^+ ion levels in new CSF squirting out of the lateral aperture of the fourth ventricle.

Sleeping and wakefulness are influenced by serotonin and norepinephrine neurons, and by cholinergic neurons in the upper pons. The ascending reticular activating system is a physiological concept based on brainstem neuronal networks having an arousal effect on the brain as seen in EEG traces. An important component is a set of pontine cholinergic neurons having an excitatory effect on thalamocortical neurons.

Supraspinal antinociception is a function of the medullary nucleus raphe magnus (NRM) and lateral reticular nucleus, and of the locus ceruleus. NRM is activated from hypothalamus and midbrain, and serotonin from NRM terminals in substantia gelatinosa of posterior horn and of spinal V activate enkephalinergic internuncials that inhibit transmission in spinothalamic neurons.

SELF TEST

Match the list of areas on the left with the transmitter substances on the right:

1	Raphe nuclei	A	Noradrenaline
2	Locus ceruleus	B	Serotonin
3	Midbrain tegmentum	C	Dopamine
4	Medullary reticular formation	D	Epinephrine
5	Substantia gelatinosa	E	GABA

Match the list of areas on the left with the functions on the right:

6	Supratrigeminal nucleus	A	Gaze control
7	Medullary chemosensitive area	B	Bladder control
8	PPRF	C	Masticatory rhythm
9	Lateral pontine tegmentum	D	Blood CO_2 regulation
10	Parabrachial nucleus	E	Respiratory rhythm

REFERENCES

Bentivoglio, M. and Steriade, M. (1990) Brainstem-diencephalic circuits as a structural substrate of the ascending reticular activation concept. In *The Diencephalon and Sleep* (Mancia, M. and Marini, G., eds), pp. 7-29. New York: Raven Press.

Bianchi, A.L., Denavit-Saube, M. and Champagnet, J. (1995) Central control of breathing. *Physiol. Rev.* **75**: 1-45.

Chalmers, J. and Pilowski, P. (1991) Brainstem and bulbospinal systems in the control of blood pressure. *J. Hypertens.* 9: 675-694.

De Keyser, J., Ebinger, G. and Vauquelin, G. (1989) Evidence for a widespread dopaminergic innervation of the human cerebral neocortex. *Neurosci. Lett.* 104: 281-285.

Gonzalez, C., Almaraz, L., Obeso, A. and Rigual, R. (1994) Carotid body chemoreceptors:from natural stimuli to sensory discharges. *Physiol. Rev.* **74**: 829-898.

Jensen, T.S. and Gebhart, G.F. (1988) General anatomy of antinociceptive systems. In *Basic Mechanisms of Headache* (Olesen, J. and Edvinsson, L., eds), pp. 189-198. Amsterdam: Elsevier.

Rosenfeld, J.P. (1994) Interacting brain components of opiate-activated, descending, pain-inhibitory systems. *Neurosci. Behav. Rev.* **18**: 403-409.

Siddall, P.J. (1995) Pain mechanisms and management. *Clin. Exp. Pharm. Physiol.* **22**: 679-688.

20

CEREBELLUM

Chapter Summary

Introduction

Functional anatomy

Microscopic anatomy
Spatial effects of mossy fiber
  activity

Representation of body parts

Afferent pathways
Olivocerebellar tract

Efferent pathways

**The cerebellum and higher
  brain function**

**Clinical disorders of the
cerebellum**
Posturography

CLINICAL PANELS
Midline lesions: truncal ataxia
Anterior lobe lesions: gait
  ataxia
Neocerebellar lesions:
  incoordination of voluntary
  movement

Study Guidelines

1 The cerebellar cortex has much the same microscopic structure throughout.
2 Afferents to the cortex enter from spinal cord and brainstem. They are excitatory, whereas the cortical outputs are inhibitory, and are exclusively from Purkinje cells.
3 The outputs from the cerebellum as a whole are in general excitatory. This is because they originate from deep, excitatory nuclei which are only partially inhibited by Purkinje cells.
4 Of special research interest are the roles played by the inferior olivary and red nuclei in relation to novel motor programs.
5 Clinically, cerebellar disease is characterized by incoordination of movement, with some differences being evident depending on the mediolateral position of the lesion where this is discrete (e.g. a tumor).

INTRODUCTION

Phylogenetically, the initial development of the cerebellum (in fishes) took place in relation to the vestibular labyrinth. With development of quadrupedal locomotion the anterior lobes (in particular) became richly connected to the spinal cord. Assumption of the erect posture and achievement of a whole new range of physical skills has been accompanied by the appearance of massive linkages between the posterior lobes and the cerebral cortex. In general, cerebellar connections with the labyrinth, spinal cord, and cerebral cortex are arranged such that each cerebellar hemisphere is primarily concerned with the co-ordination of movements *on its own side*.

The gross anatomy of the cerebellum is described briefly in Chapter 3, where it may be reviewed at this time.

FUNCTIONAL ANATOMY

Phylogenetic and functional aspects can be combined (to an approximation) by dividing the cerebellum into strips, as shown in *Figure 20.1*. The

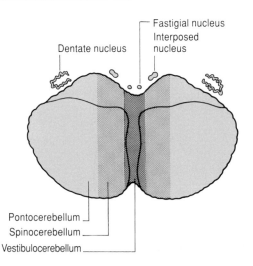

Figure 20.1 Zonation of cerebellum. The central nuclei are represented separately.

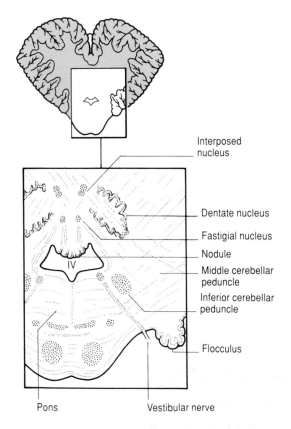

Figure 20.2 Transverse section of lower pons and cerebellum showing the position of the central and vestibular nuclei.

median strip contains the cortex of the vermis, together with the **fastigial nucleus** in the white matter close to the nodule (*Figure 20.2*). This strip is the *vestibulocerebellum*; it has two-way connections with the vestibular nucleus. It controls the responses of that nucleus to signals from the vestibular labyrinth. The fastigial nucleus also projects to the gaze centers of the brainstem. (Chapter 19).

A paramedian strip, the *spinocerebellum*, includes the paravermal cortex and the **nucleus globosus** and **nucleus emboliformis** *(Figure 20.2)*. The two nuclei are together called the **interposed nucleus.** The spinocerebellum is rich in spinocerebellar connections. It is involved in the control of posture and gait.

The remaining, lateral strip is much the largest and takes in the wrinkled **dentate nucleus** *(Figure 20.2)*. This strip is the *pontocerebellum*, because it receives a massive input from the contralateral nuclei pontis. It is also called the **neocerebellum** because the nuclei pontis convey information from large areas of the cerebral neocortex (phylogenetically the most recent). The neocerebellum is uniquely large in the human brain.

MICROSCOPIC ANATOMY

The structure of the cerebellar cortex is uniform throughout. From within outward, the cortex comprises granular, piriform, and molecular layers (*Figure 20.3*).

The **granular layer** contains billions of **granule cells,** whose somas are about the size of erythrocytes. Their short dendrites receive so-called **mossy fibers** from all sources except the inferior olivary nucleus. Before reaching the cerebellar cortex the mossy fibers, which are excitatory in nature, give off collateral branches to the deep nuclei.

The axons of the granule cells penetrate to the molecular layer where they divide in a T-shaped manner to form **parallel fibers.** The parallel fibers run parallel to the axes of the folia. They make excitatory contacts with Purkinje cells.

The granular layer also contains Golgi cells (see later).

The **piriform layer** consists of very large **Purkinje cells.** The fan-shaped dendritic trees of the Purkinje cells are the largest dendritic trees in the entire nervous system. The fans are disposed at right angles to the parallel fibers.

The dendritic trees of Purkinje cells are penetrated by huge numbers of parallel fibers, each one making successive single synapses upon dendritic spines of about 400 Purkinje cells. Not

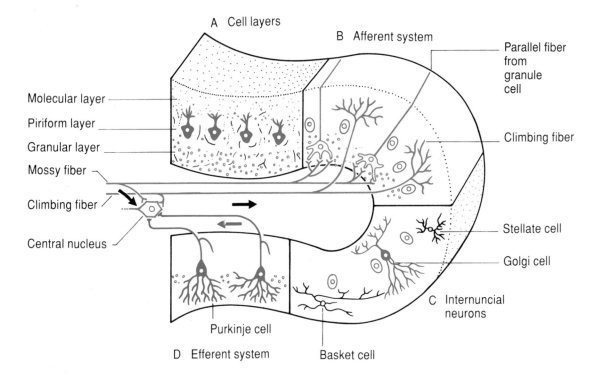

A Cell layers

B Afferent system

Parallel fiber from granule cell

Molecular layer

Piriform layer

Granular layer

Mossy fiber

Climbing fiber

Central nucleus

Climbing fiber

Stellate cell

Golgi cell

C Internuncial neurons

Purkinje cell

D Efferent system

Basket cell

Figure 20.3 Cerebellar cortex. **(A)** Cell layers; **(B)** afferent system; **(C)** internuncial neurons; **(D)** efferent system.

surprisingly, stimulation of small numbers of granule cells by mossy fibers has a merely facilitatory effect upon Purkinje cells. Many thousands of parallel fibers must act simultaneously to bring the membrane potential to firing level.

Each dendritic tree also receives a single **climbing fiber** from the contralateral inferior olivary nucleus. In stark contrast to the one-per-cell contacts of parallel fibers, The olivocerebellar fiber divides at the Purkinje dendritic branchpoints and makes thousands of synaptic contacts with dendritic spines. A single threshold pulse applied to one climbing fiber is sufficient to elicit a short burst of action potentials from the client Purkinje cell. Climbing fiber effects on Purkinje cells are so powerful that, for some time after they cease firing, the synaptic effectiveness of bundles of parallel fibers is reduced. In this sense, the Purkinje cells *remember* that they have been excited by olivocerebellar fibers.

The axons of the Purkinje cells are the only axons to emerge from the cerebellar cortex. Remarkably, they are entirely inhibitory in their effects. Their principal targets are the central nuclei. They give off collateral branches as well, mainly to Golgi cells.

The **molecular layer** is almost entirely taken up with Purkinje dendrites, parallel fibers, support-

ing neuroglial cells, and blood vessels. However, two sets of inhibitory neurons are also found there, lying in the same plane as the Purkinje cell dendritic trees. Near the cortical surface are small, **stellate cells,** and close to the piriform layer are larger, **basket cells.** Both sets are contacted by parallel fibers, and they both synapse on Purkinje cells. The stellate cells synapse upon dendritic shafts whereas the basket cells form a 'basket' of synaptic contacts around the soma, as well as forming axo-axonic synapses upon the initial segment of the axon. A single basket cell synapses upon some 250 Purkinje cells.

The final cell type in the cortex is the **Golgi cell,** whose dendrites are contacted by parallel fibers and whose axons divide extensively before synapsing upon the short dendrites of granule cells. The synaptic ensemble that includes a mossy fiber terminal, granule cell dendrites, and Golgi cell boutons, is known as a **glomerulus** (*Figure 20.4*).

SPATIAL EFFECTS OF MOSSY FIBER ACTIVITY (*FIGURE 20.5*)

As already noted, cerebellar afferents other than olivocerebellar ones form mossy fiber terminals after giving off excitatory collaterals to one of the

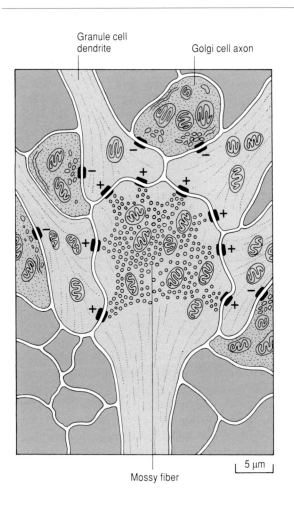

Figure 20.4   A synaptic glomerulus. +/- indicates excitation/inhibition.

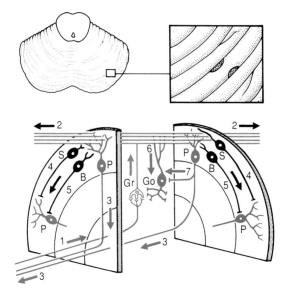

Figure 20.5   Scheme of effects of mossy fiber activity. **(1)** Mossy fiber stimulating a granule cell (Gr). **(2)** Beam of parallel fiber activity follows activation of granule cells. **(3)** Activation of on-beam Purkinje cells (P). **(4, 5)** Activation of stellate (S) and basket cells (B) inhibits off-line Purkinje cells (P). **(6)** Golgi cells (Go) terminate granule cell activity. **(7)** Intense on-line activity can be sustained by inhibition of Golgi cells.

deep nuclei. The afferents excite groups of granule cells, which in turn facilitate many hundreds of Purkinje cells. Along most of the beam of excitation, known as a *microzone,* the Purkinje cells begin to fire, and to inhibit patches of cells in one of the deep nuclei. At the same time, weakly facilitated Purkinje cells along the edges of the microzone are shut off by stellate and basket cells. As a result, the beam of excitation is sharply focused. The excitation is terminated by Golgi cell inhibition of the granule cells that initiated it. Powerful excitation will last longer because highly active Purkinje cells inhibit underlying Golgi cells through their collateral branches.

REPRESENTATION OF BODY PARTS

Representation of body parts in the human cerebellar cortex is currently under investigation by means of positron emission tomography (PET). These investigations, along with some evidence from clinical cases, indicate the presence of somatotopic maps in the anterior and posterior lobes (*Figure 20.6*).

The maps have been worked out in some detail in laboratory animals during movements. The maps for movement match up with maps of skin, eye, ear, and visceral representation worked out by stimulation of body parts.

See also Higher Brain Functions, page 201.

AFFERENT PATHWAYS

From the muscles and skin of the trunk and limbs, afferent information travels in the posterior spinocerebellar and the cuneocerebellar tract and enters the inferior cerebellar peduncle on the same side. Comparable information from the territory served by the trigeminal nerve enters all three cerebellar peduncles.

Afferents from spinal reflex arcs run in the anterior spinocerebellar tract, which reaches the

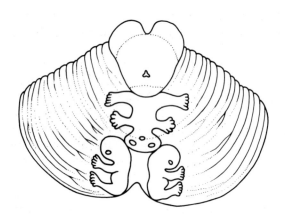

Figure 20.6 Upper surface of cerebellum showing position of somatotopic maps.

upper pons before looping into the superior cerebellar peduncle.

Special sense pathways comprise tectocerebellar fibers entering the superior peduncle from the ipsilateral midbrain colliculi, and vestibulocerebellar fibers from the ipsilateral vestibular nucleus.

Two massive pathways enter from the contralateral brainstem. The pontocerebellar tract enters through the middle peduncle, and the olivocerebellar tract enters through the inferior peduncle.

Reticulocerebellar fibers enter the inferior peduncle from the paramedian and lateral reticular nuclei of the medulla oblongata.

Finally, aminergic fibers enter all three peduncles from noradrenergic and serotonergic cell groups in the brainstem. Under experimental conditions, both kinds of neurons appear to facilitate excitatory transmision in mossy and climbing fiber terminals.

OLIVOCEREBELLAR TRACT

The sensorimotor cortex projects in an orderly, somatotopic manner on to the ipsilateral inferior and accessory olivary nuclei. The order is preserved in the olivary projections onto the body maps in the contralateral cerebellar cortex (from principal nucleus to the posterior map, from the accessory nuclei to the anterior map). Under resting conditions in animal experiments, groups of olivary neurons discharge synchronously at 5–10 Hz (impulses/second). The synchrony is probably

due to the observed presence of electrical synapses (gap junctions) between dendrites of neighboring neurons. In the cerebellar cortex, the response of Purkinje cells takes the form of *complex spikes* (multiple action potentials in response to single pulses), because of the spatiotemporal effects of climbing fiber activity along the branches of the dendritic tree.

When a monkey has been trained to perform a motor task, increased discharge of Purkinje cells during task performance takes the form of simple spikes produced by bundles of active parallel fibers. If an unexpected obstacle is introduced into the task (e.g. momentary braking of a lever that the monkey is operating), bursts of complex spikes occur each time the obstacle is encountered. As the animal learns to overcome the obstacle so that the task is completed in the set time, the spike bursts dwindle in number and finally disappear. This is just one of several experimental indicators that the olive has a significant *teaching function* in the acquisition of new motor skills.

The olive receives direct ipsilateral projections from the premotor and motor areas of the cerebral cortex, and from the visual association cortex, providing an apparently suitable substrate for its activities. It is also in touch with the outside world through the spino-olivary tract (Chapter 12).

In theory, the red nucleus of the midbrain could function as a *novelty detector* because it receives collaterals both from cortical fibers descending to the olive and from cerebellar output fibers ascending to the thalamus. Much the largest output from the red nucleus is to the ipsilateral olive, which it appears to inhibit. Upon detection of a mismatch between a movement intended and a movement organized, the red nucleus could release the appropriate cell groups in the olive until the two are harmonized.

EFFERENT PATHWAYS *(FIGURE 20.7)*

From the *vestibulocerebellum* (fastigial nucleus), axons project to the vestibular nuclei of both sides, through the inferior cerebellar peduncles. The contralateral projection crosses over within the cerebellar white matter.

Vestibulocerebellar outputs to the medial and superior vestibular nuclei control movements of the eyes (Chapter 15). A separate output to the lateral vestibular (Deiters') nucleus of the same

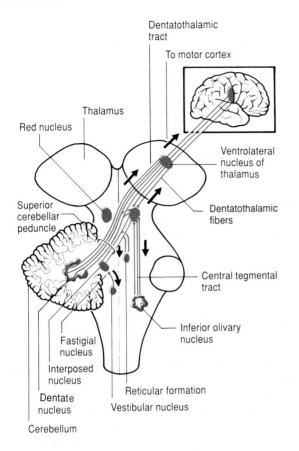

From the interposed nucleus of the *spinocerebellum*, axons emerge in the superior cerebellar peduncle. They terminate mainly in the contralateral reticular formation and red nucleus. Those reaching the pontomedullary reticular formation regulate the functions of the reticulospinal tracts in relation to posture and locomotion. Those ascending to the red nucleus may be involved in motor learning, because the output of the human red nucleus is almost entirely to the inferior olivary nucleus on that side.

From the *neocerebellum*, the massive **dentatothalamic tract** forms the bulk of the superior cerebellar peduncle. It decussates with its opposite number in the lower midbrain and later gives collaterals to the red nucleus before synapsing in the ventral lateral nucleus of the thalamus. The onward projection from the thalamus is to the motor cortex.

THE CEREBELLUM AND HIGHER BRAIN FUNCTIONS

Positron emission tomography (PET) provides information about regional changes in blood flow and oxygen consumption. 'Movement maps' such as those in *Figure 20.6* are derived from simple repetitive movements such as opening and closing a fist. A striking feature of movement maps is *how small and how medial* they are. Prior to PET, it was assumed that the lateral expansion of the human posterior lobe was necessary for manual dexterity. It now appears that the lateral expansion may be associated with

Figure 20.7 Principal cerebellar efferents. Arrows indicate directions of impulse conduction.

side controls the balancing function of the vestibulospinal tract. Some Purkinje fibers skirt the fastigial nucleus and exert tonic inhibition instead upon Deiters' nucleus.

CLINICAL PANEL 20.1

MIDLINE LESIONS: TRUNCAL ATAXIA

Lesions of the vermis occur most often in children, in the form of medulloblastomas in the roof of the fourth ventricle. These tumors expand rapidly and produce signs of raised intracranial pressure: headache, vomiting, drowsiness, papilledema. In the recumbent position there may be no abnormality of motor coordination in the limbs. Nystagmus can usually be elicited on visual tracking of the examiner's finger from side to side. Scanning movements of the eyes are also inaccurate due to poor control of the gaze centers by the vermis. A dramatic feature is an inability to stand upright without support—a state of *truncal ataxia*. This tumor, which is highly sensitive to radiotherapy, is clearly attacking the pathway from the vermis to the nucleus of the vestibular nerve. The nystagmus reflects malfunction of the medial vestibular nucleus on being deprived of its normal regulatory input. The ataxia reflects malfunction of the lateral vestibular nucleus and consequently of the vestibulospinal tract. Deficient antigravity function in this uncrossed pathway causes the child to fall to the more affected side on attempting to stand or walk.

cognitive functions (e.g. thinking), having an anatomical base in linkages with the lateral prefrontal cortex of the cerebral hemisphere. Lateral activity seems to be greatest during speech, with a one-sided predominance consistent with a possible linkage (via the thalamus) with the motor speech area of the dominant frontal cortex (Chapter 24). Something more than mere motor control may be involved, because lateral cerebellar activity is greater during functional naming,

e.g. 'dig', 'fly', than during object identification, e.g. 'shovel', 'airplane'.

CLINICAL DISORDERS OF THE CEREBELLUM

Diseases involving the cerebellum usually involve more than one lobe and/or more than one of the three sagittal strips. However, characteristic clin-

---

CLINICAL PANEL 20.2

ANTERIOR LOBE LESIONS: GAIT ATAXIA

Disease of the anterior lobe is most often observed in chronic alcoholics. Postmortem studies reveal pronounced shrinkage of the cortex of the anterior lobe, with up to 10% loss of granule cells, 20% loss of Purkinje cells, and 30% reduction in the thickness of the molecular layer. The lower limbs are most affected, and a staggering, drunken gait is evident even when the patient is sober. Some degree of correction may be exercised by voluntary control. Instability of station with the feet together, and failure to 'toe the line' on walking, are present even when the eyes are open. As the disease progresses, a peripheral sensory neuropathy may be added, giving rise to signs of sensory ataxia (Chapter 12) as well.

Tendon reflexes may be depressed in the lower limbs, due to loss of tonic stimulation of the pontine reticulospinal supply to fusimotor neurons. Reduction of monosynaptic reflex activity during walking may eventually result in stretching of soft tissues, with hyperextension of the knee joint during standing.

CLINICAL PANEL 20.3

NEOCEREBELLAR LESIONS: INCOORDINATION OF VOLUNTARY MOVEMENTS

Disease of the neocerebellar cortex, dentate nucleus or superior cerebellar peduncle leads to incoordination of voluntary movements, particularly in the upper limb. When fine purposive movements are attempted (e.g. grasping a glass, using a key) an *intention tremor* develops: the hand and forearm quiver as the target is approached, owing to faulty muscle synergies around the elbow and wrist. The hand may travel past the target ('overshoot'). Because cerebellar guidance is lost, the normal smooth trajectory of reaching movements may be replaced by stepped flexions, abductions, etc. ('decomposition of movement').

Rapid alternating movements performed under command, such as pronation/supination, become quite irregular. The 'finger-to-nose' and 'heel-to-knee' tests are performed with equal clumsiness whether the eyes are open or closed—in contrast to performance in posterior column disease (Chapter 12).

Speech is impaired both with regard to phonation and to articulation. Phonation (production of vowel sounds) is uneven and often tremulous owing to loss of smoothness of contraction of the diaphragm and intercostals. The terms 'explosive' and 'scanning' have been applied to this feature. Articulation is slurred because of faulty timing of impulses in the nerves supplying the lips, mandible, tongue, palate, and infrahyoid muscles.

Signs of neocerebellar disorder sometimes originate in the midbrain or pons rather than in the cerebellum itself. The lesion responsible (usually vascular) interrupts one or other corticopontocerebellar pathway. If the corticopontine component is interrupted, ataxia will appear in the contralateral limbs. If the pontocerebellar component is interrupted, the ataxia will be ipsilateral.

ical pictures have been described in association with lesions of the vermis (*Panel 20.1*), of the anterior lobe (*Panel 20.2*), and of the neocerebellum (*Panel 20.3*).

POSTUROGRAPHY

Posturography is the instrumental recording of the erect posture. The subject stands on a platform and spontaneous body sway is detected by strain gages beneath the corners of the platform. Linkage of the strain-gage data to a computer can yield a graphic record of anteroposterior and side-to-side sway, first with the eyes open and then with the eyes closed. This is *static posturography*, and it helps to distinguish among different causes of ataxia.

Dynamic posturography provides information on the effects of an abrupt 4° backward tilt of the supporting platform. For this phase of the examination surface EMG electrodes are applied over the calf muscles (ankle plantarflexors) and over the tibialis anterior (an ankle dorsiflexor). The normal response to the backward tilt is threefold: (a) a monosynaptic, spinal, stretch reflex contraction of the calf muscles after 45 ms; (b) a polysynaptic stretch reflex contraction of the calf muscles after 95 ms; and (c) a long-loop, reflex contraction of the ankle dorsiflexors after 120 ms. The ascending limb of the long loop is via the tibial-sciatic nerve and the posterior column–medial lemniscal pathway to the somatosensory cortex; the descending limb is via the corticospinal tract and the sciatic-peroneal nerve. Dynamic posturography helps to distinguish among a wide variety of disorders affecting different levels of the CNS and PNS.

CORE INFORMATION

The cerebellum is primarily concerned with coordination of movements on its own side. Therefore, disease in one hemisphere leads to incoordination of limb movements on that side of the body.

The cortex contains a thick inner layer of tiny granule cells, a piriform layer of Purkinje (Pj) cells, and a molecular layer containing granule cell axons and Pj dendrites. Granule cells are excitatory to Pj cells (via parallel fibers) but Pj cells — the only output cells of the cortex — are inhibitory to the central nuclei, which themselves are excitatory. Inhibitory purely cortical neurons are the stellate, basket, and Golgi cells.

Two kinds of afferents to the cortex are (a) mossy fibers from all sources except the olive — they excite granule cells; and (b) climbing fibers from the olive — they powerfully excite Pj cells.

The basic input-output circuit is: mossy fibers → granule cells → Pj cells → deep nucleus → brainstem or thalamus. Olivocerebellar neurons are most active during novel learning; they elicit poststimulus depression of the Pj cell response to mossy fiber activity — a feature surely related to motor learning. The red nucleus is in a position to match the intended input to the cerebellum with the output achieved after passage through the basic circuit.

Functional parts

Vestibulocerebellum comprises vermis and fastigial nuclei, having two-way connections with the vestibular nucleus. It may be affected by midline tumors, yielding nystagmus and truncal ataxia.

Spinocerebellum, next to vermis and including much of the anterior lobe, includes the interposed nucleus. It receives spinocerebellar pathways and it controls posture and gait. Lesions are characterized by ataxia of stance and gait.

Neocerebellum is largest and most lateral, receiving the corticopontocerebellar system. The dentate nucleus projects to the contralateral motor cortex via thalamus, and to the contralateral red nucleus. Lesions result in ipsilateral incoordination, notably of the upper limb; and to faulty phonation and articulation.

SELF TEST

Answer A if 1, 2, and 3 only are correct
        B if 1 and 3 only are correct
        C if 2 and 4 only are correct
        D if 4 only is correct
        E if all four are correct

1 **The following is/are true of the vestibulocerebellum:**

   1 It includes the entire anterior lobe
   2 The fastigial nucleus is unpaired
   3 The microscopic appearances are unique
   4 A lesion may give rise to truncal ataxia

2 **Feature(s) of the spinocerebellum:**

   1 Includes the entire posterior lobe
   2 Main target of spinocerebellar pathways
   3 Uniquely large in the human brain
   4 A lesion may result in a drunken gait pattern

3 **Feature(s) of the neocerebellum:**

   1 Efferent nucleus is the dentate
   2 Receives massive pontocerebellar input
   3 Main output is to contralateral thalamus
   4 Coordinates voluntary movements on the opposite side of the body

4 **Inhibitory neuron(s):**

   1 Basket cells
   2 Stellate cells
   3 Golgi cells
   4 Purkinje cells

5 **Climbing fibers:**

   1 Derived from ipsilateral inferior olivary nucleus
   2 Are excitatory
   3 Give rise to parallel fibers
   4 Have a teaching function

6 **An unsteady gait may result from disease of the:**

   1 Anterior cerebellar lobe
   2 Vestibular labyrinth
   3 Posterior columns
   4 Basilar pons

REFERENCES

Burke, D. and Gandevia, S.C. (1993) Muscle spindles, muscle tone and the fusimotor system. In *Science and Practice in Clinical Neurology* (Gandevia, S.C., Burke, D., and Anthony, M., eds), pp. 89–105. Cambridge: University Press.

Ebner, T.J. and Bloedel, J.R. (1987) Climbing fiber afferent system: intrinsic properties and role in cerebellar information processing. In *New Concepts in Cerebellar Neurobiology* (King, J.S., ed), pp. 371–386. New York: Alan R. Liss.

Fox, P.T., Raichle, M.E. and Thach, W.T. (1985) Functional mapping of the human cerebellum with positron emission tomography. *Proc. Natl Acad. Sci. USA* **82**: 7462–7466.

Gilbert, P.F.C. and Thach, W.T. (1977) Purkinje cell activity during motor learning. *Brain Res.* **128**: 309–328.

Horne, M.K. and Butler, E.G. (1995) The role of the cerebello-thalamocortical pathway in skilled movements. *Progr. Neurobiol.* **46**: 190–213.

Houk, J.C. and Gibson, A.R. (1987) Sensorimotor processing through the cerebellum. In *New Concepts in Cerebellar Neurobiology* (King, J.S., ed), pp. 387–416. New York: Alan R.Liss.

Kennedy, P.R. (1979) The rubro-olivo-cerebellar teaching circuit. *Med. Hypoth.* **5**: 799–807.

Leiner, H.C., Leiner, A.L. and Dow, R.S. (1991) The human cerebro-cerebellar system: its computing, cognitive, and language skills. *Behav. Brain Res.* 44: 113–128.

21

HYPOTHALAMUS

Chapter Summary

Introduction

Gross anatomy
Boundaries
Subdivisions and nuclei

Functions
Hypothalamic control of the
    pituitary gland
Other hypothalamic
    connections and functions

CLINICAL PANELS
Hypothalamic disorders
Major depression

Study Guidelines

1. Hypothalamic neuroendocrine cells fulfill the basic criteria both for neurons and for endocrine cells. Small neuroendocrine cells control release of hormones by the purely endocrine cells of the anterior pituitary gland into the cavernous sinus. Large ones have their terminals in the posterior pituitary where they release hormones into the cavernous sinus directly.
2. Some neurons confined to the hypothalamus are involved in control of body temperature, food and fluid intake, and sleep. Others, involved in attack and defense responses and memory, are controlled by the limbic system.

INTRODUCTION

The hypothalamus develops as part of the limbic system, which is concerned with preservation of the individual and of the species. Therefore it is logical that the hypothalamus should have significant controls over basic survival strategies including reproduction, growth and metabolism, food and fluid intake, attack and defense, temperature control, the sleep–wake cycle, and aspects of memory.

Most of its functions are expressed through its control of the pituitary gland and of both divisions of the autonomic nervous system.

GROSS ANATOMY

The hypothalamus occupies the side walls and floor of the third ventricle. It is a bilateral, paired structure. Despite its small size—it weighs only 4 g—it has major functions in homeostasis and survival. Its homeostatic functions include control of the body temperature and the circulation of the blood. Its survival functions include regu-

lation of food and water intake, the sleep–wake cycle, sexual behavior patterns, and defense mechanisms against attack.

BOUNDARIES

The boundaries of the hypothalamus are as follows (see *Figures 21.1* and *21.2*):
- *Superior:* the **hypothalamic sulcus** separating it from the thalamus.
- *Inferior:* the **optic chiasm, tuber cinereum** and **mamillary bodies**. The tuber cinereum shows a small swelling, the **median eminence**, immediately behind the **infundibulum** ('funnel') atop the pituitary stalk.
- *Anterior:* the lamina terminalis.
- *Posterior:* the tegmentum of the midbrain.
- *Medial:* the third ventricle.
- *Lateral:* the internal capsule.

SUBDIVISIONS AND NUCLEI

In the sagittal plane, it is customary to divide the hypothalamus into three regions: *anterior* (supraoptic), *middle* (tuberal) and posterior

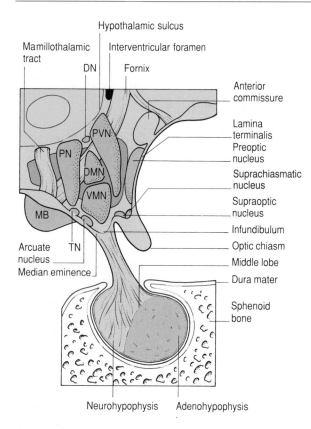

Figure 21.1 Hypothalamic nuclei and hypophysis, viewed from the right side. DN, dorsal nucleus; DMN, dorsomedial nucleus; LN, lateral nucleus (in red); MB, mamillary body; PN, posterior nucleus; PVN, periventricular nucleus; TN, tuberomamillary nucleus; VMN, ventromedial nucleus. The lateral hypothalamic nucleus is shown in dark red.

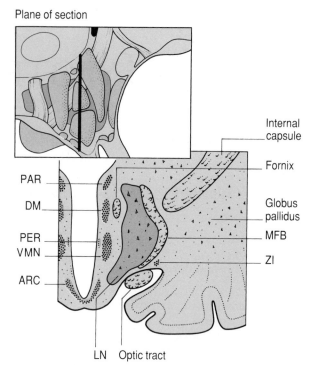

Figure 21.2 Hypothalamic nuclei, and related neural pathways, in a coronal section. ARC, arcuate nucleus; DM, dorsomedial nucleus; LN, lateral nucleus; MFB, medial forebrain bundle; PAR, paraventricular nucleus; PER, periventricular nucleus; VMN, ventromedial nucleus; ZI, zona incerta.

(mamillary). The descriptive use of 'regions' has been convenient for animal experiments involving placement of lesions. Named nuclei in the three regions are listed in *Table 21.1.*

In the coronal plane, the hypothalamus can be divided into *lateral, medial,* and *periventricular* regions. The full length of the lateral region is occupied by the **lateral hypothalamic nucleus.** Merging with the lateral nucleus is the **medial forebrain bundle,** carrying aminergic fibers to

the hypothalamus as well as to the cerebral cortex.

FUNCTIONS

HYPOTHALAMIC CONTROL OF THE PITUITARY GLAND

The arterial supply of the pituitary gland comes

Table 21.1 Hypothalamic nuclei

Anterior	Intermediate	Posterior
Preoptic	Arcuate (infundibular)	Mamillary
Supraoptic	Tuberal	Posterior
Suprachiasmatic	Lateral	Paraventricular
Dorsal	Anterior	Dorsomedial
Ventromedial	Posterior	Periventricular

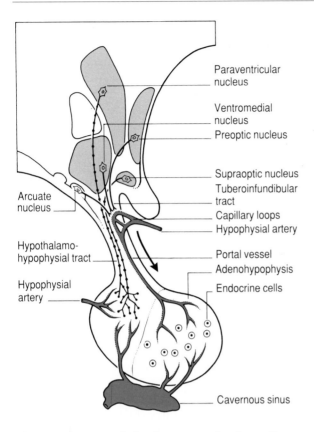

Figure 21.3 Hypothalamic neuroendocrine cells. The blood supply to the hypophysis, including the endocrine cells of the adenohypophysis, is also shown (arrow indicates direction of blood flow in the portal system).

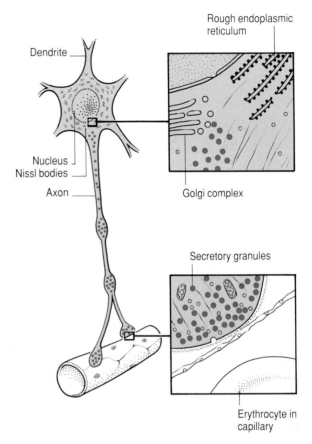

Figure 21.4 Morphology of a peptide-secreting neuroendocrine cell.

from hypophysial branches of the internal carotid artery (*Figure 21.3*). One set of branches supplies a capillary bed in the wall of the infundibulum. These capillaries drain into **portal vessels** which pass into the adenohypophysis. There they break up to form a second capillary bed which bathes the endocrine cells and drains into the cavernous sinus.

The neurohypophysis receives a direct supply from another set of hypophyseal arteries. The capillaries drain into the cavernous sinus, which delivers the secretions of the anterior and posterior lobes into the general circulation.

Secretions of the pituitary gland are controlled by two sets of **neuroendocrine cells**. Neuroendocrine cells are true neurons in having dendrites and axons and in conducting nerve impulses. They are also true endocrine cells because they liberate their secretions into capillary beds (*Figure 21.4*). With one exception (mentioned below), the secretions are peptides,

synthesized in clumps of granular endoplasmic reticulum and packaged in Golgi complexes. The peptides are attached to long-chain polypeptides called *neurophysins*. The capillaries concerned are outside the blood-brain barrier, and are fenestrated.

The somas of the neuroendocrine cells occupy the *hypophysiotropic area* in the lower half of the preoptic and tuberal regions. Contributory nuclei are the **preoptic, supraoptic, paraventricular, ventromedial,** and **arcuate** (infundibular). Two classes of neurons can be identified: **parvocellular** (small) **neurons** reaching the median eminence, and **magnocellular** (large) **neurons** reaching the posterior lobe of the pituitary gland.

The parvocellular neuroendocrine system

Parvocellular neurons of the hypophysiotropic area give rise to the **tuberoinfundibular** tract, which reaches the infundibular capillary bed.

Table 21.2 Hypothalamic parvocellular releasing/inhibiting hormones (RH/IH)

RH/IH	Anterior lobe hormone
Corticotropin RH	ACTH
Thyrotropin RH	Thyrotropin
Growth hormone RH	Growth hormone
Growth hormone IH	Growth hormone
Prolactin RH	Prolactin
Prolactin IH	Prolactin
Gonadotropic hormone RH	FSH/LH

Action potentials traveling along these neurons result in calcium-dependent exocytosis of *releasing hormones* from some and *inhibiting hormones* from others, for transport to the adenohypophysis in the portal vessels. The cell types of the adenohypophysis are stimulated/inhibited in accordance with *Table 21.2*. In the left–hand column, the only non-peptide parvocellular hormone is the prolactin-inhibiting hormone, which is *dopamine*, secreted from the arcuate (infundibular) nucleus.

The releasing/inhibiting hormones are not wholly specific: they have major effects on a single cell type, and minor effects on one or two others.

Multiple controls exist for parvocellular neurons of the hypophysiotropic area. The controls include: depolarization by afferents entering from the limbic system and from the reticular formation; hyperpolarization by local-circuit GABA neurons, some of which are sensitive to circulating hormones; and inhibition of transmitter release by opiate-releasing internuncials, which are numerous in the intermediate region of the hypothalamus. The picture is further complicated by the fact that opiates and other modulatory peptides may be released into the portal vessels and activate receptors on the endocrine cells of the adenohypophysis.

The magnocellular neuroendocrine system

Magnocellular neurons in the supraoptic and paraventricular nuclei give rise to the **hypothalamohypophysial tract,** which descends to the posterior lobe (*Figure 21.3*). Minor contributions to the tract are received from opiatergic and other peptidergic neurons in the periventricular region of the hypothalamus, and from aminergic neurons of the brainstem.

Two hormones are secreted by separate neurons located in both the supraoptic and paraventricular nuclei: *antidiuretic hormone (vasopressin)* and *oxytocin*. Axonal swellings containing the secretory granules for these hormones make up nearly half the volume of the neurohypophysis. The largest swellings, called **Herring bodies,** may be as large as erythrocytes. The Herring bodies provide a local depot of granules for release by smaller, terminal swellings into the capillary bed.

Antidiuretic Hormone

Antidiuretic hormone (ADH) continuously stimulates water uptake by the distal convoluted tubules

---

CLINICAL PANEL 21.1

HYPOTHALAMIC DISORDERS

The most dramatic disorder of hypothalamic function is *diabetes insipidus,* which is brought about by interruption of the hypothalamohypophyseal pathway—sometimes by tumors in the region, sometimes by head injury. The patient drinks upwards of 10 liters of water per day, and excretes a similar amount of urine. Historically, the term insipidus refers to the absence of taste sensation from the urine, in contrast to *diabetes mellitus,* in which the urine is sweet-tasting (mellitus) owing to its sugar content.

Hypophysectomy (surgical removal of the pituitary gland) can be performed in the treatment of other diseases, without causing more than temporary diabetes insipidus, provided the pituitary stalk is sectioned at a low level. Within a short period, sufficient ADH is secreted into the capillary bed of the median eminence to ensure adequate water conservation.

A wide variety of hypothalamic dysfunctions have been reported in the clinical literature. Causes are also varied, and include tumors, congenital malformations, and head injury. Clinical manifestations include gross obesity, disturbances of autonomic control, excessive sleepiness, and memory loss.

CLINICAL PANEL 21.2

MAJOR DEPRESSION

Major depression is a state of depressed mood occurring without an adequate explanation in terms of external events. The condition affects about 4% of the adult population, and there is a genetic predisposition: about 20% of first-degree relatives have it too. Phases of depression may begin in childhood or adolescence.

Major depression is characterized by at least several of the following features:

- Depressed general mood, with loss of interest in normal activities and outside events.
- Diminished energy, easy fatigue, loss of appetite and of sex drive, constipation.
- Impairment of self-image, with a feeling of personal inadequacy.
- Disturbance of the sleep–wake cycle, typically shown by early morning wakefulness.
- Aches and pains. Recurrent abdominal pains may simulate organ disease.
- Periods of agitation, with restlessness and perhaps suicidal tendency.

Involvement of *monoamines* was first indicated by the chance observation that the use of reserpine in treatment of hypertension produced depression as a side-effect. Reserpine depletes monoamine stores (serotonin, norepinephrine, dopamine).

The symptoms listed above are also characteristic of *chronic stress.* It is therefore not surprising to find that the suprarenal cortex is hyperactive in depressed patients. Serum cortisol levels are elevated. Normally, a rising serum cortisol level inhibits production of corticotropin-releasing-hormone (CRH) by the hypothalamus, with consequent reduction of ACTH release from the adenohypophysis. In depressed patients, this negative feedback circuit fails at the level of the hypothalamus, where CRH release is no longer checked by cortisol.

Some of the CRH neurons send branches into the brain itself — notably to the midbrain — where CRH acts as an inhibitory transmitter. These neurons inhibit mesocortical dopaminergic neurons (which are normally associated with positive motivational drive). They also inhibit rostral serotonergic neurons critically involved with diurnal rhythms, mainly through intense innervation of the suprachiasmatic nucleus. Because the noradrenergic neurons of locus ceruleus are activated by stress, and because they innervate the CRH neurons, a transmitter/receptor mismatch is a possibility.

The front line of therapy is completely occupied by drugs that enhance serotonergic transmission. The range of antidepressants is large and their sites of action vary, e.g. some inhibit reuptake from the synaptic cleft, others inhibit degradation by monoamine oxidase (Chapter 10). They take several weeks to take effect; the latent interval is taken up with desensitizing (inhibitory) autoreceptors on serotonergic cell membranes.

Electroconvulsive therapy (ECT) is at least as effective as the antidepressants. Its seems to desensitize autoreceptors, to sensitize (excitatory) serotonin receptors on target neurons, and to depress noradrenergic transmission.

---

and collecting ducts of the kidneys. The chief regulator of electrical activity in the ADH-secreting neurons is the osmotic pressure of the blood. A rise of as little as 1% in the osmotic pressure causes the plasma to be diluted to normal levels by means of increased water uptake. The neurons are themselves sensitive to osmolar changes, but they are facilitated by inputs from osmolar and volume detectors elsewhere, notably a small **organum vasculosum** behind the lamina terminalis.

Some ADH neurons also synthesize *corticotropin–releasing hormone*, the two hormones being released together from collateral branches, into the capillary pool of the infundibulum. It is of interest that ADH neuronal activity is increased when the body is stressed, and that the output of ACTH is boosted by the presence of ADH in the adenohypophysis.

Withdrawal of ADH secretion results in *diabetes insipidus (Panel 21.1)*

A prevalent disorder, *major depression*, is chemically characterized by reduced production of bioamines and excessive release of corticotropin releasing hormone (*Panel 21.2*).

Oxytocin

The principal function of oxytocin is to participate in a *neurohumoral reflex* when an infant is suckling at the breast. The afferent limb of this reflex is provided by impulses traveling from the nipple to the hypothalamus via the spinoreticular tract. Oxytocin is liberated by magnocellular neurons in response to suckling. Having entered the general circulation, it causes the expression of milk by stimulating myoepithelial cells surrounding the lactiferous ducts of the breast.

Oxytocin also has a mild stimulating action on uterine muscle during labor. The afferent stimulus in this case originates in the genital tract once labor gets under way.

OTHER HYPOTHALAMIC CONNECTIONS AND FUNCTIONS

Autonomic centers

In animals, stimulation of the anterior hypothalamic area produces *parasympathetic effects:* slowing of the heart, constriction of the pupil, salivary secretion, and intestinal peristalsis. On the other hand, stimulation of the posterior hypothalamic area produces sympathetic effects: increase in heart rate and blood pressure, pupillary dilatation, and intestinal stasis. Axons from both areas project to autonomic nuclei in the brainstem and spinal cord. In the midbrain and pons, this projection occupies a small **posterior longitudinal fasciculus** in the central gray matter.

Temperature regulation

The hypothalamus contains *thermosensitive neurons* which initiate appropriate responses to changes in the core temperature of the body. Activity of these neurons is reinforced by thermal information received (via the spinoreticular tract) from thermosensitive neurons supplying the skin (Chapter 9).

A slight change in the core temperature can usually be corrected by directing blood flow into or away from the skin, as appropriate. The requisite control of the sympathetic nervous system resides in the region of the posterior nucleus of the hypothalamus, which sends axons all the way to the lateral horn of the spinal cord.

Hypothalamic control of the sympathetic system diminishes with age. For this reason, the elderly are particularly prone to develop hypothermia in cold weather.

Hyperthermia is characteristic of *fevers.* Infectious agents (bacteria, viruses, parasites) cause tissue macrophages to liberate *endogenous pyrogen,* a protein that causes the hypothalamic 'thermostat' to be reset to a higher value. The chief mechanisms used to raise the body temperature to the new set point are cutaneous vasoconstriction and shivering.

Drinking

The chief center controling the intake of water appears to be a ribbon of cells alongside the lateral nucleus known as the **zona incerta** (*Figure 21.2*). Stimulation of this region may produce excessive drinking; lesions may result in refusal to drink, with consequent severe dehydration.

Eating

Eating habits have obvious social and cultural components, causing dietary practise to vary widely between individuals and between communities. The hypothalamus provides a baseline for caloric and nutrient intake, in the form of interplay between the lateral and ventromedial nuclei. Together, they constitute the *appestat* (appetite set point). Stimulation of a lateral hypothalamic *feeding center* causes a cat or rat to eat excessively, whereas destruction of this center results in refusal to eat. Conversely, stimulation of a ventromedial *satiety center* inhibits the urge to eat, and bilateral ventromedial lesions result in persistent overeating and gross obesity. The satiety center is normally very sensitive to glucose levels in the blood.

Rage and fear

The lateral and ventromedial nuclei are concerned with *mood* as well as food. Cats that are overweight in consequence of ventromedial lesions tend to be highly aggressive. Conversely, animals rendered underweight by ventromedial stimulation tend to be unduly docile. (See also the amygdala, in Chapter 26.)

Sleeping and waking

A tiny (0.25 mm^3) **suprachiasmatic nucleus** embedded in the upper surface of the optic chiasm receives a direct input from the retina. It participates in setting the normal sleep-wake cycle, through connections with the **pineal gland**

(Chapter 22). For reasons unknown, this nucleus contains peptidergic (vasopressin) neurons which are twice as numerous in homosexual men than in heterosexuals of either sex.

Lesions of the posterior hypothalamic area may cause hypersomnolence or even coma. This area contains the **tuberomamillary nucleus** (*Figure 21.1*), housing hundreds of *histaminergic neurons,* which project widely to the gray matter of the brain and spinal cord. Some of the fibers run rostrally within the medial forebrain bundle, in company with aminergic fibers of brainstem origin. Histaminergic fibers destined for the cerebral cortex fan out below the genu of the corpus callosum. They branch within the superficial layers of the frontal cortex, and run back to supply the cortex of the parietal, occipital, and temporal lobes.

In animals, there is abundant physiological evidence in support of an *arousal function* for the histaminergic system.

Memory

The mamillary bodies belong to a limbic circuit involving the fornix, which sends fibers to it, and the mamillothalamic tract which projects to the anterior nucleus of the thalamus. This circuit may have a function in relation to memory (Chapter 26).

Note on circumventricular organs

Patches of brain tissue close to the third and fourth ventricles have fenestrated capillaries. These patches include the organum vasculosum, the median eminence and neurohypophysis, and the **area postrema** located in the roof of the fourth ventricle at its posterior tip. The area postrema is the *chemoreceptor trigger zone,* which is sensitive to many toxic substances which are unable to cross the blood–brain barrier; the trigger zone responds by activating the underlying vomiting center.

CORE INFORMATION

The hypothalamus is a bilateral structure beside the third ventricle. In the sagittal plane, it can be divided into an anterior (supraoptic) region containing six nuclei, an intermediate (tuberal) region with eight nuclei, and a posterior (mamillary) region with two. In the coronal plane, lateral, medial and periventricular regions are described.

The pituitary gland is controlled by hypothalamic neuroendocrine cells, which are characterized by impulse transmission and hormonal secretion into capillary beds. Small (parvocellular) neuroendocrine cells project only as far as the capillary bed of the median eminence. They release several kinds of releasing/inhibiting hormones into the capillary bed, whence they are carried to the adenohypophysis in a portal system of vessels. Large (magnocellular) neuroendocrine cells form the hypothalamohypophyseal tract, which liberates antidiuretic hormone and oxytocin into the capillary bed of the neurohypophysis.

Anterior and posterior regions of the hypothalamus contain neurons that activate the parasympathetic and sympathetic system, respectively. Thermoregulatory neurons maintain the body temperature set point, mainly by manipulating the sympathetic system.

Stimulation of the lateral hypothalamic area (in animals) provokes an increase in food and water consumption. Destruction of this area, or stimulation of a ventromedial satiety center results in refusal to eat. In these experiments, overweight animals tend to be aggressive, underweight ones docile.

The suprachiasmatic nucleus participates in control of the sleep–wake cycle. Afferents come from the retina, and efferents stimulate sympathetic neurons supplying the pineal gland, provoking secretion of melatonin.

The mamillary bodies receive inputs from the limbic system via the fornix, having a function in relation to memory.

SELF TEST

For questions 1 - 5,

Answer A if the item is associated with A only
          B if associated with B only
          C if associated with both A and B
          D if associated with neither A nor B

A Tuberoinfundibular tract
B Hypothalamohypophyseal tract
C Both
D Neither

1 Origin from hypophysiotropic area
2 Composed of neuroendocrine cells

3 Secretion is into a capillary bed
4 Function depends upon a portal system of vessels
5 Involved in a neurohumoral reflex

Connect the nucleus to the function:

6 Tuberomamillary nucleus   A Sweating
7 Suprachiasmatic nucleus   B Sleeping
8 Zona incerta   C Drinking
9 Mamillary bodies   D Remembering
10 Posterior   E Alerting

REFERENCES

Akil, H. and Watson, S.J. (1987) Neuropeptides in brain and pituitary: overview. In *Psychopharmacology: The Third Generation of Progress* (Meltzer, H.Y., ed.), pp. 367–371. New York: Raven Press.

Gordon, C.J. (1986) Integration and central processing in temperature control. *Ann. Rev. Physiol.* **48:** 595–612.

Hatton, G.L. (1990) Emerging concepts of structure-function dynamics in adult brain: the hypothalamo-neurohypophysial system. *Prog. Neurobiol.* **34:** 337–504.

Kordon, C. (1985) Neural mechanisms involved in pituitary control. *Neurochem. Int.* **7:** 917–925.

Lutten, P.G.M., ter Horst, T.J., and Steffens, A.B. (1986) The hypothalamus: intrinsic connections and outflow pathways to the endocrine system in relation to the control of feeding and metabolism. *Prog. Neurobiol.* **28:** 1–54.

Rothwell, N.J. (1994) CNS regulation of thermogenesis. *Crit. Rev. Neurobiol.* **8:** 1–10.

Schwartz, J-C., Arrang, J-M., Garbarg, M., Pollard, H. and Ruat, M. (1991) Histaminergic transmission in the mammalian brain. *Physiol. Rev.* 71: 1–51.

Swaab, D.F. and Hofman, M.A. (1994) Age, sex and light: variability in the human suprachiasmatic nucleus in relation to its functions. *Prog. Brain Res.* **100:** 261–265.

22

THALAMUS, EPITHALAMUS

Chapter Summary

Thalamus
Thalamic nuclei
Synaptic interplay in the
    ventral thalamus
Thalamic peduncles

Epithalamus
Pineal gland

Study Guidelines

1   The thalamus is an assembly of largely independent nuclear groups. *Motor* thalamic nuclei receive inputs from basal ganglia and cerebellum and project to motor and premotor areas of the cerebral cortex. *Sensory* nuclei receive inputs from somatic and special senses and project to primary sensory cortical areas. *Cognitive* nuclei are strongly linked to the prefrontal cortex. *Association* nuclei are connected to association areas, and *non-specific* nuclei are involved in cortical arousal.
2   The epithalamus contains the pineal gland which is of current interest in conection with the sleep-inducing hormone, melatonin.

THALAMUS

The thalamus is the largest nuclear mass in the entire nervous system. It is a prominent feature in MRI scans in each of the three planes in which slices are taken. The afferent and efferent connections of the twelve main nuclear groups are so diverse that the thalamus cannot be said to have a unitary function.

As noted in Chapter 2, the two thalami lie at the center of the brain. Their medial surfaces face one another across the third ventricle and their lateral surfaces are in contact with the posterior limb of the internal capsule. The upper surface of each occupies the floor of a lateral ventricle. The under aspect receives sensory and cerebellar inputs as well as an upward continuum of the reticular formation.

THALAMIC NUCLEI

All thalamic nuclei except one (the reticular nucleus) have reciprocal excitatory connections with the cerebral cortex. The Y-shaped **internal medullary lamina** of white matter divides the thalamus into three large cell groups: *mediodorsal, anterior,* and *lateral (Figure 22.1A)*. The lateral group comprises *dorsal and ventral nuclear tiers*. At the back of the thalamus are the **medial** and **lateral geniculate nuclei**. The **external medullary lamina** separates the thalamus from the shell-like **reticular nucleus**.

The thalamic nuclei may be categorized into three functional groups: *specific* or *relay nuclei, association nuclei,* and *non-specific nuclei*.

Specific nuclei

The specific or relay nuclei are reciprocally connected to specific motor or sensory areas of the cerebral cortex. They comprise the nuclei of the ventral tier and the geniculate nuclei. Their afferent and efferent connections are indicated in *Figure 22.1B*.

The **ventral anterior nucleus** (VA) receives afferents from the globus pallidus, and it projects to the prefrontal cortex.

The anterior part of the **ventral lateral nucleus** (VL) receives afferents from the globus pallidus and projects to the supplementary motor area. The posterior part of VL is the principal target of the contralateral superior cerebellar peduncle, which originates in the dentate nucleus of the cerebellum; the posterior VL projects to the motor cortex.

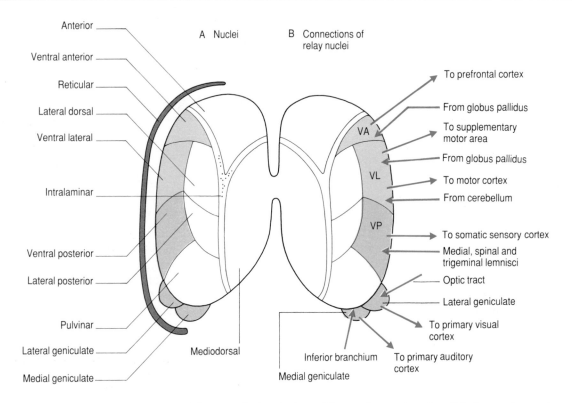

A Nuclei

B Connections of relay nuclei

Figure 22.1 Schematic illustration of the two thalami, viewed from above, showing **(A)** the twelve main nuclei; **(B)** connections of the relay nuclei. VA, ventral anterior nucleus; VL, ventral lateral nucleus; VP, ventral posterior nucleus.

The **ventral posterior nucleus** (VP) receives all of the fibers of the medial, spinal, and trigeminal lemnisci (*Figure 22.2*). It projects to the somatic sensory cortex (SI). A smaller projection is sent to the second somatic sensory area (SII) at the foot of the postcentral gyrus (see Chapter 24).

The VP is somatotopically arranged, as indicated in *Figure 22.3*. The portion of the nucleus devoted to the face and head is called the **ventroposteromedial nucleus** (VPM), that for the trunk and limbs the **ventroposterolateral nucleus** (VPL). Modality segregation is a feature of both nuclei, with proprioceptive neurons most anterior, tactile neurons in the mid-region, and nociceptive neurons at the back. The nociceptive region is sometimes called the *posterior nucleus*.

There is no evidence in the VP of an antinociceptive mechanism comparable to that found in the substantia gelatinosa region of the spinal cord and spinal trigeminal nucleus. An unexplained disorder, the *thalamic syndrome*, may follow a vascular lesion that disconnects the posterior thalamic nucleus from the somatic sensory cortex. In this condition a period of complete sensory loss may occur on the contralateral side of the body, to be replaced by bouts of severe pain occurring either spontaneously or in response to tactile stimuli.

The **medial geniculate nucleus** (medial geniculate body) is the thalamic nucleus for hearing. It receives the inferior brachium, and it projects to the primary auditory cortex.

The **lateral geniculate nucleus** (lateral geniculate body) is the principal thalamic nucleus for vision. It receives retinal inputs from both eyes by way of the optic tract, and it projects to the primary visual cortex. The visual pathways are described in Chapter 23.

Association nuclei

The association nuclei are reciprocally connected to the association areas of the cerebral cortex.

The **anterior nucleus** receives the mamillothalamic tract and projects to the cingulate cortex. It is involved in a limbic circuit and seems to have a function in relation to memory (Chapter 26).

The **mediodorsal nucleus** receives inputs from

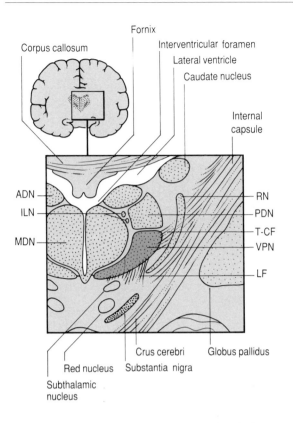

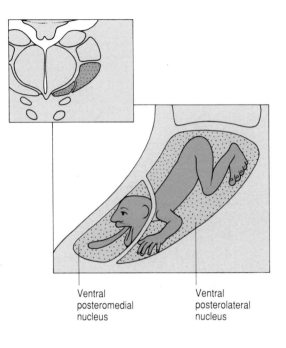

Figure 22.3 Somatic sensory map in the ventral posterior thalamic nucleus. (Redrawn and modified from Ohye (1990) with permission.)

Figure 22.2 Coronal section through the thalamus and related structures. ADN, anterior dorsal nucleus; ILN, intralaminar nucleus; LF, lemniscal fibers; MDN, mediodorsal nucleus; PDN, posterior dorsal nucleus; RN, reticular nucleus; T-CF, thalamocortical fibers; VPN, ventral posterior nucleus.

the olfactory and limbic systems and is reciprocally connected with the entire prefrontal cortex. It has poorly understood functions in relation to cognition (thinking), judgement, and mood.

The **lateral posterior nucleus** and the **pulvinar** belong to a single nuclear complex. They receive afferents from the superior colliculus and project to the entire visual association cortex and to the entire parietal association cortex. An 'extrageniculate visual pathway' runs from the optic tract to the visual association cortex by way of the superior colliculus and the pulvinar. It seems to have the function of drawing attention to objects of interest in the peripheral field of vision, but it is not itself a source of conscious visual perception.

A further projection, from pulvinar to the posterior part of the cingulate cortex, is described in Chapter 26.

Non–specific nuclei

The non–specific nuclei are so called because they

are not specific to any one sensory modality. They include the intralaminar and reticular nuclei.

The **intralaminar nuclei** are contained within the internal medullary lamina of white matter. They can be regarded as a rostral continuation of the reticular formation of the midbrain (see Ascending Reticular Activating System in Chapter 19). They project widely to the cerebral cortex, as well as to the corpus striatum.

The **reticular nucleus** is shaped like a shield around the front and lateral side of the thalamus. It is separated from the main thalamus by the external medullary lamina. All of the thalamocortical projections pass through the reticular nucleus and give collateral branches to it. The nucleus reciprocates by sending a matching, inhibitory (GABAergic) supply to the corresponding thalamic nucleus—both to the projection neurons and to a set of GABAergic internuncials within the nucleus.

Synaptic interplay in the ventral thalamus

Figure 22.4 shows synaptic relationships in the ventral posterior nucleus. Specific afferents (the medial, lateral and trigeminal lemnisci) synapse upon the inhibitory internuncials as well as on

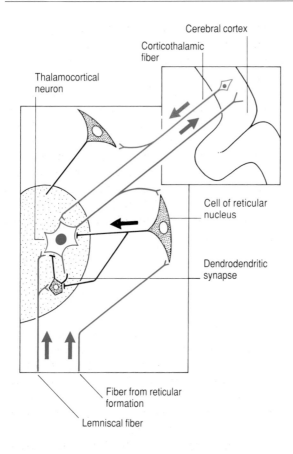

Figure 22.4 Synaptic relationships of a relay neuron in the ventral posterior nucleus of the thalamus. Arrows indicate directions of impulse transmission. Inhibitory neurons are shown in black.

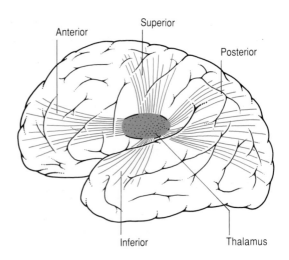

Figure 22.5 The thalamic peduncles (left hemisphere).

the thalamocortical neurons. A feature (of uncertain significance) in all of the ventral tier nuclei is an abundance of inhibitory, dendrodendritic synapses between the internuncials and the projection cells.

Some non-specific afferents from the midbrain reticular formation synapse in the reticular nucleus. Others pass to the intralaminar nuclei and to the nucleus of Meynert in the basal forebrain (Chapter 26).

In animal experiments (cat), thalamocortical neurons are inhibited by the reticular nucleus during sleep, exhibiting only intermittent short bursts of activity. During wakefulness, thalamocortical neurons fire continuously, apparently because of disinhibition: the reticular nucleus is still active, but its effect seems to be shifted to the inhibitory internuncials.

Not represented in *Figure 22.4* are *aminergic*

afferents passing to the ventral and intralaminar nuclei, from the midbrain raphe (serotonin) and locus ceruleus (norepinephrine). The proven value of tricyclic antidepressants in the therapy of chronic pain may be related to drug-induced prolongation of aminergic effects on thalamocortical neurons.

THALAMIC PEDUNCLES

The reciprocal connections between the thalamus and the cerebral cortex travel in four thalamic peduncles, as shown in *Figure 22.5*. The **anterior thalamic peduncle** passes through the anterior limb of the internal capsule to reach the prefrontal cortex and cingulate gyrus. The **superior thalamic peduncle** passes through the posterior limb of the internal capsule to reach the premotor, motor, and somatic sensory cortex. The **posterior thalamic peduncle** passes through the retrolentiform part of the internal capsule to reach the occipital lobe and the posterior parts of the parietal and temporal lobes. The **inferior thalamic peduncle** passes below the lentiform nucleus to reach the anterior temporal and orbital cortex. Each of the four fans becomes incorporated into the corona radiata.

EPITHALAMUS

The epithalamus includes the pineal gland,

habenula, and stria medullaris. The latter two are included with the limbic system in Chapter 26.

PINEAL GLAND

The pineal gland synthesizes *melatonin,* an amine hormone implicated in the sleep-wake cycle. Melatonin is synthesized from serotonin, the requisite enzymes being unique to this gland. Melatonin is liberated into the pineal capillary bed at night and has a sleep-inducing effect; it may have other benefits including clearance of harmful free radicals liberated from tissues during the aging process. Daytime secretion is suppressed by activity in sympathetic fibers reaching it from the superior cervical ganglia by way of the walls of the straight venous sinus. The relevant central pathway is from the paired suprachiasmatic nuclei via the posterior longitudinal fasciculus.

From the third decade onward, calcareous deposits ('pineal sand') accumulate within astrocytes in the pineal. Calcification is often detectable in plain radiographs of the head. A shift of the gland may denote a space-occupying lesion within the skull. However, a normal pineal may lie slightly to the left because the right cerebral hemisphere is usually a little wider than the left at this level.

CORE INFORMATION

Thalamus

The internal medullary lamina divides the thalamus anatomically into mediodorsal, anterior, and lateral nuclear groups, the lateral being separable into dorsal and ventral tiers. The thalamus may be divided functionally into specific, association, and non-specific nuclear groups. Of the specific nuclei: (1) ventral anterior receives inputs from globus pallidus and projects to prefrontal cortex; (2) the anterior part of ventral lateral receives inputs from globus pallidus and projects to supplementary motor area whereas the posterior part receives from contralateral cerebellum and projects to motor cortex; (3) ventral posterior receives the somatic sensory pathways and projects to the somatic sensory cortex; (4) the medial geniculate nucleus receives the inferior brachium and projects to the primary auditory cortex; and (5) the lateral geniculate nucleus receives from the optic tract and projects to the primary visual cortex. Of the association nuclei: (1) the anterior receives the mamillothalamic tract and projects to the cingulate cortex; (2) the mediodorsal is reciprocally connected to all parts of the prefrontal cortex; and (3) the lateral posterior-pulvinar complex receives from the superior colliculus and projects to the parietal association cortex. Of the non-specific nuclei: (1) the intralaminar receive inputs from the reticular formation and project widely to the cerebral cortex, also to the corpus striatum; (2) the reticular nucleus (outside the thalamus proper) receives excitatory collaterals from all thalamocortical and corticothalamic neurons, and returns inhibitory fibers to all nuclei within the thalamus. Reciprocal connections between thalamus and cortex travel in four thalamic peduncles which become incorporated into the corona radiata.

Epithalamus

The pineal gland secretes melatonin by night, with soporific effect. By day, sympathetic activity in the gland inhibits secretion, perhaps by blocking melatonin synthesis from precursor serotonin. The sympathetic fibers are activated by projections from the suprachiasmatic nuclei, which are activated by light.

SELF TEST

Match thalamic nuclei on the left with functions on the right:

1	Ventral lateral		**A**	Somatic sensation
2	Ventral posterior		**B**	Movement
3	Lateral geniculate		**C**	Cognition
4	Intralaminar		**D**	Vision
5	Mediodorsal		**E**	Consciousness

REFERENCES

Guillery, R.W. (1995) Anatomical evidence concerning the role of the thalamus in corticocortical communication: a brief review. *J. Anat.* **187**: 583-592.

Jones, E.G. (1985) *The Thalamus*. New York: Plenum Press.

Kultas-Ilinsky, K. and Ilinsky, I.A. (1986) Neuronal and synaptic organization of the motor nuclei of mammalian thalamus. In *Current Topics in Research on Synapses, Vol. 3*, pp. 77–145. New York: Alan R. Liss

Lenz, F.A. (1992) Ascending modulation of thalamic function and pain. In *Advances in Pain Research and Therapy* (Sicuteri, F. et al, eds), pp. 177–196. New York: Raven Press.

Mahe, V. and Chevalier, F. (1995) Human circadian clock in disease. *Presse Med.* 24: 1041–1046.

Ohye, C. (1990) Thalamus. In *The Human Nervous System* (Paxinos, G., ed.), pp. 439–468. San Diego: Academic Press.

Steriade, M. and Llinas, R.R. (1988) The functional states of the thalamus and the associated neuronal interplay. *Physiol. Rev.* **68**: 649–742.

23

VISUAL SYSTEM

Chapter Summary

Introduction

Retina
Lesions of the visual pathways

Central visual pathways
Optic nerve, optic tract
Geniculocalcarine tract and
    primary visual cortex
    Structure of the retina

Study Guidelines

1 The great length of the visual pathways makes them vulnerable to disease at widely separate locations. The pattern of visual defect differs in accordance with the site of damage.
2 Visual defects can often be detected merely by wiggling a finger in different parts of the visual field of each eye in turn.
3 The most important item of anatomical information concerns the representations of the visual fields at successive steps along the visual pathways.

INTRODUCTION

The visual system is of outstanding importance in clinical neurology. It extends from the retina of the eye to the occipital lobe of the brain. Its great length makes it especially vulnerable to demyelinating diseases such as multiple sclerosis; to tumors of the brain or pituitary gland; to vascular lesions in the territory of the middle or posterior cerebral artery; and to head injuries.

The visual system comprises the retinas, the visual pathways from the retinas to the brainstem and visual cortex, and the cortical areas devoted to higher visual functions. The retinas and visual pathways are described in this chapter. Higher visual functions are described in Chapter 24.

RETINA

The retina and the optic nerves are part of the central nervous system. In the embryo, the retina is formed by an outgrowth from the diencephalon called the optic vesicle (Chapter 1). The optic vesicle is invaginated by the lens and becomes the two-layered optic cup.

The outer layer of the optic cup becomes the pigment layer of the mature retina. The inner, nervous layer of the cup gives rise to the retinal neurons.

Figure 23.1 shows the general relationships in the developing retina. The nervous layer contains three principal sets of neurons: **photoreceptors,** which become applied to the pigment layer when the intraretinal space is resorbed; **bipolar neurons;** and **ganglion cells** which give rise to the optic nerve and project to the thalamus and midbrain. (The fibers of the optic nerve grow along

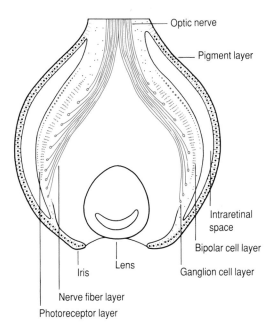

Figure 23.1 Embryonic retina.

the walls of a fissure which invaginates the under surface of the optic cup.)

Note that the retina is *inverted*: light must pass through the layers of optic nerve fibers, ganglion cells, and bipolar neurons to reach the photoreceptors. At the point of most acute vision, the **fovea centralis,** the inner layers lean away all around a cental pit (fovea), and light strikes the photoreceptors directly. In the mature eye, the fovea is about 1.5 mm in diameter and occupies the center of the **macula lutea** ('yellow spot'). The fovea is the point of most acute vision and lies in the *visual axis*—a line passing from the center of the visual field of the eye, through the center of the lens, to the fovea (*Figure 23.2*). To *fixate* or *foveate* an object is to gaze directly at it so that light reflected from its center registers on the fovea.

The visual fields of the two eyes overlap across two-thirds of the total visual field. Outside this *binocular field* is a *monocular crescent* on each side (*Figure 23.3*). During passage through the lens, the image of the visual field is reversed, with the result that, for example, objects in the left part of the binocular visual field register on the right half of each retina and objects in the upper part of the visual field register on the lower half. This arrangement is preserved all the way to the visual cortex in the occipital lobe.

From a clinical standpoint, it is essential to appreciate that *vision is a crossed sensation*. The visual field on one side of the visual axis registers on the visual cortex of the other side. In effect, the right visual cortex 'sees' the left visual field. Only half of the visual information crosses in the optic chiasma, for the simple reason that the other half has already crossed the midline in space.

Visual defects caused by interruption of the visual pathway are always described *from the patient's point of view,* i.e. in terms of the visual fields, and not in terms of retinal topography.

STRUCTURE OF THE RETINA

The retina contains three sets of neurons arranged in series: photoreceptors, bipolar neurons, and ganglion cells. It also contains two sets of neurons arranged transversely: horizontal cells, and amacrine cells (*Figure 23.4*).

Action potentials are generated by the ganglion cells, providing the requisite speed for conduction to the thalamus and midbrain. For the other cell types, distances are very short and passive electrical change (electrotonus) is sufficient for

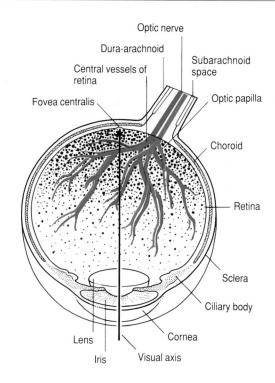

Figure 23.2 Horizontal section of the right eye, showing the visual axis.

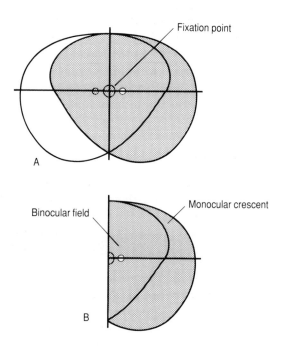

Figure 23.3 (A) Visual fields. Both eyes are targeted on the fixation point. The visual field of the right eye is shaded. The white spot represents the blind spot of the right eye. (B) The right visual field.

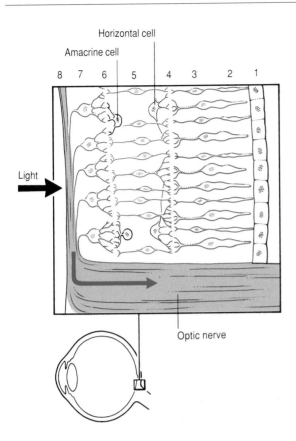

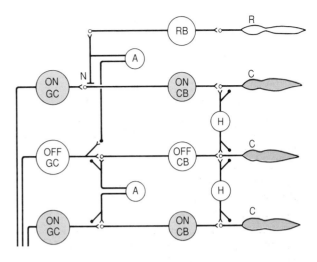

Figure 23.5 Retinal circuit diagram. (Adapted from Massey and Redburn (1987).) A, amacrine cell; C, cone; CB, cone bipolar neuron; GC, ganglion cell; H, horizontal cell; N, nexus (gap junction); R, rod; RB, rod bipolar.

Figure 23.4 The layers of the retina. (1) pigment layer; (2) photoreceptor layer; (3) outer nuclear layer; (4) outer plexiform layer; (5) inner nuclear layer; (6) inner plexiform layer; (7) ganglion cell layer; (8) nerve fiber layer.

intercellular communication, whether by gap-junctional contact or transmitter release.

Photoreceptors

The photoreceptor neurons comprise **rods** and **cones**. Rods function only in dim light and are not sensitive to color. They are absent from the fovea. Cones respond to bright light, are sensitive to color (received in the form of electromagnetic wavelength energy) and to shape, and are most numerous in the fovea.

Each photoreceptor has an outer and an inner segment and a synaptic end-foot. In the outer segment the plasma membrane is folded to form hundreds of membranous discs which incorporate visual pigment formed in the inner segment. The synaptic end-foot makes contact with bipolar neurons and horizontal cell processes in the outer plexiform layer.

A surprising feature of the photoreceptors is

that they are hyperpolarized by light. During darkness Na^+ channels are opened, creating sufficient positive electrotonus to cause leakage of transmitter from the end-feet. Illumination causes the Na^+ channels to close.

Cone and rod bipolar neurons

Cone bipolar neurons
Cone bipolar neurons are of two types. ON bipolars are switched on (depolarized) by light, being inhibited by transmitter released in the dark. They converge onto ON ganglion cells. OFF bipolars have the reverse response and converge onto OFF ganglion cells (*Figure 23.5*).

Rod bipolar neurons
Rod bipolar neurons are all hyperpolarized by light. They activate ON and OFF ganglion cells indirectly, by way of amacrine cells.

Horizontal cells

The dendrites of horizontal cells are in contact with photoreceptors. The peripheral dendritic branches give rise to axon-like processes which make inhibitory contacts with bipolar neurons.

The function of horizontal cells is to inhibit bipolar neurons, of similar kind, outside the immediate zone of excitation. The excited bipolars and ganglion cells are said to be on-line; the inhibited ones are off-line.

Amacrine cells

Amacrine cells have no axons. Their appearance is octopus-like, the dendrites all emerging from one side of the cell. Dendritic branches come into contact with bipolar neurons and ganglion cells.

More than a dozen different morphological types of amacrine cells have been identified, as well as several different transmitters including acetylcholine, dopamine, and serotonin. Possible functions include contrast enhancement and movement detection. For the rods, they convert large numbers of rods from OFF to ON with respect to ganglion cells.

Ganglion cells

The ganglion cells receive synaptic contacts from bipolar neurons in the inner plexiform layer. The typical response of ganglion cells to bipolar activity is 'center-surround'. An ON ganglion cell is excited by a spot of light, and inhibited by a surrounding annulus (ring) of light. The inhibition is caused by horizontal cells. OFF ganglion cells give the reverse response.

Coding for color

There are three types of cone with respect to spectral sensitivity. One is sensitive to red, one to green, and one to blue. Groups of each type are connected to ON or OFF ganglion cells.

The characteristic response of ganglion cells is one of *color opponency*:

- Ganglion cells that are on-line for green are off-line for red.
- Ganglion cells that are on-line for red are off-line for green.
- Ganglion cells that are on-line for blue are off-line for yellow, i.e. for green and red cones acting together.

Coding for black and white

White light is a mixture of green, red, and blue. In bright conditions it is encoded by the three corresponding cones, all of them converging onto common ganglion cells. Both ON and OFF ganglion cells are involved in black-and-white vision, just as in color vision.

In very dim conditions, e.g. starlight, only rod photoreceptors are active, and objects appear in varying shades of gray. The rods are subject to the same rules as cones, showing center-surround antagonism between white and black, and being connected to ON or OFF ganglion cells.

Most ganglion cells are small (parvocellular or 'P') having small receptive fields and being responsive to color and shape. A minority are large (magnocellular or 'M') having large receptive fields and being especially responsive to movements within the visual field.

CENTRAL VISUAL PATHWAYS

OPTIC NERVE, OPTIC TRACT

The optic nerve is formed by the axons of the retinal ganglion cells. The axons acquire myelin sheaths as they leave the optic disc.

The number of ganglion cells varies remarkably between individuals, from 800 000 to 1.5 million. Since every ganglion cell contributes to the optic nerve, the number of axons in the optic nerve is correspondingly variable.

The retinal ganglion cells are homologous with the projection neurons of the spinal cord. The optic nerve is homologous with spinal cord white matter, and is not a peripheral nerve. As explained in Chapter 7, peripheral nerves, whether cranial or spinal, contain Schwann cells and collagenous sheaths, and are capable of regeneration. The optic nerve contains neuroglial cells of central type (astrocytes and oligodendrocytes) and is not capable of regeneration in mammals. As well, the nerve is invested with meninges containing an extension of the subarachnoid space—a feature largely responsible for the changed appearance of the fundus oculi when the intracranial pressure is raised (Chapter 4).

At the optic chiasm, fibers from the nasal hemiretina enter the contralateral optic tract whereas those from the temporal hemiretina remain uncrossed and enter the ipsilateral tract.

As already noted in Chapter 21, some optic nerve fibers enter the suprachiasmatic nucleus of the hypothalamus. This connection has been invoked to account for the beneficial effect of bright artificial light, for several hours per day, in the treatment of wintertime depression.

The optic tract winds around the midbrain and divides into a medial and a lateral root.

Medial root of optic tract

The medial root contains 10% of the optic nerve

fibers. It enters the side of the midbrain. It contains four distinct sets of fibers:

1 Some fibers, mainly from retinal M cells, enter the superior colliculus and provide for automatic scanning, e.g. in reading this page.
2 Some fibers are relayed from the superior colliculus to the pulvinar of the thalamus; they belong to the extra-geniculate visual pathway to the visual association cortex (Chapter 22).
3 Some fibers enter the pretectal nucleus and serve the pupillary light reflex (Chapter 18).

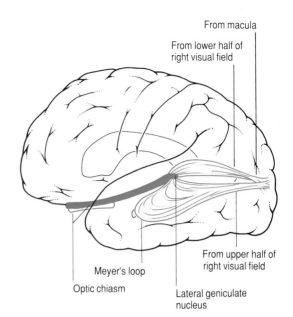

Figure 23.6 Left optic radiation visualized from the left side.

Figure 23.7 A dissection of the visual pathways, viewed from below. (Photograph reproduced from The Human Brain, by N. Gluhbegovic and T.W. Williams, by kind permission of the authors and of J.B. Lippincott, Inc.)

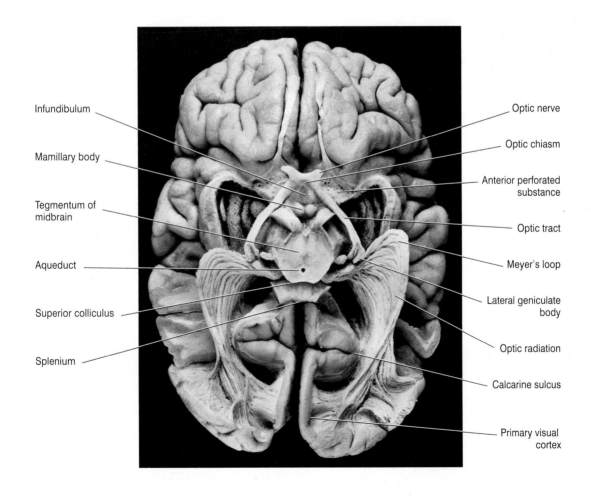

223

4 Some fibers enter the parvocellular reticular formation, where they have an arousal function (Chapter 19).

Lateral root of the optic tract and lateral geniculate nucleus

The lateral root of the optic tract terminates in the lateral geniculate nucleus (body) of the thalamus (LGN). The LGN shows six cellular laminae, three of which are devoted to crossed fibers and three to uncrossed fibers. The two deepest laminae (one for crossed and one for uncrossed fibers) are magnocellular and receive axons from retinal 'M' ganglion cells concerned with detection of *movement*. The other four are parvocellular and receive the axons of 'P' cells concerned with *particulars*, namely visual detail and color.

The circuitry of the LGN resembles that of other thalamic relay nuclei, and includes inhibitory (GABA) terminals derived from internuncial neurons and from the thalamic reticular nucleus. (The portion of the reticular nucleus serving the LGN is called the **perigeniculate nucleus**.) Corticogeniculate axons arise in the primary visual cortex and synapse upon distal dendrites of relay cells as well as upon inhibitory internuncials. Cortical synapses on relay cells are twice as numerous as those derived from retinal ganglion cells. Cortical stimulation usually enhances the response of relay cells to a given retinal input. A likely, but unproven function could be that of selective enhancement of particular features of the visual scene, e.g. when searching for an object of known shape or color.

GENICULOCALCARINE TRACT AND PRIMARY VISUAL CORTEX

The **geniculocalcarine tract**, or **optic radiation**, is

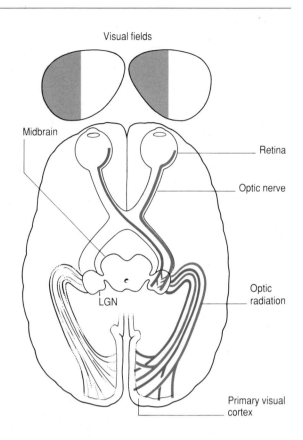

Figure 23.8   Diagram of the visual pathways. The two visual fields are represented separately, without the normal overlap.

of major clinical importance because it is frequently compromised by vascular disorders or tumors in the posterior part of the cerebral hemisphere. It travels from the lateral geniculate nucleus to the primary visual cortex.

The anatomy of the optic radiation is shown in *Figures 23.6-23.8*. Fibers destined for the lower half of the primary visual cortex sweep forward into the temporal lobe, as *Meyer's loop*, before turning back to accompany those traveling to the

---

CLINICAL PANEL 23.1

view from various directions, with the index finger wiggling.

- In a blind area, the patient does not see blackness; the patient does not see anything. (We are normally unaware of the 'blind spot' created by the optic nerve head, even with one eye closed.)
- Visual defects are described from the patient's viewpoint, in terms of the visual fields.
- Possible sites of injury to the visual pathways are shown in *Figure CP 23.1.1*. The effects produced correspond to the numbers in the following list.

Lesions	Field defects
1 Partial optic nerve	Ipsilateral scotoma[a]
2 Complete optic nerve	Blindness in that eye
3 Optic chiasm	Bitemporal hemianopia
4 Optic tract	Homonymous[b] hemianopia
5 Meyer's loop	Homonymous upper quadrant anopia
6 Optic radiation	Homonymous hemianopia
7 Visual cortex	Homonymous hemianopia
8 Macular cortex	Central scotomas (bilateral)

[a]A scotoma is a patch of blindness.
[b]Matching.

Notes on the numbered lesions

1. Eccentric lesions of the optic nerve produce scotomas in the nasal or temporal field of the affected eye. When a young adult presents with a scotoma, multiple sclerosis must always be suspected.
2. Total conduction blockage may follow head injury.
3. Compression of the middle of the chiasm is most often caused by an adenoma (benign tumor) of the pituitary gland.
4. Lesions of the optic tract are rare. Although homonymous (matching) visual fields are affected, the outer, exposed half of the tract tends to be more affected than the inner half, and the hemianopia is then described as incongruous.
5. Meyer's loop may be selectively caught by a tumor in the temporal lobe.

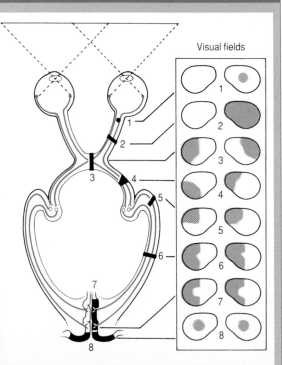

Figure CP 23.1.1 Visual field defects following various lesions of the visual pathways.

6. Lesions involving the optic radiation include tumors arising in the temporal, parietal, or occipital lobe. The visual fields of both eyes tend to be affected to an equal extent (congruously). Tumors impinging on the radiation from below produce an upper quadrantic defect at first whereas tumors impinging from above produce a lower quadrantic defect. The stem of the radiation occupies the retrolentiform part of the internal capsule and is often compromised for some days by edema, following hemorrhage from a branch of the middle cerebral artery (classical stroke, Chapter 27).
7. Thrombosis of the posterior cerebral artery produces a homonymous hemianopia. The notches in field chart no. 7 represent macular sparing. Sparing of the macular hemifields is inconstant.
8. Bilateral central scotomas are most often caused by a backward fall with occipital concussion.

upper half. The tract enters the retrolentiform part of the internal capsule and continues in the white matter underlying the lateral temporal cortex. It runs alongside the posterior horn of the lateral ventricle before turning medially to enter the occipital cortex.

The **primary visual cortex** occupies the walls of the calcarine sulcus along its entire length (the sulcus is 10 mm deep). It emerges onto the medial surface of the hemisphere for 5 mm both above and below the sulcus, and on to the occipital pole of the brain for 10 mm. Its total area is about 25 cm^2. In the freshly cut brain it is easily identified by a thin band of white matter (the *visual stria* of Gennari) within the gray matter—hence an alternative term, *striate cortex*. The left and right eyes are represented in the cortex in alternating stripes called *ocular dominance columns* (see Chapter 24).

Retinotopic map

The contralateral visual field is represented upside down. The plane of the calcarine sulcus represents the horizontal meridian. Retinal representation is posteroanterior, with a greatly magnified foveal representation in the posterior half and the monocular crescent close to the corpus callosum.

The clinical effects of various lesions of the visual pathway are described in *Panel 23.1*.

The visual cortex and higher visual areas are described in Chapter 24.

CORE INFORMATION

The embryonic retina is an outgrowth of the diencephalon. The embryonal optic cup is composed of an outer, pigment layer, an inner, nervous layer, with an intraretinal space between. The nervous layer contains three sets of radially disposed neurons, viz. photoreceptors, bipolar cells, and ganglion cells, and two tangential sets, viz. horizontal cells and amacrine cells. Except at the fovea centralis, light must pass through the other layers to reach the photoreceptors. The visual image is inverted and reversed by the lens. Two-thirds of the visual field is binocular, the outer one-sixth on each side being monocular. Visual defects are described in terms of visual fields.

Rod photoreceptors function in dim light and are absent from the fovea. Cones are most numerous in the fovea; they are responsive to shape and have three kinds of sensitivity to color. Ganglion cell responses are concentric, showing center-surround color opponency. M ganglion cells are relatively large, are movement detectors and project their axons to the two magnocellular layers of the lateral geniculate nucleus (LGN). P cells signal particular features of the image as well as color and project to the four parvocellular layers of LGN. LGN is binocular, receiving signals from the contralateral nasal hemiretina (via the optic chiasm) and from the ipsilateral temporal hemiretina. Both sets of axons arrive by the optic tract, which also gives offsets to the midbrain for low-level visual reflexes.

The geniculocalcarine tract (optic radiation) arises from M and P cells of LGN and swings around the side of the lateral ventricle to reach the primary visual cortex, in the walls of the calcarine sulcus.

Distinctive visual field defects occur following damage at any of the five major components of the visual pathway (optic nerve, chiasm, tract, radiation, visual cortex).

SELF TEST

Select the best response:

1 The nervous layer of the (embryonic) optic cup contains the following cell types, *except:*

A Pigment cells
B Photoreceptors
C Bipolar neurons
D Amacrine cells
E Ganglion cells

2 In the mature retina, impulse conduction occurs in the:

A Outer nuclear layer
B Outer plexiform layer
C Inner nuclear layer
D Inner plexiform layer
E Nerve fiber layer

3 Fibers in the medial root of the optic tract target the:

A Superior colliculus
B Pretectal nucleus
C Reticular formation
D All of the above
E A and B only

4 Match the lesion site with the visual defect:

1 Right optic nerve
2 Optic chiasm
3 Right Meyer's loop
4 Left visual cortex
5 Occipital concussion

A Bitemporal hemianopia
B Left upper quadrant hemianopia
C Right homonymous hemianopia
D Scotoma, right eye
E Bilateral central scotoma

REFERENCES

Bynke, H. (1984) The visual fields. In *Neuro-ophthalmology, Vol. 3* (Lessell, S. and van Dalen, J.T.W., eds), pp. 348-357. Amsterdam: Elsevier.

Celesia, G.G. and DeMarco, P.J. (1994) Anatomy and Physiology of the visual system. *J. Clin. Neurophysiol.* **11**: 482-492.

Curcio, C.A. and Kimberly, A.A. (1990) Topography of ganglion cells in human retina. *J. Comp. Neurol.* **300**: 5-25.

Frisen, L. (1980) The neurology of visual acuity. *Brain* **103**: 639-670.

Karten, H.J., Keyser, K.T. and Brecha, N.C. (1990) Biochemical and morphological heterogeneity of retinal ganglion cells. In *Vision and the Brain* (Cohen, B. and Bodis-Wollner, I., eds), pp. 19-33. New York: Raven Press.

Koch, C. (1987) The action of the corticofugal pathway on thalamic nuclei: a hypothesis. *Neuroscience* **23**: 399-406.

Massey, S.C. and Redburn, D.A. (1987) Transmitter circuits in the vertebral retina. *Prog. Neurobiol.* **28**: 55-96.

Vaney, D.I. (1994) Patterns of neuronal coupling in the retina. *Prog. Retl Eye Res.* **13**: 301-355.

Wu, S.M. (1994) Synaptic transmission in the outer retina. *Ann. Rev. Physiol.* **56**: 141-168.

24

CEREBRAL CORTEX

Chapter Summary

Structure
Laminar organization

Cortical areas
Sensory areas
Motor areas
Prefrontal cortex

Hemispheric asymmetries
Handedness and language
Cognitive style
Parietal lobe

CLINICAL PANELS
Frontal lobe dysfunction
The aphasias
Developmental dyslexia
Schizophrenia
Parietal lobe dysfunction

Study Guidelines

1   The cerebral cortex is the part of the body that makes us truly human. Its structure is enormously complex, and assignment of functions to different parts is made difficult, and often unrealistic, by the multiplicity of interconnections.
2   Sensory, motor, and cognitive areas of the cortex are taken in turn.
3   Although damage often leads to permanent disability, the plasticity of the cortex is of special interest to all concerned with neurorehabilitation. Examples are taken from sensory and motor areas.
4   Language functions, with their strikingly asymmetrical distribution in the great majority of the population, are of great significance in the contexts of clinical diagnosis and speech rehabilitation.
5   Also asymmetrical as a rule are the functional emphases of the parietal lobes, which are taken last because of their complex relationships.
6   Cortical functions are most often deranged by vascular lesions. For this reason, Chapters 5 (vascular anatomy), 24 (cortical functions), and 27 (clinical effects of vascular pathologies) are highly interrelated. A first reading of Chapter 27 will help to consolidate much of the new information presented here.

STRUCTURE

The cerebral cortex varies in thickness from 2 to 4 mm, being thinnest in the primary sensory areas and thickest in the motor and association areas. More than half is hidden from view in the walls of the sulci. The cortex contains about 50 billion neurons; about 500 billion neuroglial cells; and a dense capillary bed.

The cortex has both a laminar and a columnar structure. The general cytoarchitecture varies in detail from one region to another, permitting the cortex to be mapped into dozens of histologically different 'areas.' Although considerable progress has been achieved in relating individual 'areas' to specific functions, they are merely nodal points having widespread connections with other parts of the brain.

LAMINAR ORGANIZATION

A laminar (layered) arrangement of neurons is apparent in sections taken from any part of the cortex. Phylogenetically old elements, including limbic cortex in the medial temporal lobe, are trilaminar whereas six cellular laminae are seen in the **neocortex** covering the remainder of the brain.

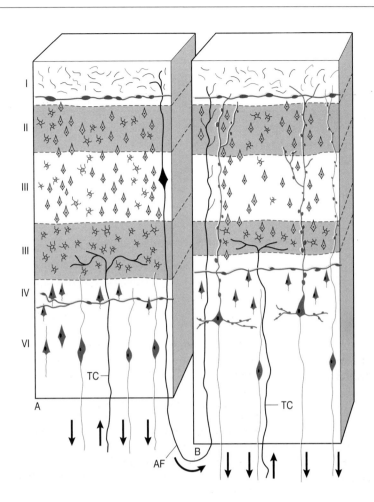

Figure 24.1 Cerebral isocortex. (A) Primary sensory cortex (somatic, visual, auditory); (B) primary motor cortex (area 4). Projection neurons are shown in red; their dendrites reach lamina I. AF, association fiber; TC, thalamocortical fiber.

Cellular laminae of the neocortex
(Figure 24.1A)

I   The **molecular layer** contains the most distal dendritic branches of the pyramidal cells, and the most distal branches of axons projecting from the intralaminar nuclei of the thalamus.

II   The **outer granular layer** contains small pyramidal and stellate cells.

III   The **outer pyramidal layer** contains medium-sized pyramidal cells projecting to other parts of the cortex.

IV   The **inner granular layer** contains stellate cells receiving afferents from the thalamic relay nuclei. Stellate cells are especially numerous in the primary somatic, primary visual, and primary auditory cortex. The term *granular cortex* is applied to these

areas. In contrast, the primary motor cortex contains relatively few stellate cells in lamina IV and is called *agranular.*

V   The **inner pyramidal layer** contains large pyramidal cells projecting to the corpus striatum, brainstem, and spinal cord.

VI   The **fusiform layer** contains modified pyramidal cells projecting to the thalamus.

Columnar organization *(Figure 24.1A)*

In the somatic sensory cortex, the neurons were discovered (in monkeys) to be arranged functionally in terms of *columns* 50-100 μm in diameter extending radially through all laminae. Within each column, all of the cells are modality-specific. For example, a given column may respond to movement of a particular joint but not to stimulation of the overlying skin. Subsequent research has shown that cell columns comprising several hundred neurons are the functional units or *modules* of the cortex. Some modules are activated by specific thalamo-cortical inputs, others by cortico-cortical inputs from the same hemisphere, others again by inputs from the opposite hemisphere. Aggregates of modules create a *cortical mosaic*.

Cell types *(Figure 24.1B, C)*

The three principal morphological cell types are pyramidal cells, spiny stellate cells, and smooth stellate cells.

- **Pyramidal cells** have cell bodies ranging in height from 20-30 μm in laminae II and III to more than twice that height in lamina V. Tallest of all, at 80-100 μm, are the *giant cells of Betz* in the motor cortex. The apical and basal dendrites of pyramidal cells branch freely and are studded with spines. The axon gives off recurrent branches before leaving the gray matter. All pyramidal cells are excitatory, and use glutamate or closely related aspartate as transmitter.
- **Spiny stellate cells** have spiny dendrites and in general are excitatory. They receive most of the afferent input from the thalamus and from other areas of the cortex, and they synapse upon pyramidal cells.
- **Smooth stellate cells** have non-spiny dendrites and in general are inhibitory. They receive recurrent collateral branches from pyramidal cells and they synapse upon other pyramidal cells. Inhibitory, GABA-secreting neurons make up about 25% of all neurons in the cerebral cortex. Some synapse upon the bases of dendritic spines, some synapse upon the somas, and some synapse upon initial axonal segments. As is the case in the cerebellar cortex (Chapter 20), the GABA neurons exert a focusing action by silencing weakly active cell columns.

Bipolar cells are found mainly in the outer laminae. Most contain one or more peptides, such as VIP (vasoactive intestinal polypeptide), CCK (cholecystokinin), or somatostatin. Peptides are also co-liberated with GABA from many smooth stellate cells.

Human cortical neurons can be captured in fragments of biopsies taken for other purposes. They can be kept alive for several hours and examined for responses to transmitters and transmitter analogs. It appears that a single pyramidal cell may have as many as ten different kinds of receptor scattered over its surface. It also appears that the response of the neuron to a particular transmitter is not completely predictable being modified by concurrent effects of other transmitters.

Afferents

Afferents to a given region of the cortex are derived from five sources:

1 Long and short **association fibers** from other parts of the ipsilateral hemisphere.
2 **Commissural fibers** from the matching region of the opposite hemisphere.
3 **Thalamocortical fibers** from the appropriate specific or association nucleus.
4 **Non-specific thalamocortical fibers** from the intralaminar nuclei.
5 **Neuraxial fibers** from the hypothalamus and brainstem. Nuclei and transmitters are as follows:

- tuberoinfundibular
  (hypothalamus):   histamine
- tegmentum (midbrain):   dopamine
- raphe nucleus (midbrain): serotonin
- locus ceruleus (pons):   norepinephrine

Targets of pyramidal neurons

- *Association fibers* are composed of axons of small pyramidal cells that loop from one part of the cortex to another within a hemisphere. Short association fibers interconnect neighboring gyri. Long association fibers, including the superior and inferior longitudinal fasciculi and the arcuate fasciculus, link different lobes of the brain. The cingulum underlying the cingulate cortex contains short and long association fibers and belongs to the limbic system (Chapter 26).
- *Commissural fibers* are composed of axons of medium-sized pyramidal cells that link matching areas of cortex on the two sides of the brain. The corpus callosum is much the largest of the commissures. Other commissures are the anterior, posterior, habenular, and hippocampal.
- *Projection fibers* are axons of large pyramidal cells that project to the basal ganglia, brainstem, and spinal cord.

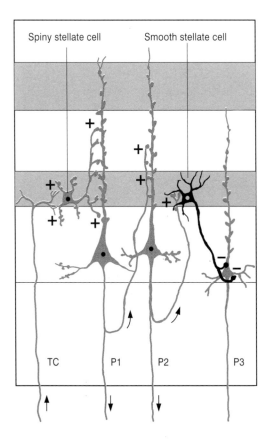

Figure 24.2 Input-output connections. Arrows indicate directions of impulse traffic. +/- signs denote excitation/inhibition. TC, thalamocortical fiber. Pyramidal cell P1 is excited by the spiny stellate cell; it excites P2 within its own cell column; P3 within a neighboring column is inhibited by the smooth stellate cell.

CORTICAL AREAS

The most widely used reference map is that of Brodmann, who divided the cortex into 47 areas on the basis of cytoarchitectural differences. Most of these areas are shown in *Figure 24.2*.

Two dominant methods are in use for localization of functions in the human cortex and other parts of the brain. Both techniques depend upon the local increases in blood flow that meet the additional oxygen demand imposed by localized neural activity.

■ *Positron emission tomography (PET)* utilizes rapid injection of water labeled with ^{15}O into a forearm vein; the positrons in the ^{15}O react with nearby electrons in the blood to create

gamma-rays which are counted by gamma-ray detectors. *Functional magnetic resonance imaging (fMRI)* does not require introduction of any extraneous material. It depends upon the different magnetic susceptibility of oxygenated versus deoxygenated blood. As it happens, the local increases in blood flow are more than sufficient to meet oxygen damands, and it is the relative excess of oxyhemoglobin that is exploited to generate the NMR signal.

SENSORY AREAS

Somatic sensory cortex (areas 3, 1, 2)

The somatic sensory or *somesthetic cortex* occupies the entire postcentral gyrus including its anterior and posterior surfaces. Representation of contralateral body parts is inverted and the hand, lips and tongue have disproportionately large representations. Separate body maps can be constructed for different modalities of sensation. Thus, slowly adapting cutaneous receptors relay to area 3, rapidly adapting ones to area 1, and articular receptors to area 2. A fourth area (called 3a), in the floor of the central sulcus, receives information relayed from muscle spindles.

In addition to thalamic afferents from the ventral posterior nucleus, the somesthetic cortex receives commissural fibers from its opposite number through the corpus callosum, and short association fibers from the motor cortex. Many of the fibers from the motor cortex are collaterals of corticospinal fibers traveling to the anterior horn of the spinal cord, and they may contribute to the *sense of weight* when an object is lifted.

Efferents from the somesthetic cortex pass to the motor cortex, to the opposite somesthetic cortex, and to area 5 of the posterior parietal cortex. In addition, projection fibers descend to sensory relay nuclei, namely the ventral posterior nucleus of the thalamus, the posterior column nuclei, and the posterior gray horn of the spinal cord. The fibers targeting the posterior column nuclei and posterior horn are incorporated in the pyramidal tract.

On the medial surface of the parietal operculum is a small *secondary somatic sensory area* (SII). It receives a larger nociceptive projection from the thalamus than does SI, and it is highlighted during PET scans of the brain during peripheral painful stimulation (Chapter 25). SII

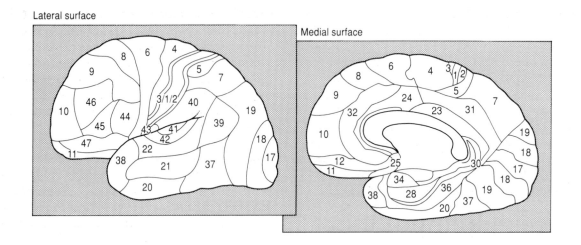

Lateral surface

Medial surface

Figure 24.3 Cytoarchitectural areas of Brodmann. (Redrawn, and slightly modified, from Zilles (1990), with permission.)

also collaborates with SI in aspects of tactile discrimination.

Area 5 is called the *supplementary sensory area* by some workers, and the *somesthetic association area* by others. In animal experiments, individual cortical modules have peripheral receptive fields covering several body segments. Many modules are *multimodal*, responding to both cutaneous and proprioceptive stimuli. Multimodal cell columns seem to provide the necessary basis for *stereognosis*—the ability to identify a three-dimensional object held in the hand without looking at it.

Plasticity of the somatic sensory cortex

In monkeys, cortical sensory representations of the individual digits of the hand can be defined very exactly by recording the electrical response of cortical cell columns to tactile stimulation of each digit in turn. These digital maps can be altered by peripheral sensory experience, as the following experiments indicate:

■ The median nerve supplies the ventral surface of the outer three digits of the hand whereas the radial nerve supplies their dorsal surfaces. If the median nerve is crushed, the representation of the dorsal surface on the digital map increases at the expense of the ventral representation. The increase begins within hours and progresses slowly over a period of weeks. With regeneration of the median nerve, the cortical map reverts to normal.

■ If the middle digit is denervated, the corresponding cortical area is unresponsive for a few hours, then becomes progressively (over weeks) taken over by expansion of the representations of the second and fourth digits.

■ If the pad skin of a digit is chronically stimulated, e.g. by having to press a rotating sanded disc in order to release pellets of food, representation of the pad may increase to twice its original size over a period of weeks, reverting to normal after the experiment is discontinued.

These experiments show that somatic sensory maps are *plastic*, being modified by peripheral events. A purely anatomical explanation (for example, sprouting of nerve branches within the CNS, or peripherally) is not appropriate for the earliest changes, which begin within hours. Instead, they can be accounted for on the basis of sensory competition.

Sensory competition

Sensory maps made at the level of the posterior gray horn, posterior column nuclei, thalamus, and somesthetic cortex all show evidence of anatomical overlap. For example, the thalamocortical somesthetic projection for the third digit overlaps its projections for the second and fourth. Within the zone of overlap, cortical columns are shared by afferents from two adjacent digits. As already explained, smooth stellate cells exert lateral inhibition upon weakly stimulated columns.

Under experimental conditions (in cats), the number of columns responding to a particular thalamocortical input can be increased by local infusion of a GABA antagonist drug, which suppresses lateral inhibition. The effect of removal of a peripheral sensory field may be comparable: if one set of thalamocortical neurons falls silent due to loss of sensory input, it no longer exerts lateral inhibition and cortical columns within its territory are taken over by neighboring, active sets.

In the human somatosensory body map, the the digits are represented next to the face. In several well documented cases of upper limb amputation, patients had later experiences of 'phantom finger' sensations on touching their face on that side with an implement such as a comb held in the other hand. This illusion may occur within two weeks of amputation. It can be explained on the basis of the unmasking of pre-existing overlap of thalamocortical neurons.

Visual cortex

The visual cortex comprises the *primary visual cortex* (area 17) and the *visual association cortex* (areas 18 and 19).

Primary visual cortex

As noted in Chapter 22, the primary visual cortex is the target of the geniculocalcarine tract, which relays information from the ipsilateral halves of both retinas, and therefore from the contralateral visual field. The myelinated fibers enter the cortex and create the visual stria (of Gennari). They terminate by synapsing upon spiny stellate cells of the highly granular lamina IV. The spiny stellate cells belong to *ocular dominance columns,* so named because alternating columns are dominated by inputs from the left and right eyes (*Figure 24.4*). In a surface view of the visual cortex, the columnar arrangement takes the form of whorls, resembling finger prints. The geniculocalcarine projection is so ordered that matching points from the two retinas are registered side by side in contiguous columns. This arrangement is ideal for binocular vision because modules at the edge of a column respond to inputs from both eyes.

Under experimental conditions (monkeys), spiny stellate cells of the primary visual cortex give 'simple' responses to slits of light of a particular orientation. Some of the pyramidal cells give 'complex' responses to bars (broad slits) of a

particular orientation; for many cells, the bar must be moving broadside in a specific direction. Other pyramidal cells are 'hypercomplex,' responding to L-shapes. This hierarchy of responses can be explained on the basis of convergence of several simple-cell axons onto complex cells and convergence of complex-cell axons on to hypercomplex cells.

Visual association cortex

Afferents to areas 18 and 19 are mainly from area 17 but include some direct thalamic projections from the pulvinar. Cell columns in areas 18 nd 19 are concerned with *feature extraction.* Some columns respond to geometrical shapes, some respond to movement in a particular direction, some respond to color, and some are involved in stereopsis (depth perception). Many columns have large receptive fields; some of these straddle the physiological blind spot (optic nerve

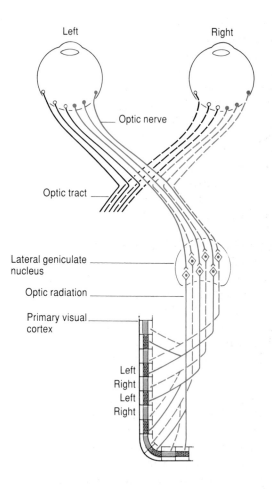

Figure 24.4 Left-eye, right-eye contributions to the ocular dominance columns in the primary visual cortex.

head) and may be responsible for 'covering up' the blind spot during monocular vision.

Outputs from the visual association cortex are mainly *dorsal* and *ventral* (*Figure 24.5*). The dorsal output (described as the 'where?' pathway) is to the posterior parietal cortex (area 7); it is concerned with stereopsis and movement and with the position of objects in relation to one another (see Parietal Lobe, later). The ventral output (the 'what?' pathway) passes to the cortex on the under surface of the temporal lobe, concerned with analysis of form and color.

The 'what?' cortex includes modules in the lingual gyrus specifically devoted to the recognition of faces. Failure of this function (*prosopagnosia*) may occur as an early and harrowing sign of Alzheimer's disease (Chapter 26): overnight, the patient may no longer recognize family members, despite retaining recognition of common objects. Lateral to the face recognition area is the color recognition area. A state of *achromatopsia* may occur following a sustained fall in blood pressure within the territory of the basilar artery (this usually includes the two posterior cerebrals); such patients see everything only in black-and-white.

How are visual association areas activated, for example in execution of a decision to look for an apple in a bowl of mixed fruit, or a particular word in a page of text? In PET studies, the frontal lobe is active whenever attention is being paid to a task at hand. The *dorsolateral frontal cortex* is particularly active during visual tasks involving form and color; the *ventrolateral frontal cortex* is particularly active during reading. During visual searching, the role of the frontal lobe seems to be to activate memory stores within the visual association areas, so that the memories are held on-line during the search. The anterior part of the cingulate cortex is also active. (The cingulate cortex is considered with the limbic system in Chapter 26.)

Plasticity of the primary visual cortex

The basic pattern and balance of ocular dominance columns is preserved in animals reared in complete darkness. On the other hand, if one eye is sealed from birth the stripes in area 17 for that eye become abnormally narrow, and those for the open eye abnormally broad. The effect can be explained on the basis of *synaptic competition*. During a critical period (6th postnatal week in monkeys), the right-eye left-eye projections from the lateral geniculate nucleus overlap extensively. As the cortex matures the redundant axonal arbors (multiple branches) are withdrawn and the column edges become sharply defined. If one eye is deprived of sensory experience from birth, the corresponding geniculocalcarine neurons branch less extensively and those from the 'experienced' eye do not withdraw.

Auditory cortex

The *primary auditory cortex* occupies the anterior transverse temporal gyrus of Heschl, as described in Chapter 16. Heschl's gyrus corresponds to areas 41 and 42 on the upper surface of the superior temporal gyrus. Columnar organization in the primary auditory cortex takes the form of *isofrequency stripes*, each stripe responding to a particular tonal frequency. Higher frequencies activate lateral stripes in Heschl's gyrus, lower frequencies activate medial stripes. Because of incomplete crossover of the central auditory pathway in the brainstem (Chapter 16), *each ear is represented bilaterally*. In experimental recordings, the primary cortex responds equally well from both ears in response to monaural stimulation but the contralateral cortex is more responsive during simultaneous binaural stimulation.

The auditory association cortex corresponds to area 22. It includes Wernicke's area for language perception (see under Language, later). Visual and auditory data are brought together in the

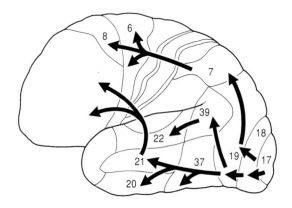

Figure 24.5 Higher visual projections. Projections to and from area 7 are concerned with location and stereopsis. Projections to and from area 20/21 are concerned with detail and color. Projections to and from area 39 are concerned with symbols including letters and numbers. Area 6 (premotor cortex) organizes motor responses to external cues. Area 8 controls contraversive visual saccades.

cortex bordering the superior temporal sulcus (junction of areas 21 and 22 in *Figure 24.2*).

Excision of the entire auditory cortex (in the course of removal of a tumor) has no obvious effect on auditory perception. The only significant defect is loss of *stereoacousis*: on testing, the patient has difficulty in appreciating the direction and distance of a source of sound.

MOTOR AREAS

Primary motor cortex

The primary motor cortex (area 4) is a strip of agranular cortex within the precentral gyrus. It gives rise to 60-80% (estimates vary) of the pyramidal tract (PT). The remaining PT fibers originate in the premotor and supplementary motor areas and in the parietal cortex, as illustrated in Chapter 13. There is an inverted somatotopic representation of contralateral body parts, with relatively large areas devoted to the hand and tongue. *Ipsilateral* body parts are also represented in the same manner, ipsilateral motoneurons being supplied by the 10% of PT fibers that remain uncrossed. The ipsilateral supply is significant in the recovery of motor function following strokes (Chapter 27).

Direct stimulation of the human motor cortex indicates that the cell columns control *movement direction*. Individual PT fibers are known to branch extensively as they approach the anterior gray horn, and to terminate on motoneuronal dendrites in nuclei serving several different muscles. The pattern of distribution of PT fibers is directed toward *movement synergy*, which in this context means the simultaneous contraction of all of the muscles concerned, with a bias among them suited to the task at hand. The act of picking up a pen, for example, requires a moderate contraction of opponens pollicis as prime mover, a matching level of contraction of the portion of flexor digitorum serving the index finger tendon, and lesser levels of contraction of adductor and flexor brevis pollicis. Steadying the upper limb as a whole during any kind of manipulative activity is a function of the premotor cortex (see later).

Plasticity in the motor cortex

In monkeys and in lower mammals, small lesions of the motor cortex produce an initial paralysis of the corresponding body part, followed within a few days (sometimes within hours) by progressive recovery. The recovery is attributable to a change of allegiance of cell columns close to the lesion, which take on the missing motor function. Instead of inflicting a lesion, it is possible to enlarge the motor territory of a patch of cortex merely by injecting a GABA antagonist drug locally into the cortex. Expansion of motor territories at spinal cord level is already provided for by extensive overlap of projections from area 4 to the motor cell columns in the ventral gray horn.

Sources of afferents to the primary motor cortex

1   *The opposite motor cortex,* through the corpus callosum. The strongest commissural linkages are between matching cell columns that control the vertebral and abdominal musculature. This is to be expected since these muscle groups routinely act bilaterally in maintaining the upright position of the trunk and head. The weakest commissural linkages are between cell columns controling the distal limb muscles, where the two sides tend to act independently.

2   *Somatosensory cortex. Cutaneous* cell columns in areas 1, 2 and 3 feed forward via short association fibers. Linkages for the hand are especially numerous; the distance is short because the hand areas of the motor and somatic sensory cortex mainly occupy the corresponding walls of the central sulcus. *Proprioceptive* cell columns in area 3a receive afferent relays from the annulospiral endings of muscle spindles; they send short association fibers to the corresponding motor columns for participation in the long-loop stretch reflex (Chapter 20).

3   *Contralateral dentate nucleus.* The cerebellum assists in the selection of appropriate muscles for synergic activities, and in the timing and strength of their contractions.

4   *Premotor cortex (PMC, area 6 on the lateral surface of the hemisphere).* The PMC is about six times larger than the primary motor cortex. It receives cognitive inputs from the frontal lobe in the context of motor intentions, and a rich sensory input from the parietal lobe (area 7) incorporating tactile and visuospatial signals. It is especially active when motor routines are run in response to visual or somatic sensory cues, e.g. reaching for an object in full view or identifying an object out of sight by manipulation. The PMC is always active bilaterally if at all. One

explanation is the need for interhemispheric transfer of motor plans through the corpus callosum. It is also the case that the PMC has a major projection to the brainstem nuclei that give origin to the reticulospinal tracts (and a minor one to the pyramidal tract). Lesions confined to the human PMC are rare, but they are characterized by postural instability of the contralateral shoulder and hip. A significant function of the PMC therefore seems to be that of bilateral postural fixation – for example, to fixate the shoulders during bimanual tasks or to stabilize the hips during walking.

5 *Supplementary motor area (SMA, area 6 on the medial surface of the hemisphere)*. In contrast to the PMC's responsiveness to external cues, the SMA responds to internal cues. In particular, it is involved in motor planning, as exemplified by the fact that SMA is activated by the frontal lobe the moment we *intend* to make a movement, even if the movement is not performed. The principal function of SMA seems to be that of preprogramming movement sequences that have already been built into motor memory. It functions in collaboration with a motor loop passing through the basal ganglia (Chapter 25) and projects to area 4 as well as contributing directly to the pyramidal tract. Unilateral lesions of SMA are associated with *akinesia* (difficulty in initiating movement) of the contralateral arm and leg. Bilateral lesions are accompanied by total akinesia, including akinesia for speech initiation.

Like PMC, the SMA is always activated bilaterally, and the interhemispheric transfer function may be the same. For example, novel motor skills learned for the right hand can be mastered relatively quickly later on by the left hand — but not if the corpus callosum has been cut.

The significance of an input to SMA from the cingulate cortex is described in Chapter 26.

Frontal eye field (*Figure 24.5*)

The frontal eye field (FEF) is mainly located in area 8, directly in front of the premotor cortex, but there is some overlap on to the precentral gyrus. The FEF is responsible (under control by the prefrontal cortex) for voluntary saccadic eye movements (Chapter 18). Both clinical and experimental (monkey) observations indicate that:

- ■ The FEFs are tonically active, bilaterally.
- ■ Increased activity in the midregion of the FEF on one side causes a horizontal saccade toward the contralateral visual hemispace (a *contraversive saccade*).
- ■ Increased activity in the upper region on one side produces an obliquely downward contraversive saccade; bilateral upper region activation causes both eyes to look straight down.
- ■ Increased lower region activity has corresponding effects with respect to upward gaze.

PREFRONTAL CORTEX

The prefrontal cortex has two-way connections with all parts of the isocortex except the primary motor and sensory areas, with its fellow through the genu of the corpus callosum, and with the mediodorsal nucleus of the thalamus. It is uniquely large in the human brain and is concerned with the highest brain functions including abstract thinking, decision making, anticipating the effects of particular courses of action, and social behavior. Any or all of these may be compromised by frontal lobe disease (*Panel 24.1*).

HEMISPHERIC ASYMMETRIES

The two cerebral hemispheres are *asymmetrical* in certain respects. Some of the asymmetries have to do with handedness, language, and complex motor activities; other, more subtle differences come under the general rubric of *cognitive style*.

HANDEDNESS AND LANGUAGE

Handedness indicates the hemisphere that is dominant for motor control. Left hemisphere/ right hand dominance is the rule. The best indicator available for population estimates of handedness is the preferred hand for writing; this criterion indicates a right hemisphere dominance for motor control in about 10% — at any rate for literate communities!

In 90% of subjects the left hemisphere is dominant for language. In 5% the right hemisphere is dominant, and in 5% the two hemispheres have an equal share. Although the left hemisphere is dominant in respect of both motor control and language, the two features are not interdependent; many lefthanders have their language areas in the left hemisphere.

FRONTAL LOBE DYSFUNCTION

General symptoms of frontal lobe disease include loss of short-term memory, lack of foresight (failure to anticipate the consequences of a course of action), and distractibility (poor concentration). These symptoms often signal the onset of Alzheimer's disease (Chapter 26). Local symptoms may be added to the general picture, if the disease process is predominantly in the dorsolateral or orbital parts of the prefrontal cortex.

Large *dorsolateral lesions* are associated with hypokinesia and apathy, with indifference to surrounding events. The picture resembles that of the 'withdrawn' type of schizophrenia, and it is of interest that in 'withdrawn' schizophrenic patients cortical blood flow may not show the anticipated increase in the dorsolateral region, in response to appropriate psychological tests.

Large *orbitofrontal* lesions are associated with hyperkinesia, with increased instinctual drives in relation to food and sexual behavior, and often with rather puerile jocularity. Hyperkinetic frontal lobe disorders have been treated in the past by means of leukotomy—a surgical procedure in which the white matter above the orbital cortex was severed through a supraorbital incision.

Language areas

Although several areas of the cortex, notably in the frontal lobe, are active during speech, two areas are specifically devoted to this function.

Broca's area (Figure 24.6)
The French pathologist Pierre Broca assigned a motor speech function to the inferior frontal gyrus of the left side in 1861. The principal premotor area for speech occupies areas 44 and 45 of Brodmann, in the inferior frontal gyrus (*Figure 24.2*). The main output of Broca's area is to cell columns in the face and tongue areas of the motor cortex. Lesions involving Broca's area are associated with expressive aphasia (see *Panel 24.2*). Some workers believe that expressive aphasia requires that the lesion should also include the lower end of the precentral gyrus.

Wernicke's area (Figure 24.6)
The German neurologist Karl Wernicke made extensive contributions to language processing in the late nineteenth century. He designated the posterior part of area 22 in the superior temporal gyrus of the left hemisphere as a sensory area concerned with understanding the spoken word. The upper surface of Wernicke's area is called the **temporal plane** (*Figure 24.7*). In the dominant hemisphere the volume of cerebral cortex in the temporal plane is much larger on that side. The lateral fissure is longer in consequence — a feature readily identified on MRI scans. Lesions involving Wernicke's area in adults are associated with receptive aphasia (see *Panel 24.2*).

Wernicke's area is linked to Broca's area by the **arcuate fasciculus,** which curves around the posterior end of the lateral fissure within the white matter deep to the supramarginal gyrus.

Right hemisphere contribution
During normal conversation there is some increase in blood flow in areas of the right hemisphere matching those of the left (*Figure 24.5*). These areas are believed to be concerned with melodic aspects of speech—the cadences, emphases, and nuances, collectively called *prosody*. Disturbances of the melodic function are called *aprosodias* (*Panel 24.2*).

Angular gyrus
The angular gyrus (area 39) belongs descriptively to the inferior parietal lobule. The *left* angular gyrus receives a projection from the inferior part of area 19 (the lingual gyrus), and itself projects to the temporal plane. It is commonly included as a part of Wernicke's area.

The angular gyrus seems to contain a neural lexicon of words, syllables, and numerical or other symbols, which can be retrieved by visual inputs—or even by visual imagery—and forwarded in the form of impulse trains to area 22. During reading, it is engaged in the conversion of written syllables ('graphemes') into the corresponding sound equivalents ('phonemes').

Modular organization of language

In alert subjects, electrical studies of the cortex exposed during neurosurgical procedures indicate the presence of a vast cortical mosaic for language. The mosaic of language modules extends along the entire length of the frontoparietal operculum above the lateral sulcus and of the temporal operculum below the sulcus. The frontoparietal operculum is predominantly concerned with the motor functions of speaking and writing, and the temporal operculum with the sensory functions of hearing and reading.

Where the planum temporale of the two hemispheres is of equal size, language functions may be bilaterally distributed. Alternatively, the planum may be underdeveloped in the language-dominant hemisphere. Maldevelopment of the planum temporale is a significant feature in cases of developmental dyslexia (*Panel 24.3*) and schizophrenia (*Panel 24.4*).

COGNITIVE STYLE

Hemispheric specializations in relation to

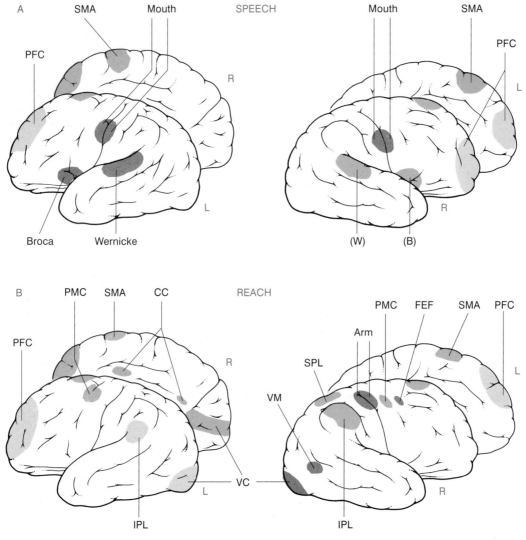

Left arm reaching into left hemispace

Figure 24.6 Areas of increased cortical metabolic activity: (A) during speech; (B) while reaching with the left arm into the left visual hemispace. CC, cingulate gyrus; FEF, frontal eye field; IPL, inferior parietal lobule; PFC, prefrontal cortex; PMC, premotor cortex; SMA, supplementary motor area; VC, visual cortex; VM, visual motion detection area. (B), (W), right hemisphere partners of Broca's and Wernicke's areas.

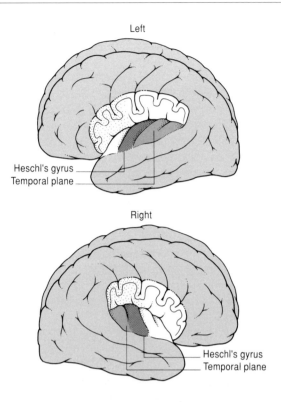

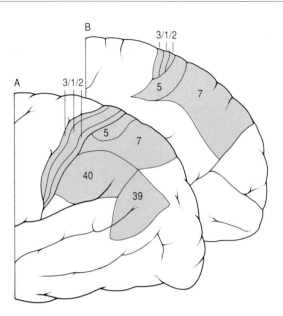

Figure 24.8 Brodmann's areas in the parietal lobe. (A) Lateral view; (B) medial view. 3/1/2, somesthetic cortex; 5, somesthetic association area; 7, posterior parietal cortex; 39, angular gyrus; 40, supramarginal gyrus.

Figure 24.7 Views of the temporal lobe, showing Heschl's gyrus (shaded) and the temporal plane (red). Both areas are on the upper surface of the temporal lobe.

information processing have been revealed by various forms of visual, auditory, and tactile tests. Results show that the left hemisphere is superior in processing information that is susceptible to *sequential analysis* of its parts whereas the right is superior in respect of *shapes* and of *spatial relationships*. Accordingly, the left hemisphere is described as being *analytical* and the right as being *holistic*. The right is also musical: there is a relative increase in blood flow in the right auditory association area when listening to music, versus a left-sided increase for words.

PARIETAL LOBE (*FIGURE 24.8*)

The parietal lobe—especially the *right* one—is of prime importance for appreciation of spatial relationships. There is also evidence that the parietal lobe—especially the left one—is concerned with initiation of movement.

Posterior parietal lobe and covert attention

Clinically, the term *posterior parietal lobe* refers

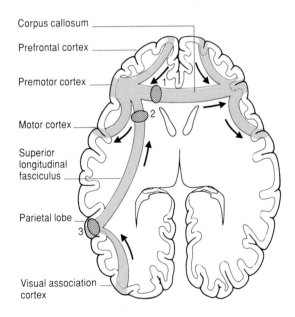

Figure 24.9 Pathways serving motor responses to sensory cues. (Adapted from Kertesz and Ferro (1984) *Brain* **107**: 921-933.) The premotor cortex is under higher control by the prefrontal cortex. For the numbers, see text.

THE APHASIAS

Aphasia is a disturbance of language function caused by a lesion of the brain. The usual cause is a stroke produced by vascular occlusion in the anterior cortical territory of the left middle cerebral artery. (Vascular lesions of the forebrain are described in Chapter 27.)

Expressive aphasia

Patients having a lesion that includes Broca's area suffer from expressive aphasia. These patients have difficulty in expressing what they want to say. Speech is slow, labored, and characteristically 'telegraphic' in style. The important nouns and verbs are spoken but prepositions and conjunctions are omitted. The patient comprehends what other people are saying and is well aware of being unable to speak fluently. There is usually an associated agraphia (inability to express thoughts in writing). If the lesion involves a substantial amount of the cortical territory of the middle cerebral artery, there will be a motor weakness of the right lower face and right arm. Because the lips are affected, the patient will also have *dysarthria* (difficulty in speech articulation) in the form of slurring of certain syllables.

Receptive aphasia

A lesion in Wernicke's area is accompanied by a deficit of auditory comprehension. (If the lesion includes the angular gyrus, the ability to read will be compromised also.) In addition to their difficulty in understanding the speech of others, these patients lose the ability to monitor their own conversation, and usually have difficulty in retrieving correct descriptive names. Speech fluency is normal but two kinds of abnormality occur in the use of nouns:

- Verbal paraphrasia (use of words usually of allied meaning): instead of 'use a knife', 'use a fork'.
- Phonemic paraphrasia (use of made-up but similar-sounding syllables): instead of 'knife and fork', 'bife and dork'.

The most striking feature of Wernicke's aphasia is that, despite garbling to the point of being unintelligible, the patient may be quite unaware of making mistakes.

Aprosodia

Lesions of the right hemisphere may affect speech in subtle ways. Lesions that include area 44 on the right tend to change the patient's speech to a dull monotone. On the other hand, lesions that involve area 22 may lead to listening errors—for example, being unable to detect inflections of speech, the patient may not know whether a particular remark is intended as a statement or as a question.

---

to area 7, which forms the bulk of the superior parietal lobule. Area 7 receives the dorsal visual outputs of the visual association cortex, concerned with stereopsis and movement. It also receives inputs from the extrageniculate visual pathway, via the pulvinar (Chapter 22), and a substantial limbic input from the anterior cingulate gyrus. It projects via the superior longitudinal fasciculus to the ipsilateral frontal eye field and premotor cortex.

In monkeys, cell columns in area 7 are activated when a significant object (e.g. fruit) appears in the contralateral visual hemifield. Through association fibers, the active cell columns increase the resting firing rate of columns in the frontal eye field and premotor cortex, but without producing movement. The effect is called *covert attention*, or *covert orientation*. It becomes *overt* when the animal responds with a saccade with or without a reaching movement directed toward the object. (The scales may be tipped by an additional input from the prefrontal cortex.) Following a lesion to area 7, the motor responses to significant targets occur late, and are inaccurate.

In human volunteers, patches of increased cortical metabolism occur in area 7 and area 24 (anterior cingulate cortex) in response to objects of interest (or to any moving object) in the contralateral visual hemifield. The right

CLINICAL PANEL 24.3

DEVELOPMENTAL DYSLEXIA

It is generally agreed that reading is a more skilled activity than speech, because it requires an exquisite level of integration of visual scanning and auditory (inner speech) comprehension. Reading is thought to activate two pathways in parallel: one passes via the angular gyrus to Wernicke's area and accesses a phonological representation of every syllable in a temporal lobe memory store; the other passes to the left dorsolateral prefrontal cortex and accesses a semantic (meaning) memory store for every word.

Developmental dyslexia affects 3-4% of literate populations. The characteristic feature is a specific and pronounced reading difficulty in children who are the match of their peers in other respects. The performance of dyslexic children can often be improved by special training. Nevertheless, severe dyslexia is known to be associated with significant developmental deficiencies in relevant parts of the brain.

■ MRI images reveal that the temporal plane of dyslexic children is smaller than average on the dominant (language) side.

■ The magnocells (M cells) of the ganglionic layer of the retina and lateral geniculate nucleus are smaller than normal and their (smaller) axons conduct more slowly. One consequence is that the scanning movements used in reading, controlled by M cell inputs to the superior colliculus (Chapter 23) are so inefficient that written syllables tend to run together and individual letters may appear to be transposed. The eyes may even be seen to wobble in an unstable manner during reading.

■ The magnocellular neurons of the medial geniculate nucleus, which project to the primary auditory cortex (Chapter 16) are also smaller than normal. The effect is one of reduced detection of the frequency and amplitude of sounds, leading to below-normal perception of words that are read aloud.

Explanations for these three developmental abnormalities are speculative. An autoimmune response to surface antigens known to be present on the surface of developing ganglion cells of the visual and auditory pathways, with consequent retardation of their growth, has been proposed. (See also Insula, in Chapter 25.)

---

hemisphere is more responsive than the left, and lesions of the right parietal lobe are more often accompanied by contralateral visual neglect (*Panel 24.5*).

Inferior parietal lobule and the body schema

Clinically, the term *inferior parietal lobule* refers to area 40, which includes the supramarginal gyrus. Area 40 receives visual information from area 7 and tactile information from area 5; also a limbic input from the posterior cingulate cortex (area 23).

The term *body schema* refers to an awareness of the existence and spatial relationships of body parts, based on previous (stored) and current sensory experience. The reality of body schema has been established by the astonishing condition known as *anosognosia* (Greek, 'unawareness of disease') in which a patient who has suffered a massive stroke involving the parietal lobe as well

as the descending motor pathways, denies ownership of the contralateral, hemiplegic side of the body. A relatively common disorder is that of *hemineglect,* where the contralateral side is ignored but can be used if attention is drawn to it (see *Panel 24.5*). Hemineglect is much commoner with a right parietal lobe lesion than a left one.

Parietal lobe and movement initiation

There are several sites for movement initiation in different behavioral contexts. The present context is the performance of learned movements of some complexity: examples would include turning a door knob, combing one's hair, blowing out a match, and clapping. It is logical to anticipate a starting point within the dominant hemisphere, because they can all be performed in response to verbal command (oral or written). This notion receives support from the observation that, if the corpus callosum has been severed surgically, the patient can perform a learned movement on

CLINICAL PANEL 24.4

SCHIZOPHRENIA

Schizophrenia occurs in about 1% of the population in all countries where the incidence has been studied. In about 10% of cases there is some evidence of a schizophrenic personality in one or more close relatives. MRI brain imaging studies reveal some degree of atrophy of frontal and temporal parts of the cortex, especially on the left side. There is a reduction or even a reversal of the usual left-right difference in the size of the planum temporale on the upper surface of the temporal lobe. In postmortem studies a substantial failure of development of the neurons that project from the medial geniculate nucleus to the primary auditory cortex on the left side has also been detected; this may be attributed to failure of the lost cells to establish proper connections with target neurons in the primary auditory cortex. The various anatomical changes can be accounted for, theoretically, on a basis of disordered cell migrations into the developing cortex during the middle trimester of gestation, with consequent failure to establish a full range of connectivities during postnatal growth.

The mode of presentation is quite variable but the behavioral changes permit most patients to be categorized into two classes: those in whom positive symptoms predominate, and those in whom negative symptoms predominate.

- *Positive symptoms* include hallucinations, delusions, and bizarre behavior. Hallucinations are typically auditory (the patient hears voices, and commonly converses with them aloud). Delusions often take a paranoid form, with a belief that one's thoughts and actions are being controlled by some outside agency. Bizarre behavior may include physical aggression in response to the hallucinations or delusions. The positive symptoms are believed to originate in the temporal lobe. Although positive symptoms may cause great alarm, they are much more responsive to treatment than the negative ones.

- *Negative symptoms* are those of withdrawal from society into a private world. The patient has little to say, and in conversation rambles from one inconsequential theme to another. There is a loss of emotional responsiveness ('flattening of affect'). Personal hygiene is a matter of indifference. The negative symptoms are attributed to 'hypofrontality,' i.e. to diminished frontal lobe function. PET scans support this idea, by demonstrating failure of the normal response of the left dorsolateral prefrontal cortex to standard tests of cognitive function.

Treatment of schizophrenia is by means of one of the antipsychotic drugs that block dopamine receptors (for example, chlorpromazine or haloperidol). These drugs are very effective in terminating bouts of bizarre behavior and in reducing the likelihood of their recurrence. A side-effect of these drugs is a tendency to provoke some of the physical symptoms of Parkinson's disease, which is known to be preceded by substantial loss of nigrostriatal dopaminergic neurons (Chapter 25). This is one reason why overactivity of the mesocortical/mesolimbic dopaminergic system (Chapter 19) is considered significant in schizophrenia, although it does not account for the mainly left-sided pathology. Another reason is the fact that symptoms closely resembling the positive ones of schizophrenia may be induced by a 'binge' of amphetamine ('speed'); amphetamine is known to increase the release of dopamine in the brain and to inhibit its re-uptake into the nerve endings that released it.

In schizophrenia, dopaminergic overactivity seems not to be a matter of overproduction but of greater effectiveness through an increased number of postsynaptic dopamine receptors on the neurons in the cerebral cortex.

command using the right hand, but not on attempting it with the left hand.

Failure to perform a learned movement on request is called *ideomotor apraxia*. It has been repeatedly observed immediately following vascular lesions at the sites shown in *Figure 24.9*.

CLINICAL PANEL 24.5

PARIETAL LOBE DYSFUNCTION

Damage to one or more parts of the parietal lobe may result from vascular occlusion within the territory of the middle cerebral artery, or from a tumor.

Somesthetic cortex

The somesthetic cortex (Brodmann's areas 3, 1, and 2) is most often compromised by rupture of a striate branch of the middle cerebral artery (classical stroke, Chapter 27). 'Cortical-type' sensory loss is shown by reduction in sensory acuity on the opposite side of the body (raised sensory threshold, poor point localization, poor two-point discrimination, loss of vibration sense and of position sense).

Sensory association cortex

Area 5 may be damaged from behind, by a tumor or vascular lesion. The classical picture is that of a patient with normal sensory acuity who cannot identify an object such as a key on palpation alone. This sign is called *astereognosis*.

Posterior parietal cortex

Lesions confined to area 7 are rare. They are associated with delayed and inaccurate saccading toward objects presented to the contralateral visual hemifield. Reaching movements into contralateral space are also inaccurate (the patient tends to knock things over).

Supramarginal gyrus

Lesions affecting area 40 are usually vascular (middle cerebral artery) and are usually concomitant with contralateral hemiplegia with or without hemianopia. However, the blood supply to this area is sometimes selectively occluded.

The characteristic result of damage to the supramarginal gyrus is *hemineglect*. The patient ignores the opposite side of the body unless attention is specifically drawn to it. A male patient will shave only the ipsilateral side of the face; a female patient will comb her hair only on the ipsilateral side. The patient will acknowledge a tactile stimulus to the contralateral side when tested alone; simultaneous testing of both sides will only be acknowledged ipsilaterally (*sensory extinction*).

Aspects of posterior parietal lobe function are affected as well. The patient tends to ignore the contralateral visual hemispace, even if the visual pathways are intact, and there is *visual extinction* (contralaterally) to simultaneous bilateral stimuli.

Hemineglect is at least five times commoner following lesions on the *right* side, irrespective of handedness.

Angular gyrus

An isolated vascular lesion of the left angular gyrus (very rare) usually produces *alexia* (complete inability to read) and *agraphia* (inability to write), because letters on the page are suddenly without any meaning. If the temporal plane has survived, patients can still name words spelt aloud to them. For *ideomotor apraxia*, see main text.

Lesions at site 1 effectively sever the corpus callosum and produce ipsilateral limb apraxia (left lesion, left limb). Lesions at either site 2 (superior longitudinal fasciculus) or site 3 (angular gyrus) may produce *bilateral* limb apraxia. In practice, right-limb apraxia may be impossible to assess because of associated right hemiplegia or receptive aphasia.

Ideomotor apraxia can be accounted for if the dominant parietal lobe is considered to contain a repertoire of learned movement programs which,

on retrieval, elicit appropriate responses by the premotor cortex on one or both sides under directives from the prefrontal cortex. (The basal ganglia would be involved as well, as described in Chapter 25.)

Ideomotor apraxia is a transient phenomenon. Because parietal blood flow increases almost equally on both sides during reaching movements (*Figure 24.5*), the right hemisphere seems to be able to assume a full role for the left arm when no longer overshadowed.

CORE INFORMATION

The cerebral cortex has both a laminar and a columnar organzation. The two basic cell types are pyramidal and stellate. Pyramidal cells occupy all of the cellular layers except lamina IV, which is rich in spiny stellate cells. Small pyramidal cells link the gyri within the hemisphere; medium-sized pyramidal cells link matching areas of the two hemispheres; the largest ones project to thalamus, brainstem, and spinal cord. Spiny stellate cells are excitatory to pyramidal cells, smooth ones are inhibitory. Columnar organization takes the form of cell columns 50-100 μm wide.

The somatic sensory cortex contains an inverted representation of body parts. Important inputs come from the VP nucleus of thalamus; important outputs go to the primary motor cortex. The primary visual cortex receives the geniculocalcarine tract. Cellular response of differing complexity depend upon convergence of simpler on to more complex cell types. The visual association areas are characterized by feature extraction e.g. motion, color, shape. Form and color extraction continues into the cortex on the under side of the temporal lobe, motion into the posterior parietal lobe. The primary auditory cortex occupies the upper surface of the superior temporal gyrus and the auditory association cortex is lateral to it.

The primary motor cortex occupies the precentral gyrus. It gives rise to most of the pyramidal tract, the body parts being represented upside down. Its main inputs are from the somatosensory cortex, cerebellum via VL nucleus of thalamus, and the premotor and supplementary motor areas. The premotor area operates mainly in response to external cues, the suppplementary motor area in response to internally generated ones. The frontal eye field is in front of the premotor cortex. Under control of the prefrontal cortex it causes contraversive conjugate movement of the eyes.

Hemispheric asymmetries mainly concern handedness, language and cognitive style. Some 10% of people are lefthanders. Language areas are leftsided in 90%, rightsided in 5% and bilateral in 5%. Broca's motor speech area occupies the inferior frontal gyrus; lesions here give rise to expressive aphasia with difficulty in writing. Wernicke's receptive speech area in the planum temporale is required for understanding the spoken word; lesions here result in receptive aphasia, and difficulty in reading if the angular gyrus is involved. The left hemisphere is usually superior in processing information susceptible to sequential analysis; the right hemisphere is superior for analysis of shapes and spatial relationships. Spatial sense requires the right posterior parietal lobe in particular. The inferior parietal lobule is concerned with the body schema; lesions here may result in neglect of personal and extrapersonal space on the opposite side. Finally, the left parietal lobe may initiate complex motor programs; lesions here may be associated with ideomotor apraxia.

SELF TEST

Answer **A** if 1, 2, and 3 only are correct
B if 1 and 3 only are correct
C if 2 and 4 only are correct
D if 4 only is correct
E if all four are correct

1 The somesthetic cortex receives direct inputs from the:

1 Thalamus
2 Opposite motor cortex
3 Ipsilateral motor cortex
4 Primary visual cortex

2 The primary visual cortex of the right side receives visual information from the:

1 Temporal field of the left eye
2 Nasal field of the left eye
3 Nasal field of the right eye
4 Temporal field of the right eye

3 Visual information forwarded to the posterior parietal cortex mainly concerns:

1 Color
2 Motion
3 Texture
4 Location

4 Pyramidal tract fibers originate from the:

1 Primary motor cortex
2 Primary sensory cortex
3 Premotor cortex
4 Supplementary motor area

5 Expressive aphasia is usually accompanied by:

1 Agraphia
2 Fluent speech
3 Dysarthria
4 Aprosodia

6 Receptive aphasia may feature:

1 Alexia
2 Slow, labored speech
3 Made-up words
4 Deafness

7 Characteristic(s) of right parietal lobe dysfunction:

1 Astereognosis
2 Contralateral neglect
3 Sensory extinction
4 Ideomotor apraxia

REFERENCES

Alexander, M.P., Baker, E., Naeser, M.A., Kaplan, E. and Palumbo, C. (1992) Neuropsychological and neuroanatomical dimensions of ideomotor apraxia. *Brain* 115: 87–107.

Ashe, J. and Ugurbil, K. (1994) Functional imaging of the motor system. *Current Opin. Neurobiol.* 4: 832–839.

Cumming, W.J.K. (1988) The neurobiology of the body schema. *Br. J. Psychiat.* 153 (Suppl. 2): 7–11.

Donoghue, J.P. and Saines, J.N. (1994) Motor areas of the cerebral cortex. *J. Clin. Neurophysiol.* 11: 382-396.

Elliott, Lois L. (1994) Functional brain imaging and hearing. *J. Acoust. Soc. Am.* 96: 1397–1408.

Celesia, C.G. (1994) Anatomy and physiology of the visual system. *J. Clin. Neurophysiol.* 11: 482–492.

Desomone, R. and Duncan, J. (1995) Neural mechanisms of selective attention. *Ann. Rev. Neurosci.* 18: 193–222.

Fuster, J.M. (1989) *The Prefrontal Cortex.* New York: Raven Press.

Galaburda, A.M., Menard, M.T. and Rosen, T.D. (1994) Evidence for aberrant auditory anatomy in developmental dyslexia. *Proc. Natl Acad. Sci. USA* 91: 8010-8013.

Halsband, U. and Freund, H.-J. (1993) Motor learning. *Current Opin. Neurobiol.* 3: 940–949.

Innocenti, G. (1994) Some new trends in the study of the corpus callosum. *Behav. Brain Res.* 64: 1–8.

Jncke, L., Schlaug, G., Huang, Y. and Steinmetz, H. (1994) Asymmetry of the planum temporale. *Neuroreport* 5: 1161–1163.

Kaas, J. H. (1991) Plasticity of sensory and motor maps in adult mammals. *Ann. Rev. Neurosci.* 14: 137–167.

Kertesz, A., Polk, M., Black, S.E. and Howell, J. (1992) Anatomical asymmetries and functional laterality. *Brain* 115: 589–605.

Lang, W., Hollinger, P., Eghker, A. and Lindinger, D. (1994) Functional localization of motor processes in the primary and supplementary motor areas. *J. Clin. Neurophysiol.* 11: 397–419.

Liotti, M., Gay, C.T. and Fox, P.T. (1994) Functional imaging and language. *J. Clin. Neurophysiol.* **11:** 175–190.

McCormick, D.A. and Williamson, A. (1989) Convergence and divergence of transmitter action in human cerebral cortex. *Proc. Natl Acad. Sci. USA* **86:** 8098–8102.

Naas, R. (1994) Advances in reading difficulties. *Current Opin. Neurol.* **7:** 179–186.

Perelle, I.B. and Ehrman, N.D. (1994) An international study of human handedness: the data. *Behav. Genet.* **24:** 217–225.

Posner, M.J. (1994) Attention: the mechanisms of consciousness. *Proc. Natl Acad. Sci. USA* **91:** 7398–7403.

Sakata, H. and Taira, M. (1994) Parietal control of hand action. *Current Opin. Neurobiol.* **4:** 847–856.

Salin, P.-A. and Bullier, J. (1995) Corticocortical connections in the visual system: structure and function. *Physiol. Rev.* **75:** 107–154.

Schwartz, A.B. (1994) Distributed motor processing in cerebral cortex. *Current Opin. Neurobiol.* **4:** 840–846.

Silbersweig, D.A. *et al.* (1995) A functional neuroanatomy of hallucinations in schizophrenia. *Nature* **378:** 176–179.

Stein, J.F. (1994) Developmental dyslexia, neural timing, and hemispheric lateralisation. *Intl J. Neurophysiol.* **18:** 241–249.

Tanji, J. (1994) The supplementary motor area in the cerebral cortex. *Neurosci. Res.* **19:** 251–268.

Ungerlieder, L.G. (1995) Functional brain imaging studies of cortical mechanisms for memory. *Science* **270:** 769–775.

Weinberger, N.M. (1995) Dynamic regulation of receptive fields and maps in the adult sensory cortex. *Ann. Rev. Neurosci.* **18:** 129–158.

Zilles, K. (1990) Cortex. In *The Human Nervous System* (Paxinos, G., ed) , pp. 757–802. San Diego: Academic Press.

Zilles, K. *et al.* (1995) Mapping of human and macaque sensorimotor areas by integrating architectonic, transmitter receptor, MRI and PET data. *J. Anat.* **187:** 515-538.

25

BASAL GANGLIA

Chapter Summary

Introduction

Basic circuits
Motor loop
Associational loop
Limbic loop
Oculomotor loop

CLINICAL PANELS
Hypokinesia: Parkinson's
    disease
Hyperkinesia

Study Guidelines

The contributions of the basal ganglia to motor control systems is the subject of intense research at basic and clinical levels. In this account, the open-loop pathways linking different areas of the cerebral cortex through the basal ganglia are highlighted. Particular emphasis is placed on the braking and release mechanisms inherent in the arrangement of sequential sets of inhibitory neurons.

Pathological changes within the basal ganglia are associated with several kinds of motor disorders, both in children and adults.

INTRODUCTION

The term 'basal ganglia' is used to designate the areas of basal forebrain and midbrain known to be involved in the control of movement (*Figure 25.1*). It includes:

- The **striatum** (mainly the caudate nucleus and the putamen of the lentiform nucleus, but also including the nucleus accumbens which belongs to the limbic system).
- The **pallidum** (globus pallidus), which comprises an *external part* and an *internal part* (the internal part has a midbrain extension known as the **pars reticulata** of the **substantia nigra**).
- The **subthalamic nucleus.**
- The main, pigmented component of **substantia nigra** known as the **pars compacta.**

Thalamic nuclei specifically devoted to basal gangliar function are the **ventral anterior nucleus** and the anterior part of the **ventral lateral nucleus.** The thalamic **mediodorsal nucleus** is involved in a cognitive pathway.

BASIC CIRCUITS

It is possible to demonstrate at least four open-loop circuits. All four commence in the cerebral cortex, traverse the basal ganglia and return to different areas of the cortex. They comprise:

1 a *motor loop*, concerned with learned movements;
2 a *cognitive loop*, concerned with motor intentions;
3 a *limbic loop*, concerned with emotional aspects of movement;
4 an *oculomotor loop*, concerned with voluntary saccades.

MOTOR LOOP

The clinically important motor loop commences in the sensorimotor cortex and returns to the supplementary motor area.

Figure 25.2 is derived from *Figure 25.1A*, representing a coronal section through the posterior part of the striatum. The figure depicts

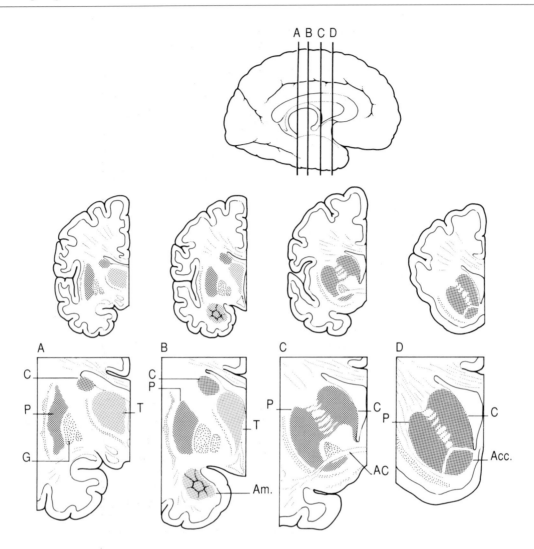

Figure 25.1 Four coronal sections of the brain, viewed from behind. Ventral parts enlarged below. Acc., nucleus accumbens; AC, anterior commissure; Am., amygdala; C, caudate nucleus; G, globus pallidus; P, putamen; T, thalamus.

component parts of the motor loop which include the putamen, pallidum and ventral lateral nucleus of the thalamus.

Figure 25.3 is a schematic representation of the component elements. Note that the middle part of the loop splits into two pathways from striatum to thalamus: a one-station *direct* pathway via the internal part of the pallidum (GPi), and a three-station *indirect* pathway via the external part of the pallidum (GPe), the subthalamic nucleus (STN), and the internal part of the pallidum (GPi). GPi is common to both pathways. The onward projection to the ventrolateral nucleus of the thalamus runs partially superficial to the crus cerebri, as the **ansa lenticularis** (*Fig. 25.2*) and partially through the crus as the **lentic-**

ular fasciculus. Notice that the projections from striatum (shown in black) to both segments of pallidum are *inhibitory* (GABAergic) as are the onward projections from the pallidum.

The *nigrostrial pathway* projects from substantia nigra, pars compacta to the striatum, where it makes two kinds of synapses upon the projection neurons. Those upon direct pathway neurons are facilitatory, by way of dopaminergic type 1 receptors (D1) on the dendritic spines; those upon indirect pathway neurons are inhibitory, by way of D2 receptors. The cholinergic internuncials are excitatory to projection neurons; they are inhibited by dopamine.

A healthy substantia nigra is tonically active, favoring activity in the direct pathway.

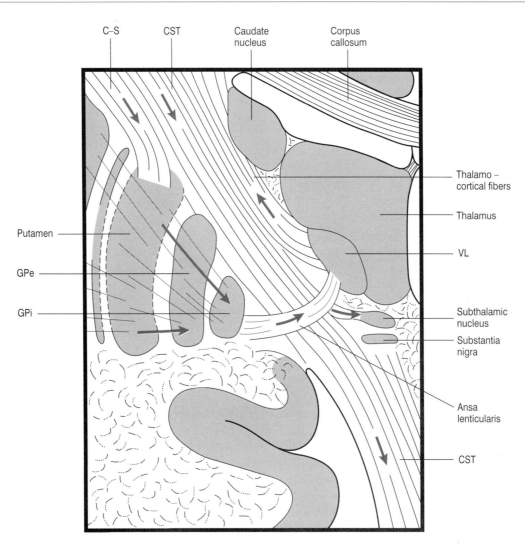

C–S   CST   Caudate nucleus   Corpus callosum

Thalamo – cortical fibers

Thalamus

Putamen

VL

GPe

GPi

Subthalamic nucleus

Substantia nigra

Ansa lenticularis

CST

Figure 25.2 Coronal section through the motor loop, based on *Figure 25.1A*. Arrows indicate directions of impulse traffic. *Note* the following:

1   Corticostriate fibers (C-S) are running from the somatic sensory and primary motor cortex to the putamen.
2   The corticospinal tract (CST) gives fibers to the subthalamic nucleus.
3   The putamen projects into the external and internal segments of the globus pallidus (GPe and GPi). GPi projects to the ventrolateral (VL) nucleus of thalamus. VL projects to the supplementary motor area, as shown in *Figure 25.3*.

Facilitation of the direct pathway is necessary for the supplementary cortex (SMA) to become active before and during movement. SMA activity immediately prior to movement can be detected by means of recording electrodes attached to the scalp. This activity is known as the (electrical) *readiness potential,* and it is produced by silencing of GPi neurons with consequent liberation (by *disinhibition*) of thalamocortical neurons traveling to SMA, with follow-through to the sensorimotor cortex for the initiation of movement.

There is a somatotopic organization of the projections from the putamen and globus pal-

lidus, permitting selective facilitation of neurons relevant to (say) arm movements via the direct route, with simultaneous disfacilitation of unwanted (say) leg movements via the indirect route. For suppression of unwanted movements, the subthalamic nucleus (STN), acting upon the body map in GPi, is especially important, since we know that destruction of STN results in uncontrollable spontaneous movements on the opposite side of the body.

A fall in dopamine production by substantia nigra, pars compacta results in facilitation of the *indirect* pathway, because of withdrawal of D1

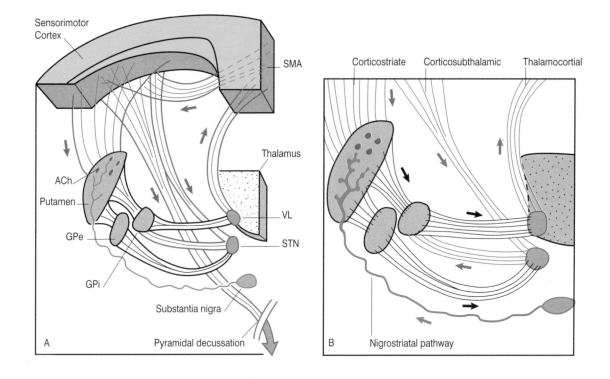

Figure 25.3   Details of the motor loop. Pink/red = excitatory; gray/black = inhibitory. Arrows indicate directions of impulse traffic. **(A)** General scheme. **(B)** Enlargement from A omitting the corticospinal tract. Note that the direct pathway from the sensorimotor cortex and back again involves five projections in sequence; the indirect pathway involves seven.

facilitation of the direct pathway and of D2 inhibition of the indirect pathway. Increased activity of the (inhibitory) striatum-GPe connection suppresses activity in the GPe-STN connection. The subthalamic nucleus is thereby disinhibited (liberated), with consequent excitation of the (inhibitory) neurons of GPi; followthrough inhibition of the ventral lateral nucleus of the thalamus; and (in consequence) reduced activity in SMA and motor cortex. This is a feature of *Parkinson's disease*, described in *Panel 25.1*.

Although movements can be produced on the opposite side of the body by direct electrical stimulation of the healthy putamen, the basal ganglia do not normally initiate movements. Nevertheless, they are active during all kinds of movement, whether fast or slow. They seem to be involved in *scaling the strength* of muscle contractions and, in collaboration with SMA, in *organizing the requisite sequences* of excitation of cell columns in the motor cortex. They come into action after the corticospinal tract has already been activated by 'premotor' areas including the cerebellum. Because patients with

Parkinson's disease have so much difficulty in performing internally generated movement sequences, it is believed that the putamen provides a reservoir of learned motor programs which it is able to assemble in appropriate sequence for the movements decided upon, and to transmit the coded information to SMA.

There is some uncertainty about a role for the basal ganglia in motor learning, i.e. in the acquisition of new motor skills. In monkey experiments, single-cell recordings from the putamen indicate that motor learning is likely. On the other hand, PET scans in human volunteers demonstrate increased blood flow through the putamen, of much the same magnitude whether a contralateral movement is new or routine, fast or slow, internally generated or in response to external cues — or even when a movement is only being imagined. In the cerebellum, by contrast, blood flow is significantly greater during procedural learning (acquisition of a new motor skill). Since the basal ganglia are concerned with optimizing patterns of muscular activity during motor performance, this know-how could be dis-

CLINICAL PANEL 25.1

HYPOKINESIA: PARKINSON'S DISEASE

Parkinson's disease (PD) affects about 1% of people over 50 years of age in all countries. The primary underlying pathology is degeneration of nigrostriatal neurons, causing an increase of striatal activity with a shift from the direct to the indirect motor pathway. The main line of treatment is by intake of *levodopa,* which is metabolized to dopamine during passage through the blood–brain barrier. The following symptoms/signs are characteristic, although not all are expressed in every patient: akinesia, bradykinesia, rigidity, tremor, and impairment of postural reflexes.

■ *Akinesia* is defined as a difficulty in movement initiation. It takes major voluntary effort to begin to get up from a chair. Akinesia is explained on the basis of inadequate direct-pathway activation of SMA, with consequent reduction in amplitude of the readiness potential and reduced input to the motor cortex.

■ *Bradykinesia* means slowness of movement. Patients report that routine activities, such as opening a door, require deliberate planning and consciously guided execution. Electromyographic studies of the limb musculature show a reduction of the 'initial agonist burst' of electrical change accompanying the first contraction of relevant prime movers. Normally, the basal gangliar contribution to movement comes on stream some milliseconds after the premotor cortex and cerebellum have raised the firing rate of motor-cortex neurons to threshold at spinal motoneuron level. In PD the boost to lower motorneuron activation is weak, because of the weakened contribution from SMA. Exaggerated proprioceptive feedback from the musculature (see below) may contribute to bradykinesia by falsely indicating the level of muscular performance.

■ *Rigidity.* Rigidity affects all of the somatic musculature simultaneously, but a predilection for flexors imposes a stooped posture. Passive flexion and extension of the joints show resistance through the full range of movement. The term 'lead pipe rigidity' is used to distinguish it from the 'claspknife rigidity' of the spastic state that accompanies upper motor neuron lesions.

Rigidity in Parkinson's disease is caused by an exaggerated response to the normal proprioceptive inflow from the muscles. Historically, it has been abolished by section of dorsal nerve roots, thus proving its peripheral sensory origin. It can also be alleviated by a surgical lesion of the pallidum or of the VL nucleus of the thalamus.

It is a maltter of current debate whether there is loss of an inhibitory influence descending direct to the reticular formation from some cells in GPi, or whether the striatum is abnormally responsive to a long-loop proprioceptive reflex relayed to the sensori-motor cortex and fed into the motor loop.

■ *Tremor.* Tremor at 3-6 Hz is usual and may be the leading clinical feature. Typically, it involves muscle groups at rest, fading during voluntary movement and during sleep. (Cerebellar tremor, in contrast, is usually absent at rest and is brought out by voluntary movement.) Rhythmic head-nodding and rhythmic movements of the fingers and hands may be obvious. During passive movement of the joints, a subtle underlying tremor may give rise to ratchety 'cogwheeling'.

Tremor is associated with rhythmic bursting activity of cells in the striatum, pallidum and VL nucleus of thalamus, and in anterior horn cells of the spinal cord. Because bursting activity can be abolished by rigid fixation of the tremulous body part, the explanation would seem to lie in release of spinal reflex arcs from tonic inhibition (perhaps from GPi), with the effect of setting up a flip-flop reciprocal inhibition of opposing muscle groups.

■ *Impairment of postural reflexes.* Patients go off balance easily, and tend to fall stiffly ('like a telegraph pole') in response to a mild accidental push. The underlying fault is an impairment of anticipatory postural adjustments: normally, a push to the upper part of the body elicits immediate contraction of lower limb muscles appropriate for the maintenance of equilibrium.

Two other symptoms, oculomotor hypokinesia and dementia, are mentioned in the main text.

tributed through SMA to the motor cortex and perhaps to the cerebellum, for storage in the form of facilitated cell assemblies.

COGNITIVE LOOP

The caudate nucleus receives inputs from all of the association areas of the cortex. From the caudate, the loop passes through the pallidum and the ventral anterior (VA) nucleus of the thalamus. The VA nucleus projects to the prefrontal cortex. The cortical connections of the caudate suggest that it participates in planning ahead, particularly with respect to complex motor intentions.

LIMBIC LOOP

The limbic loop passes from the cingulate gyrus and amygdala through the nucleus accumbens (ventral striatum) and the ventral pallidum, returning via the mediodorsal thalamic nucleus to the premotor cortex and SMA. The limbic loop is likely to be involved in giving motor expression to emotions, for example through

---

CLINICAL PANEL 25.2

HYPERKINESIA

Hyperkinetic states are characterized by spontaneous (involuntary) muscle contractions. They are most often seen in children, in association with cerebral palsy.

CEREBRAL PALSY

Cerebral palsy is an umbrella term covering a variety of motor disorders arising from damage to the brain in the perinatal period. The incidence is about 2 per 1000 live births in all countries. The most frequent association is with *prematurity* at the time of birth. Immaturity of the lungs may result in insufficient oxygenation of the brain. Immaturity of the thyroid gland may also be significant (thyroxine is required for normal development of the cerebral cortex). The pathology usually takes the form of softening of the white matter surrounding the ventricles, probably in consequence of some circulatory disturbance. Patients having involuntary movements also have damage to the basal ganglia.

During the early postnatal months affected children are usually 'floppy' (atonic), changing to a spastic state by the end of the first year. Remarkably, about half of children who are spastic at the age of two will be completely normal by the age of five, while most of the remainder 'grow into their disability' and become more severely affected.

Choreoathetosisis is a consequence of basal gangliar damage (*Figure 25.4*). *Chorea* refers to spontaneous twitching of various muscle groups in a more or less random manner, which interferes with voluntary movements.

Athetosis refers to writhing movements which may be so severe as to prevent sitting or standing. Waxing and waning of muscle tone commonly cause the head to roll about. Spontaneous movements are regarded as an escape phenomenon resulting from damage to the striatum and/or subthalamic nucleus. Such damage would cause GPi to become relatively silent, allowing the VL nucleus of thalamus the freedom to fire spontaneously.

HEMIBALLISM

Hemiballism (or hemiballismus) tends to occur in the elderly. It is known to result from thrombosis of a small branch of the posterior cerebral artery supplying the subthalamic nucleus. The condition is perhaps the most remarkable one in the whole of clinical neurology. It is marked by the abrupt onset of wild, flailing movements of the contralateral arm, sometimes of the leg as well. The appearances suggest that the thalamocortical pathway from VL to SMA has gone completely out of control.

HUNTINGTON'S CHOREA

Huntington's chorea is an autosomal (chromosome 4) dominant, inherited disease which occurs in 50% of the offspring of affected families. Onset of symptoms is usually delayed until the forties. The clinical history is one of chronic, progressive chorea, often with athetoid movements superimposed. Sooner or later, a progressive dementia sets in.

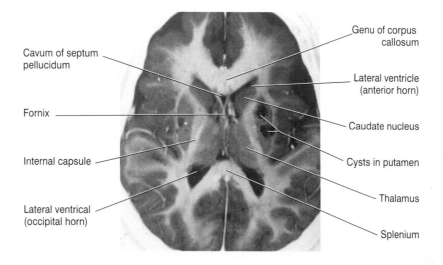

Cavum of septum
pellucidum

Fornix

Internal capsule

Lateral ventrical
(occipital horn)

Genu of corpus
callosum

Lateral ventricle
(anterior horn)

Caudate nucleus

Cysts in putamen

Thalamus

Splenium

Figure 25.4 Horizontal MRI 'slice' at the level of the corpus striatum from a 2-year-old girl suffering from severe choreoathetosis as a result of intrauterine infection (toxoplasmosis). The putamen on both sides is partly replaced by cysts. (Photograph kindly provided by Dr Paul Finn, Director, MR Research and Development, Siemens Medical Systems Inc., Iselin, New Jersey)

smiling or gesturing, or adoption of aggressive or submissive postures. The loop is rich in dopaminergic nerve endings, and their decline may account for the mask-like facies and absence of spontaneous gesturing characteristic of Parkinson's disease; also (in part) for the *dementia* which may set in after several years.

OCULOMOTOR LOOP

The oculomotor loop commences in the **frontal eye field** (area 8) and **posterior parietal cortex** (area 7). It passes through the caudate nucleus and through the substantia nigra, pars reticulata (SNpr). It returns via the ventral anterior nucleus of the thalamus to the frontal eye field and prefrontal cortex. SNpr sends an inhibitory (GABA) projection to the superior colliculus, where it synapses upon the cells controlling automatic saccades (Chapter 18). When the eyes are at rest, SNpr is tonically active.

Whenever a deliberate saccade is made toward an object of interest, the appropriate gaze center is activated by the direct projection from the frontal eye field. The oculomotor loop is activated at the same time and the superior colliculus is disinhibited (just as the VL nucleus is disinhibited when the somatic motor loop is activated). The superior colliculus then discharges to reinforce the activity of the direct pathway. Maximum speed (80 km/h) is achieved instantly.

In Parkinson's disease, *oculomotor hypokinesia* can be revealed by special tests. Saccades toward targets in the peripheral visual field tend to be slow, and sometimes inadequate. The hypokinesia can be explained on the basis of faulty disinhibition of the superior colliculus following associated degeneration of SNpr.

Other disorders involving the basic ganglia include several *hyperkinetic states* briefly described in *Panel 25.2*.

CORE INFORMATION

The basal ganglia are nuclear groups involved in movement control. They comprise the striatum, the nucleus accumbens, the pallidum; the subthalamic nucleus (STN), the substantia nigra pars compacta, and motor nuclei of the thalamus. The bulk of the pallidum is divided into an external segment (GPe) and an internal segment (GPi), the latter tapering into the midbrain as the substantia nigra, pars reticulata. Four open-loop circuits commence in the cerebral cortex, pass through the basal ganglia, and return to different areas of the cortex. The substantia nigra, pars compacta stands to one side of the circuits but influences them by way of the nigrostriatal pathway.

Cortical inputs to the striatum and STN are excitatory. Striatal outputs are inhibitory to the pallidum so, as the pallidal outputs to STN and thalamus. STN is excitatory to GPi.

The direct pathway, striatum → GPi is facilitated by the normal tonic activity of nigrostriatal dopaminergic neurons. The indirect pathway, striatum GPe → STN → GPi is inhibited. For the motor circuit, facilitation of the direct pathway is necessary for the SMA to become active before and during movement. SMA activity immediately prior to movement appears on EEG as the readiness potential, and it is produced by silencing of GPi neurons with consequent liberation (disinhibition) of thalamocortical neurons to SMA, with follow-through to SMC for the initiation of movement.

Striatum and pallidum are somatotopically organized, permitting selective activation of body parts; STN is especially important for inhibition of unwanted movements.

The main function of the motor loop seems to be the appropriate sequencing of serial order actions for the execution of learned motor programs. In Parkinson's disease, the loss of nigrostriatal dopaminergic neurons means that the indirect pathway becomes dominant, with follow-through suppression of VL and reduced SMA activity, thus accounting for the characteristic akinesia. Bradykinesia, rigidity, tremor, and impairment of postural reflexes are explained in the Clinical Panel.

The cognitive loop begins in association cortex, and returns via VA nucleus of thalamus to the premotor cortex and prefrontal areas. It seems to be concerned with advance planning for later movements. The limbic loop begins in cingulate cortex and amygdala, passes through nucleus accumbens and returns to SMA; it is probably involved in giving physical expression to the current emotional state. The oculomotor loop involves the frontal eye field and the substantia nigra, pars reticulata. It acts to liberate the superior colliculus for execution of saccadic movents of the eyes.

Hyperkinetic states include many cases of cerebral palsy; also Huntington's chorea and hemiballism.

SELF TEST

Answer **A** if the item is associated with A only
B if associated with B only
C if associated with both A and B
D if associated with neither A nor B

A Putamen
B Globus pallidus
C Both
D Neither

1 In receipt of excitatory inputs from sensorimotor cortex A
2 Chief transmitter is GABA A
3 Contain(s) cholinergic neurons
4 Inhibitory to motor nuclei of thalamus B

5 Part of a motor circuit traversing the basal ganglia

A Substantia nigra pars compacta
B Substantia nigra pars reticulata
C Both
D Neither

6 Contained in tegmentum of midbrain
7 Dopaminergic
8 Glutamatergic
9 Defective in Parkinson's disease
10 Inhibitory to superior colliculus

REFERENCES

Albin, R.L., Young, A.B. and Penney, J.B. (1989) The functional anatomy of basal ganglia disorders. *Trends Neurosci.* **12**: 366–375.

Alheid, G.F., Heimer, L., and Switzer, R.C. (1990) Basal ganglia. In *The Human Nervous System* (Paxinos, G., ed.), pp. 483–582. San Diego: Academic Press.

Berger, W., Discher, M., Trippel,M., Ibrahim, I.K. and Dietz, V. (1992) Developmental aspects of stance regulation, compensation and adaptation. *Exp. Brain Res.* **90**: 610–619.

Brooks, D.J. (1995) The role of the basal ganglia in motor control: contributions from PET. *J. Neurol. Sci.* **128**: 1–13.

DeLong, M.R. (1990) Primate models of movement disorders of basal ganglia origin. *Trends Neurosci.* **13**: 281–289.

Gentile, A.M. (1992) The nture of skill acquisition: therapeutic implications for children with movement disorders. In *Movement Disorders in Children* (Forssberg, H. and Hirschfeld, H., eds), pp. 31–40. Basel: Karger.

Goldman-Rakic, P.S. and Selemon, L.D. (1990) New frontiers in basal ganglia research. *Trends Neurosci.* **13**: 241–244.

Graybiel, A.M., Aosaki, T., Flaherty, W. and Kimura, M. (1994) The basal ganglia and adaptive motor control. *Science* **265**: 1826–1831.

Kuban, K.C.K. and Leviton, A. (1994) Cerebral palsy. *New Engl. J. Med.* **330**: 188–195.

Leonard, C.T. (1994) Motor behavior and neural changes following perinatal and adult-onset brain damage: implications for therapeutic interventions. *Phys. Ther.* **74**: 753–767.

Marsden, C.D. and Obeso, J.A. (1994) The functions of the basal ganglia and the paradox of stereotaxic surgery in Parkinson's disease. *Brain* **117**: 877–897.

Meara, R.J. (1994) Review: the pathophysiology of the motor signs in Parkinson's disease. *Age and ageing* **23**: 342–346.

Smith, A.D. and Bolam, J.P. (1990) The neural network of the basal ganglia as revealed by the study of synaptic connections of identified neurones. *Trends Neurosci.* **13**: 259–271.

Stanley, F.J. (1994) The aetiology of cerebral palsy. *Early Hum. Dev.* **36**: 81–88.

Summers, J.J. (1994) The pathogenesis of gait hypokinesia in Parkinson's disease. *Brain* **117**: 1169–1181.

26

OLFACTORY AND LIMBIC SYSTEMS

Chapter Summary

Olfactory system
Olfactory epithelium
Olfactory bulb

Limbic system
Parahippocampal gyrus
Hippocampal formation
Insula
Cingulate cortex and posterior parahypocampal gyrus
Septal area
Amygdala
Basal forebrain

CLINICAL PANELS
Olfactory disturbance
Temporal lobe epilepsy
Alzheimer's disease

Study Guidelines

Olfactory system
In most vertebrates the olfactory system is altogether more important than it is in humans. Clinically, its main interest is that damage to the olfactory pathway on one side is associated with anosmia on that side. Taste is the only other uncrossed sensation.
    Olfactory function is tested by inhalation of volatile substances.

Limbic system
The limbic system developed phylogenetically in close association with the olfactory system. Cortical and subcortical limbic areas are prominent features of the brain in primitive mammals, where they are intimately concerned with mechanisms of attack and defense, procreation, and feeding.
    The principal effector elements of the limbic system are the hypothalamus and the reticular formation. Studies in higher mammals have shown important relationships between limbic elements and memory.

OLFACTORY SYSTEM

The olfactory system is remarkable in four respects:

1   The somas of the primary afferent neurons occupy a surface epithelium.
2   The axons of the primary afferents enter the cerebral cortex directly; second-order afferents are not interposed.
3   The primary afferent neurons undergo continuous turnover, being replaced from stem cells.
4   The pathway to the highest cortical centers (in the frontal lobe) is entirely ipsilateral.

The olfactory system comprises the olfactory epithelium and olfactory nerves; the olfactory bulb and tract; and several patches of olfactory cortex.

OLFACTORY EPITHELIUM

The olfactory epithelium occupies the upper one-fifth of the lateral and septal walls of the nasal cavity. The epithelium contains three cell types (*Figure 26.1*):

1   **Olfactory neurons**. These are bipolar neurons, each with a dendrite extending to the epithelial surface and an unmyelinated axon contributing to the olfactory nerve. The dendrites are capped by immotile cilia containing molecular receptor sites. The axons run upward through the cribriform ('sieve-like') plate of the ethmoid bone and enter the olfactory bulb. The axons (some 3 million on each side) are grouped into fila (bundles) by investing Schwann cells. The collective fila constitute the **olfactory nerve**.

2 **Sustentacular cells** are interspersed among the bipolar neurons.

3 **Basal cells** lie between the other two cell types. Olfactory bipolar neurons are unique among mammalian neurons in that they undergo a continuous cycle of growth, degeneration and replacement. The basal cells transform into fresh bipolar neurons, which survive for about a month. Replacement declines over time, accounting for the general reduction in olfactory *acuity* with age.

OLFACTORY BULB *(FIGURE 26.1)*

The olfactory bulb consists of three-layered, allocortex surrounding the commencement of the olfactory tract. The chief cortical neurons are some 50 000 **mitral cells,** which receive the olfactory nerve fibers and give rise to the olfactory tract.

Contact between olfactory fibers and mitral cell dendrites takes place in some 2000 **glomeruli,** which are sites of innumerable synapses and have a glial investment. Glomeruli which are 'on-line' (active) inhibit neighboring, 'off-line' glomeruli through the mediation of GABAergic **periglomerular cells** (cf. the horizontal cells of the retina). Mitral cell activity is also sharpened at a deeper level by **granule cells,** which are devoid of axons (cf. the amacrine cells of the retina). The granule cells receive excitatory dendrodendritic contacts from active mitral cells and they suppress neighboring mitral cells through inhibitory (GABA) dendrodendritic contacts.

Central connections

Mitral-cell axons run centrally in the **olfactory tract** *(Figure 26.2)*. The tract divides in front of the anterior perforated substance into **medial** and **lateral olfactory striae.**

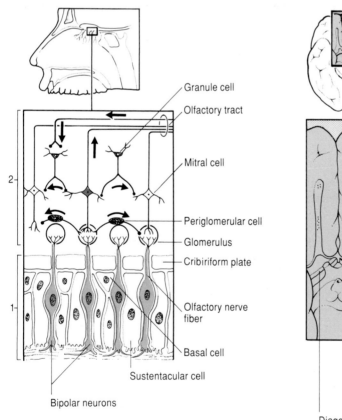

Figure 26.1 Connections of olfactory epithelium and olfactory bulb. The second glomerulus from the left is 'on line' (see text).

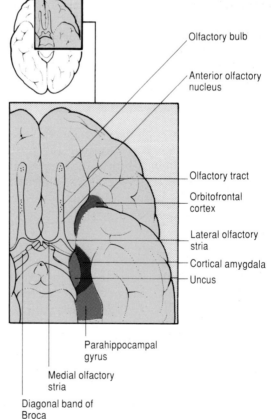

Figure 26.2 Brain viewed from below, showing cortical olfactory areas.

The medial stria contains axons from the **anterior olfactory nucleus,** which consists of multipolar neurons scattered within the olfactory tract. Some of these axons travel to the septal area via the diagonal band (see later, under Limbic System). Others cross the midline in the anterior commissure and inhibit mitral cell activity in the contralateral bulb (by exciting granule cells there). The result is a relative enhancement of the more active bulb, providing a directional cue to the source of olfactory stimulation.

The lateral olfactory stria terminates in the **piriform lobe** of the anterior temporal cortex. The human piriform lobe includes the cortical part of the amygdala, the uncus, and the anterior end of the parahippocampal gyrus. The highest center for olfactory discrimination is the posterior part of the orbitofrontal cortex, which receives connections from the piriform lobe via the mediodorsal nucleus of the thalamus.

Several pathways link the olfactory cortical areas with the hypothalamus and brainstem (for some details, see under Limbic System). These linkages trigger autonomic responses such as salivation and gastric contraction, and arousal responses through the reticular formation (Chapter 19).

Points of clinical interest are mentioned in *Panel 26.1.*

LIMBIC SYSTEM

The limbic system comprises the limbic cortex (so-called *limbic lobe*) and related subcortical nuclei. The term 'limbic' (Broca, 1878) originally referred to a *limbus* or rim of cortex immediately adjacent to the corpus callosum and diencephalon. The limbic cortex is now taken to include the three-layered *allocortex* of the hippocampal formation and septal region together with transitional *mesocortex* in the parahippocampal gyrus, cingulate gyrus, and insula. The principal subcortical component of the limbic system is the amygdala (which merges with cortex). Cortical areas closely related to the limbic system are the orbitofrontal cortex and the temporal pole (*Figure 26.3*). Closely related subcortical areas are the hypothalamus and reticular formation, and the nucleus accumbens.

PARAHIPPOCAMPAL GYRUS

The parahippocampal gyrus is a major junction-

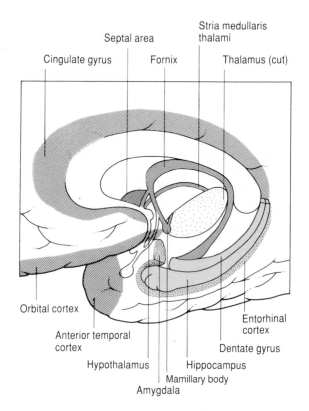

Figure 26.3 Medial view of cortical and subcortical limbic areas.

CLINICAL PANEL 26.2

TEMPORAL LOBE EPILEPSY

Next to vascular disorders, seizures (epileptic attacks) are the commonest group of problems encountered in clinical neurology. Some 3% of the population suffer two or more attacks during their lifetime.

The term 'seizure' refers to a transient alteration of behavior brought about by abnormal burst-firing of neurons in the cerebral cortex. Seizures are divided into two main categories:

- *Primary generalized tonic-clonic seizures* are characterized by sudden onset of unconsciousness with falling. The body stiffens for up to a minute (tonic stage) and then exhibits jerky movements of all four limbs and chewing movements of the mouth for a second minute (clonic stage). A third minute is spent in more relaxed unconsciousness. EEG (electroencephalographic) recordings taken at the onset of this kind of *ictus* (attack) show simultaneous bilateral burst-firing all over the cortex.
- *Primary partial seizures* are more common. They nearly always originate in a focus of run-away neural activity within the temporal lobe and spread over the general cortex within seconds to trigger a *secondary* tonic-clonic seizure. Premonitory 'auras' at the beginning of temporal lobe seizures include well-formed visual or auditory hallucinations (scenes, sound sequences), a sense of familiarity with the surrounding scene ('*déjà vu*'), a sense of strangeness ('*jamais vu*') or a sense of fear. Attacks originating in the uncus are ushered in by unpleasant olfactory or gustatory auras.

Drug treatment of seizures (see below) is not always successful, and surgery is frequently undertaken in intractable cases. Following accurate localization of the ictal focus, a tissue block including the focus may be removed, with abolition of seizures in four out of five cases. Histological examination of the surgical biopsy typically reveals *hippocampal sclerosis:* the picture is one of glial scarring, with extensive neuronal loss in CA2 and CA3 sectors. The granule cells of the dentate gyrus are relatively well preserved, and these appear to be responsible for the ictal burst-firing. Loss of inhibitory, GABA internuncials has been blamed in the past but these cells have recently been shown to persist. Instead, the granule cells appear to be *disinhibited,* because of loss of minute, excitatory, **basket cells** from among their dendrites.

Because 30% of sufferers from temporal lobe epilepsy have first-degree relatives similarly afflicted, often from childhood, a genetic influence must be significant. One possibility could be 'faulty wiring' of the hippocampus during mid-fetal life. Histological preparations may show areas of congenital misplacement of hippocampal pyramidal cells, some lying on their sides or even in the subjacent white matter.

The sclerosis is regarded as a typical CNS healing process following extensive loss of neurons. The neuronal loss in turn seems to be inflicted by *glutamate toxicity* — a known effect of excessively high rates of discharge of pyramidal cells in any part of the cerebral cortex. In temporal lobe seizures the pyramidal cells of the entorhinal cortex are blamed because of their direct input to dentate granule cells through the perforant path. Dentate granule cells are the main source of burst-firing, which is no surprise in view of their natural role in long-term potentiation and kindling (see main text).

Anticonvulsant drugs are of a broadly predictable nature. Most either enhance GABA-mediated inhibitory processes or inhibit glutamate. Some are used in order to stabilize the membranes of excitatory nerve terminals, making their ion channels less permeable to sodium and/or calcium.

al region between the cerebral isocortex and the allocortex of the hippocampal formation. Its anterior part is the **entorhinal cortex** (area 28 in *Figure 26.2*), which is six-layered but has certain peculiar features. The entorhinal cortex can be said to face in two directions. Its *neocortical face* exchanges massive numbers of afferent and efferent connections with all four association areas of the neocortex. Its *allocortical face* exchanges abundant connections with the hippocampal formation. In the broadest terms, the entorhinal cortex receives a constant stream of cognitive and sensory information from the association areas, transmits it to the hippocampal formation for consolidation (see later), retrieves it in consolidated form and returns it to to the association areas where it is encoded in the form of memory traces.

HIPPOCAMPAL FORMATION

The hippocampal formation comprises the **subiculum,** the **hippocampus proper,** and the **dentate gyrus** (*Figure 26.4*). All three are composed of temporal lobe allocortex which has tucked itself into an S-shaped scroll along the floor of the lateral ventricle. The band-like origin of the fornix from the subiculum and hippocampus is the **fimbria.** The hippocampus is also known as *Ammon's horn* (after an Egyptian deity with a ram's head); for research purposes it is divided into three CA (*cornu ammonis*) zones, of which CA1 and CA3 are the largest.

The **principal cells** of the subiculum and hippocampus are **pyramidal cells;** those of the dentate gyrus are **granule cells.** The dendrites of both granule and pyramidal cells are studded with dendritic spines. The hippocampal formation is also rich in inhibitory (GABA) internuncial neurons.

It should be mentioned that in general discussions related to memory, it is customary to use the term 'hippocampus' as synonymous with 'hippocampal formation.'

Connections

The largest *afferent* connection of the hippocampal formation is the **perforant path,** which projects from the entorhinal cortex onto the dendrites of dentate granule cells (*Figure 26.5*). (The medial part of the entorhinal cortex gives rise to a second, *alvear* path which contributes to a sheet of fibers on the surface of the hippocampus, the **alveus.** This smaller pathway terminates in CA1; it will not be mentioned further.)

The axons of the granule cells are called **mossy fibers;** they synapse upon pyramidal cells in the

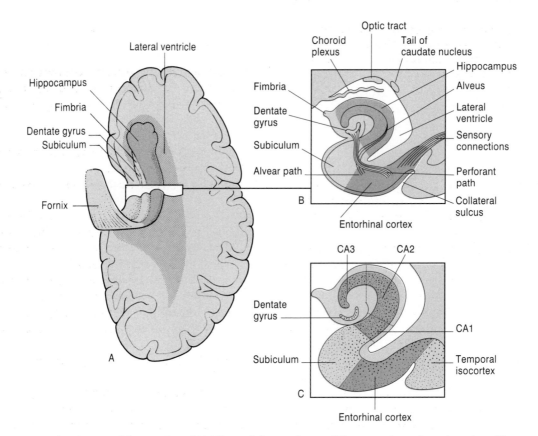

Figure 26.4   Hippocampal formation. **(A)** Viewed from above; **(B)** coronal section showing fiber pathways; **(C)** coronal section showing the three sectors of the hippocampus proper (cornu ammonis).

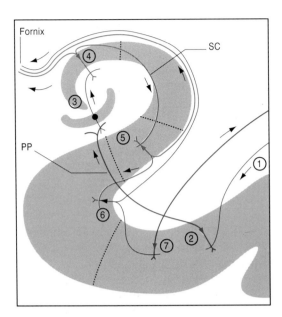

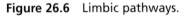

Figure 26.5 Input-output connections of the hippocampal formation.
1 Afferent from sensory association cortex.
2 Entorhinal pyramidal cell projecting perforant path (PP) fiber to dentate gyrus.
3 Dentate granule cell projecting to CA3.
4 CA3 principal neuron projecting to fornix and to entorhinal cortex.
5 CA1 principal cell projecting to fornix and giving a Schaffer collateral (SC) to CA1.
6 Subicular principal cell projecting to fornix and to entorhinal cortex.
7 Entorhinal pyramidal cell projecting to senory association cortex.

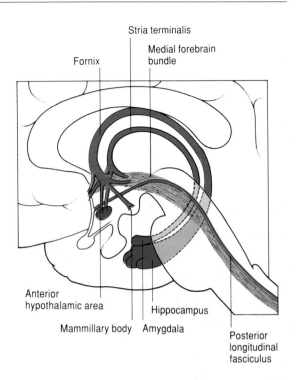

Figure 26.6 Limbic pathways.

CA3 sector. The axons of the CA3 pyramidal cells project into the fimbria; before doing so they give off *Schaffer collaterals* which run a recurrent course from CA3 to CA1. CA1 projects into the entorhinal cortex.

The largest *efferent* connection is the massive back-projection from entorhinal cortex to the association areas of the neocortex. A second, forward projection is the **fornix** (*Figure 26.6*). The fornix is a direct continuation of the **fimbria,** which receives axons from the subiculum and hippocampus proper. The **crus** of the fornix arches up beneath the corpus callosum, where it joins its fellow to form the **trunk.** Anteriorly, a **pillar** descends on each side and divides above the anterior commissure. **Precommissural fibers** enter the septal area. **Postcommissural fibers** enter the anterior hypothalamus, the mamillary bodies, and the medial forebrain bundle.

In addition to the discrete connections mentioned above, the hippocampus is diffusely innervated from several sources, mainly by way of the fornix:

- A dense *cholinergic* innervation is received from the septal nucleus.
- A *noradrenergic* innervation is received from the locus ceruleus.
- A *serotonergic* innervation enters from the raphe nuclei of the midbrain. The possible linkage between serotonin and major depression is mentioned in Chapter 21.
- A *dopaminergic* innervation enters from the ventral tegmental area of the midbrain. The supposed linkage between dopamine and schizophrenia is mentioned in Chapter 24.

Memory function of the hippocampal formation

As already mentioned, information from the neocortical association areas is channeled through area 28, consolidated in the hippocampal formation, and returned from area 28 to the association areas for long-term storage. The fornix is a second, circuitous pathway from hippocampus to neocortex.

The evidence for a *mnemonic* (memory) function in the hippocampal formation is discussed at considerable length in psychology journals. Some insights are listed below.

■ Bilateral damage or removal of the hippocampal formation is followed by *anterograde amnesia,* a term used to denote absence of conscious recall of newly acquired information for more than a few minutes. When asked to name a commonplace object the subject will have no difficulty because long-term memories are stored elsewhere, in association areas of the isocortex. However, when the same object is shown a few minutes later the subject will not remember having seen it. This is known as a loss of *declarative* (data-based) memory.

  Procedural (how-to-do) memory is preserved. If asked to assemble a jigsaw puzzle the subject will do it in the normal way. When asked to repeat the exercise the next day, the subject will do it faster although there will be no recollection of having seen the puzzle previously. *The hippocampus is not required for procedural memory.* The cerebellum appears to be the primary store for procedural memory because of the motor teaching function of the olive (Chapter 20).

■ *Long-term potentiation* (LTP) is uniquely powerful in dentate gyrus and hippocampus. It is regarded as vital for preservation (consolidation) of memory traces. Under experimental conditions, LTP is most easily demonstrated in the perforant path-dentate granule cell connections and in the Schaffer collateral-CA1 connections. A strong, brief (milliseconds) stimulus to the perforant path or Schaffer collaterals induces the target cells to show long-lasting (hours) sensitivity to a fresh stimulus. LTP is associated with a cascade of biochemical events in the target neurons, following activation of appropriate glutamate receptors. It is accompanied by the rapid (within minutes), transient appearance of new synaptic contacts and the expansion of old ones.

  LTP is described as an *associative* phenomenon, because it requires that the powerful, depolarizing stimulus must be coupled with a weak stimulus to the depolarized neuron from another source. LTP is promoted by *opioid peptides,* which are co-released from

perforant path neurons, and by *noradrenaline* and *dopamine.* The two amines may have a bearing on the attentional or motivational state at the time of learning.

■ In both human and animal experiments, *cholinergic activity in the hippocampus* seems to be significant for learning. In human volunteers, central ACh blockade (by administration of scopolamine) severely impairs memory for lists of names or numbers whereas a cholinesterase inhibitor (physostigmine) gives above-normal results. Clinically, hippocampal cholinergic activity is severely reduced in Alzheimer's disease, which is particularly associated with amnesia (see *Panel 26.3*).

■ *Kindling* ('lighting a fire') is a property unique to the hippocampal formation and amygdala, although its relationship to learning is not obvious. Kindling is the progressively increasing group response of neurons to a repetitive stimulus of uniform strength. In experimental animals it can spread from mesocortex to isocortex and cause generalized convulsive seizures (see *Panel 26.2*).

■ The contribution of the fornix projection to memory is uncertain. Indirect evidence has been adduced from *diencephalic amnesia,* a state of anterograde amnesia which may follow bilateral damage to the diencephalon. Such damage may interrupt the *Papez circuit* linking the fornix to the cingulate gyrus by way of the mamillary body and the anterior nucleus of the thalamus. Complete transection of the fornix may have the same effect, although amnesia is not an invariable result.

INSULA

(a) The anterior insula is a cortical center for pain. (b) The main part is continuous with the frontoparietal and temporal opercular cortex, and it seems to have a *language* rather than a limbic function. During language tasks, PET scans show activity there as well as in the opercular speech receptive and motor areas – but not in congenital dyslexics, where it remains silent. (c) The posterior insula is interconnected with the entorhinal cortex and the amygdala.

CINGULATE CORTEX AND POSTERIOR PARAHIPPOCAMPAL GYRUS

The cingulate cortex is part of the Papez circuit, receiving a projection from the anterior nucleus

ALZHEIMER'S DISEASE

Dementia is defined as a severe loss of cognitive function without impairment of consciousness. Alzheimer's disease (AD) is the commonest cause of dementia, afflicting 5% of people in their seventh decade and 20% of people in their ninth. AD patients fill 20% of all beds in psychiatric institutions.

The illness is ushered in by episodes of forgetfulness about names and faces, and progresses within weeks or months to amnesia for recent events (e.g. the patient may describe something within minutes of having already done so) and to general disorientation in time (days and dates) and space, and inability to manage personal affairs. Later stages are characterized by disregard for personal hygiene and nutrition.

MRI brain scans usually reveal severe atrophy of the cerebral cortex, with widening of the sulci and enlargement of the ventricular system. Postmortem histological studies of the cerebral cortex reveal:

■ Extensive loss of pyramidal neurons throughout the brain.
■ *Amyloid plaques* and *neurofibrillary tangles*, notably in the hippocampus and amygdala. The plaques begin in the walls of small blood vessels and have been explained in terms of an enzyme defect resulting in abnormal, *beta-amyloid* protein production. The tangles are made up of clumps of microtubules associated with an abnormal variant of a microtubule-associated *tau* protein. The tangles are progressively replaced by amyloid.
■ Loss of up to 90% of the cholinergic neurons from the *basal nucleus of Meynert,* together with their extensive projections through the cerebral isocortex and mesocortex. Indeed, degenerating ACh terminals seem to contribute to the neurofibrillary tangles in the temporal lobe.

The above three sets of changes are characteristic of AD, but they are not diagnostic because one set or more may be noted in other brain disorders. To date, there seems to be no effective treatment.

An unusual variant, known as *early-onset AD,* shows clear evidence of an autosomal dominant trait. The illness appears during the fourth or fifth decade. Chromosomal analyses have revealed a specific mutation in the gene coding for amyloid precursor protein on the long arm of chromosome 21. This mutation is also found in Down's syndrome, where sufferers surviving into middle age usually develop AD.

---

of the thalamus and becoming continuous with the parahippocampal gyrus behind the splenium of the corpus callosum.

The *anterior* cingulate cortex includes areas 32 and 24 (*Figure 24.3*). It belongs to the *rostral limbic system* which includes the amygdala, ventral striatum, orbitofrontal cortex and anterior insular cortex. The anterior cingulate cortex has several functional subdivisions.

■ One area receives afferents from the intralaminar nuclei of the thalamus. It is one of four cortical areas that show a pronounced increase in metabolic activity in response to a painful stimulus applied to the body surface. The other three are the primary and secondary somatic sensory areas and the anterior insula (*Figure 26.7*). Surgical undercutting (*anterior cingulotomy*) is a procedure sometimes performed for the relief of intractable pain. In successful cases the severity of the pain is not altered but the unpleasant, aversive quality is removed.

■ A second area, connected to amygdala and anterior insula, elicits autonomic and respiratory responses when stimulated electrically. This area is thought to participate in eliciting the visceral responses typical of emotional states.

■ Stimulation of a third area, connected to amygdala and orbitofrontal cortex, generates subjective emotional responses varying from fear to elation.

■ A fourth, *executive* area, linked to the ventral striatum, putamen and supplementary motor area (SMA), becomes active prior to

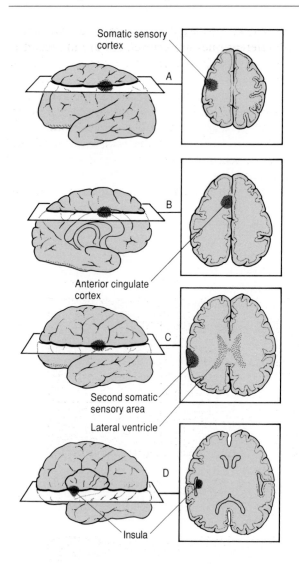

Somatic sensory cortex

A

Anterior cingulate cortex

B

Second somatic sensory area

Lateral ventricle

C

Insula

D

Figure 26.7 Cortical areas showing increased metabolic activity following application of noxious heat to the right volar forearm. (Adapted from Talbot *et al.* (1991) *Science* **251**: 1355-1358 and Coghill *et al.* (1994) *J. Neurosci.* **14**: 4095-4108.

movement — and even prior to the SMA itself. In the light of the anterior cingulate's placement within the rostral limbic system, the executive area is thought to have special significance in generating *appropriate motor plan selection* by the SMA.

The *posterior* cingulate gyrus (area 23 of Brodmann) merges with the posterior parahippocampal gyrus (area 36). This cortical complex is richly interconnected with visual, auditory and tactile/spatial association areas. They evidently contain memory stores related to these functions because PET studies reveal increased activity in one or more parts of the complex when scenes or experiences are conjured up in the mind.

SEPTAL AREA

The septal area is the chief *pleasure center* of the brain. It comprises the **septal nucleus,** merged with the cortex directly in front of the anterior commissure, together with a few cells extending into the septum pellucidum.

Afferents are received from:

- the amygdala, via the diagonal band of Broca;
- the olfactory tract, via the medial olfactory stria;
- the hippocampus, via the fornix; and
- brainstem monoaminergic neurons, via the medial forebrain bundle.

Efferent projections run to the hypothalamus, brainstem, and hippocampus. The largest projection to the brainstem is by way of the **stria medullaris thalami** and the **habenular nucleus.** The habenular nuclei of the two sides are connected through the **habenular commissure** located close to the root of the pineal gland and often calcified (Chapter 2). The habenular nucleus sends the **fasciculus retroflexus** to synapse in an **interpeduncular nucleus** of the reticular formation in the midbrain. The interpeduncular nucleus is linked to autonomic nuclei in the brainstem and spinal cord.

The *septohippocampal pathway* runs to the hippocampus by way of the fornix.

The septal area appears to participate in several different functional activities:

- Electrical stimulation of the human septal nucleus produces a most agreeable sense of well-being. In animals, the nucleus is one of several 'reward areas' of the brain, as judged by eagerness to self-stimulate by means of a lever attached to an indwelling electrode. Rats may self-stimulate the septal nucleus to the exclusion of all other activities, even to the point of death from starvation. An electrolytic lesion of the nucleus has the opposite effect: the animal shows extreme displeasure (so-called 'septal rage').
- The nucleus provides the bulk of the cholinergic nerve supply to the hippocampus, with a probable mnemonic role.
- The septohippocampal projection is responsible for rhythmic, slow-wave activity (4-7 Hz)

of hippocampal neurons. It is detectable as *theta rhythm* in the electroencephalogram. The functional significance of theta rhythm is unknown.

AMYGDALA

The amygdala (Greek, almond; also called the amygdaloid body or amygdaloid complex) is a large group of nuclei above and in front of the temporal horn of the lateral ventricle. Afferent nuclear groups are *dorsomedial* and *ventrolateral*; efferent ones are *central*. All are in receipt of monoaminergic afferents from the midbrain and pons (serotonin, dopamine, norepinephrine).

The *dorsomedial nuclei* merge with the piriform cortex and receive afferents from all parts of the olfactory cortex. The *ventrolateral nuclei* receive afferents from the auditory, visual and somatic sensory association areas; also from the hippocampus.

The *central nuclei* send some fibers to the

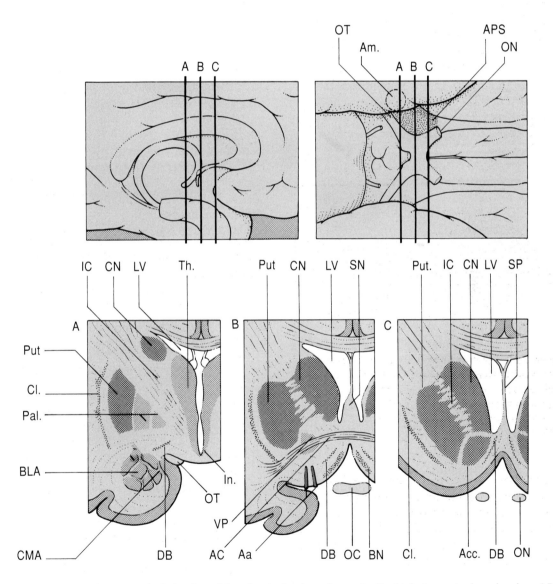

Figure 26.8 Coronal sections of the basal forebrain in the planes indicated. Aa, arteries piercing APS; Am., amygdala; Acc., nucleus accumbens; AC, anterior commissure; APS, anterior perforated substance; BLA, basolateral amygdala; BN, basal nucleus of Meynert; Cl., claustrum; CMA, corticomedial amygdala; CN, caudate nucleus; DB, diagonal band of Broca; IC internal capsule; In., infundibulum; LV, lateral ventricle; OC, optic chiasm; ON, optic nerve; OT, optic tract; Pal., pallidum; Put., putamen; SN, septal nucleus; SP, septum pellucidum; Th., thalamus; VP, ventral pallidum.

nucleus accumbens and to the premotor and pre-frontal cortex. The remaining efferents enter the stria terminalis or the ventral amygdalofugal pathway.

The *stria terminalis* (*Figure 26.6*) follows the curve of the caudate nucleus and accompanies the thalamostriate vein along the upper surface of the thalamus. It sends fibers to the septal area and hypothalamus, and, through the medial forebrain bundle, to the autonomic and respiratory nuclei of the brainstem. The *ventral amygdalofugal pathway* passes medially below the lentiform nucleus. It contains fibers going to the mediodorsal nucleus of the thalamus, and it provides an additional route to the septum, hypothalamus and brainstem.

At a functional level, the amygdala is involved in *defense* and *attack*. In lower mammals the dorsomedial nuclear group is clearly important because of its olfactory setting. In primates, the ventrolateral group is dominant because of its auditory, visual, and somatic inputs.

The central nuclear group is in a position (a) to produce movements of an instinctive nature (eg. adoption of defensive or aggressive postures) through its linkages with the ventral striatum (nucleus accumbens) and premotor cortex; (b) to have cognitive effects (influencing decisions to retreat or attack) through its linkages with the hippocampus and prefrontal cortex; (c) to influence endocrine functions of the hypothalamus — notably initiation of the stress response through the pituitary-adrenal axis; (d) and to mobilize elements of the reticular formation controlling the eye, cardiovascular system and respiration.

Electrical stimulation of the human amygdala most often produces an acute sense of *fear*, accompanied by intense sympathetic activity and sometimes by evasive movements. Bilateral ablation of the amygdala has been carried out in humans for treatment of *rage attacks*, characterized by irritability, building up over several hours to dangerous aggressiveness. The operation has been successful in eliminating such attacks. In monkeys, bilateral ablation leads to placidity, together with a tendency to explore objects orally and a state of hypersexuality (*Kluver-Bucy syndrome*). A comparable syndrome has occasionally been observed in humans.

BASAL FOREBRAIN (*FIGURE 26.8*)

The basal forebrain extends from the bifurcation of the olfactory tract as far back as the infundibulum, and from the midline to the amygdala. In its roof are the anterior commissure, the *ventral pallidum* (pierced by the commissure), and the *ventral striatum* whose anterior end contains the **nucleus accumbens**. Above and medial to the nucleus accumbens is the **septal nucleus** below the septum pellucidum. The septal nucleus has a two-way linkage with the amygdala through the **diagonal band** (of Broca), which contains a small nucleus of its own.

In the floor of the basal forebrain is the **anterior perforated substance,** pierced by central branches of the anterior and middle cerebral arteries. Here the cerebral cortex is replaced by scattered nuclear groups, of which the largest is the **nucleus basalis magnocellularis** of Meynert.

The *cholinergic neurons of the basal forebrain* have their somas mainly in the septal and basal nuclei (*Figure 26.9*). The septal nucleus gives rise to the *septohippocampal pathway,* which reaches the hippocampus through the fornix. This projection is supplemented by cholinergic fibers from the **nucleus of the diagonal band.** The basal nucleus projects to all parts of the cerebral neocortex, which also contains scattered intrinsic cholinergic neurons.

The septal, basal, and diagonal band nuclei are often called the *basal forebrain nuclei,* or 'the nucleus of Meynert' in the context of Alzheimer's disease. In the hippocampus, the cholinergic supply seems to be relevant to the consolidation of information into memory, as well as generating theta rhythm on EEG recordings. In the neocortex, the cholinergic supply is tonically active in

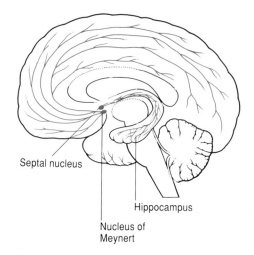

Figure 26.9 Cholinergic innervation of the cerebral cortex from the basal forebrain nuclei.

the waking state, contributing to the 'awake' pattern on EEG recordings. In animals, activation of the basal nucleus potentiates and prolongs the responsiveness of cortical cell columns to inputs from the 'specific' sensory and motor thalamic nuclei.

CORE INFORMATION

OLFACTORY SYSTEM

The olfactory system comprises the olfactory epithelium in the nose, the olfactory nerves, olfactory bulb and olfactory tract, and several patches of olfactory cortex. The epithelium comprises bipolar olfactory neurons, supporting cells, and basal cells which renew the bipolar neurons at a diminishing rate throughout life. Central processes of the bipolar neurons form the olfactory nerves, which penetrate the cribriform plate of the ethmoid bone and synapse upon mitral cells in the bulb. Mitral cell axons form the olfactory tract, which has several low-level terminations in the anterior temporal lobe. Olfactory discrimination is a function of the orbitofrontal cortex, which is reached by way of the mediodorsal nucleus of the thalamus.

LIMBIC SYSTEM

The limbic system comprises the limbic cortex and related subcortical nuclei. The limbic cortex includes the hippocampal formation, septal region, parahippocampal gyrus, cingulate gyrus, and insula. The principal subcortical nucleus is the amygdala. Closely related are the orbitofrontal cortex, temporal pole, hypothalamus and reticular formation, and the nucleus accumbens.

The anterior part of the parahippocampal gyrus is the entorhinal cortex, which receives cognitive and sensory information from the association areas, transmits it to the hippocampal formation for consolidation and returns it to the association areas where it is encoded in the form of memory traces.

The hippocampal formation comprises the subiculum, the hippocampus proper, and the dentate gyrus. Sectors of the hippocampus are called CA (cornu ammonis) 1, 2 and 3.

The perforant path projects from the entorhinal cortex on to the dendrites of dentate granule cells. Granule cell axons synapse on CA3 pyramidal cells which give Schaffer collaterals to CA1. CA1 back-projects to the entorhinal cortex which is heavily linked to the association areas.

The fornix is a direct continuation of the fimbria, which receives axons from the subiculum and hippocampus. The crus of the fornix joins its fellow to form the trunk. Anteriorly the pillars of the fornix divide into precommissural fibers entering the septal area and postcommissural fibers entering anterior hypothalamus, mamillary bodies and medial forebrain bundle.

Bilateral damage or removal of the hippocampal formation is followed by anterograde amnesia (loss of declarative memory). Procedural memory is preserved. Long-term potentiation (LTP) of granule and pyramidal cells is regarded as a key factor in the consolidation of memories.

The insula has uncertain functions in relation to the autonomic system, taste, and pain. The anterior cingulate cortex responds to noxious peripheral stimulation; the posterior cingulate responds to the emotional tone of what is seen or felt. The septal area is the chief pleasure center of the brain. It also gives rise to the septohippocampal pathway which is responsible for theta rhythm and seems to have a memory function.

The amygdala is a large group of nuclei above and in front of the temporal horn of the lateral ventricle. Afferent nuclear groups are dorsomedial and basolateral; efferent ones are central. The central nuclei send some fibers to the nucleus accumbens and to the premotor and prefrontal cortex. The remaining efferents reach hypothalamus and brainstem via the stria terminalis and ventral amygdalofugal pathway. The amygdala is involved in the emotional and motor responses associated with defense and attack.

The basal forebrain is the gray matter in and around the anterior perforated substance. It includes the cholinergic, nucleus basalis of Meynert which projects to all parts of the neocortex, and the cholinergic, septal nucleus projecting to the hippocampus. Both lose up to 90% of their neurons in Alzheimer's disease.

SELF TEST

Answer A if 1, 2, and 3 only are correct
        B if 1 and 3 only are correct
        C if 2 and 4 only are correct
        D if 4 only is correct
        E if all four are correct

1 In the olfactory system:

1 The olfactory nerves belong to bipolar neurons
2 The olfactory tract originates from mitral cells
3 Uncinate epilepsy may be preceded by olfactory auras
4 Inability to smell is called ageusia

2 The hippocampal formation includes the:

1 Hippocampus proper
2 Subiculum
3 Dentate gyrus
4 Entorhinal cortex

3 Targets of entorhinal efferents include the:

1 Dentate gyrus
2 Subiculum
3 Association areas of neocortex
4 Uncus

4 Characteristics of dentate granule cells include:

1 Inhibitory action
2 Long-term potentiation
3 Projection to parietal lobe
4 Kindling

5 Contributors to the fornix include the:

1 Subiculum
2 Hippocampus proper
3 Septal nucleus
4 Locus ceruleus

6 Long-term memories are stored in the:

1 Hippocampus proper
2 Dentate gyrus
3 Entorhinal cortex
4 Association areas of the cortex

REFERENCES

Agranoff, B.W. (1989) Learning and memory. In *Basic Neurochemistry: Molecular, Cellular, and Medical Aspects*, 4th edn (Siegel, G.J. *et al.*, eds), pp. 915–927. New York: Raven Press.

Baxendale, S.A. (1995) The hippocampus — functional and structural correlations. *Seizure* **4**: 105–117.

Dekker, A.J.A.M., Connor, D.J. and Thal, L.J. (1991) The role of cholinergic projections from the nucleus basalis in memory. *Neurosci. Behav. Rev.* **15**: 299–317.

De Lacalle, S., Lim, C., Sobreviela, T., Mufson, E.J., Hersh, L.B. and Saper, C.B. (1994) Cholinergic innervation of the human hippocampal formation including the entorhinal cortex. *J. Comp. Neurol.* **345**: 321–344.

Delacour, J. (1994) A central activation role for the hippocampus: a viewpoint. *Neurosci. Res. Comm.* **16**: 1–10.

de Olmos, J. (1990) Amygdaloid nuclear gray complex. In *The Human Brain* (Paxinos, G., ed), pp. 583–710. San Diego: Academic Press.

Devinsky, Morrell, M.J., and Vogt, B.A. (1995) Contributions of anterior cingulate cortex to behavior. *Brain* **118**: 279–306.

Eichenbaum, H., Otto, T. and Cohen, N.J. (1994) Two functional components of the hippocampal memory system. *Behav. Brain Sci.* **17**: 449–517.

Frith, C.D. *et al.* (1996) Is developmental dyslexia a disconnection syndrome? Studies with PET. *Brain* **119**: 143–158.

Garza-Trevino, E.S. (1994) Neurobiological factors in aggressive behavior. *Hosp. Commun. Psychiat.* **45**: 690–699.

Jay, V. and Becker, L.E. (1994) Surgical Pathology of epilepsy. *Pediat. Pathol.* **14**: 731–750.

LeDoux, J.E. (1995) Emotion: clues from the brain. *Ann. Rev. Psychol.* **46**: 209–235.

Leonard, B.E. (1992) *Fundamentals of Psychopharmacology*. Chichester: Wiley.

Macchi, G. (1989) Anatomical substrate of emotional reactions. In *Handbook of Neuropsychology, Vol. 3* (Boller, F. and Grafman, J., eds), pp. 283–303. Amsterdam: Elsevier.

Malenka, R.C. (1994) Synaptic plasticity in the hippocampus. *Cell* **78**: 835–838.

McDonald, A.J. (1992) Cell types and intrinsic connections of the amygdala. In *The Amygdala: Neurobiological Aspects of Emotion, Memory, and Mental Dysfunction*, pp. 67–96. New York: Wiley-Liss.

Meldrum, B.S. (1994) The role of glutamate in epilepsy and other CNS disorders. *Neurology.* **44**: (Suppl. 8) S14–S22.

Mesalum, M.M. (1995) The cholinergic contribution to neuromodulation in the cerebral cortex. *Sem. Neurosci.* **7**: 297–307.

Morris, B.J. and Johnston, H.M. (1995) A role for hippocampal opioids in long-term functional plasticity. *Trends Neurosci.* **18**: 350–354.

Prah, J.D. and Benignus, V.A. (1985) Olfaction: anatomy, physiology, and behavior. In *Toxicology of the Eye, Ear, and other Special Senses* (Hayes, A.W., ed), pp. 25–39. New York: Raven Press.

Shin, C. (1994) Mechanism of epilepsy. *Ann. Rev. Med.* **45**: 379–389.

Willis, W.D. (1995) From nociception to cortical activity. In *Advances in Pain Research and Therapy*, Vol. 22 (Brom, B. ed), pp. 1–19. Philadelphia: Lippincott–Raven.

27

CEREBROVASCULAR DISEASE

<table>
<tr><td>Chapter Summary</td><td colspan="2">Study Guidelines</td></tr>
<tr><td>

Introduction

Anterior versus posterior circulation

Occlusions within the anterior circulation
Internal carotid artery

Occlusions within the posterior circulation

Transient ischemic attacks

Aneurysms

CLINICAL PANELS
Anterior cerebral artery
   occlusion
Middle cerebral artery
   occlusion
Internal carotid artery
   occlusion
Posterior cerebral artery
   occlusion
Subarachnoid hemorrhage
</td><td>1
2
3
4
5</td><td>

This final chapter touches upon a large range of neurological symptoms and signs, because it deals with vascular damage to every part of the brain. The great majority of the symptoms and signs have been already been mentioned individually, in other contexts.

The Clinical Panels may convey the impression that clinical diagnosis is rather straightforward. However, following major vascular insults, patients are seldom alert and co-operative.

An objective of this chapter is to demonstrate the value of an understanding of the regional anatomy of the brain, because cerebrovascular accidents cause injury to regions, with consequent effects on multiple systems.

The increasing range of diagnostic aids is not diminishing the requirement for clinical acumen. The more accurate the tentative diagnosis, the more likely it is that the most appropriate technology will be selected.

A fresh recollection of material in Chapter 5 (on the blood supply) and Chapter 24 (on cortical functional anatomy) is advisable.
</td></tr>
</table>

INTRODUCTION

Cerebrovascular disease is the third leading cause of death in adults, being superseded only by heart disease and cancer. The most frequent expression of cerebrovascular disease is that of a *stroke*, which is defined as a focal neurological deficit of vascular origin which lasts for more than 24 hours if the patient survives. The most frequent example is a *hemiplegia* caused by a vascular lesion of the internal capsule. However, some

two dozen varieties of stroke symptomatologies are recognized, based upon place and size.

The three chief underlying disorders are atherosclerosis within the large arteries supplying the brain, heart disease, and hypertension.

■ *Atherosclerosis* signifies fatty deposits in the intimal lining of the internal carotid and vertebrobasilar system — most notably in the internal carotid trunk or in one of the vertebral arteries. The deposits pose a dual threat:

in situ enlargement may cause progressive occlusion of a main artery; and breakaway deposits may form emboli (plugs) blocking distal branches within the brain. However, gradual occlusion is often redeemed by routing of blood through alternative channels. For example, an internal carotid artery (ICA) may be occluded over a period of ten years or more without apparent brain damage; the contralateral ICA may utilize the circle of Willis to perfuse *both* pairs of anterior and middle cerebrals; it is not unusual in such cases for *external* carotid blood to assist, by retrograde flow from the facial artery through the ophthalmic artery on the affected side. Similarly, gradual occlusion of the stem of one of the three cerebral arteries may be compensated for through small anastomotic arteries on the brain surface, perfused by the other two cerebrals. On the other hand, all of the arteries penetrating the brain substance are *end arteries*, i.e. their communication with neighboring penetrating arteries are too fine to save brain tissue in the event of blockage, even if this is slow.

- Many cerebral emboli originate as blood clots in the left side of the heart, in association with *coronary* or *valvular disease* or atrial fibrillation.
- *Hypertension* is obviously associated with cerebral hemorrhage, which may be so massive as to rupture into the ventricular system and cause death within minutes or hours. Less obvious are *lacunae* ('small pools') up to 2 cm in diameter, derived from necrotic (dead) brain tissue around small arteries that have become occluded by mural thickening in response to the hypertension.

An area of brain destruction produced by vascular occlusion or hemorrhage is an *infarct*. Cerebral infarcts become swollen after a few days, and some become large enough to produce *distance effects* by causing subfalcal or tentorial herniation of the brain in the manner of a tumor (Chapter 4).

It is usually easy to distinguish the symptoms/signs of vascular disease from those of a tumor. A vascular stroke takes up to 24 hours to evolve whereas the time frame for tumors is usu-

---

CLINICAL PANEL 27.1

ANTERIOR CEREBRAL ARTERY OCCLUSION

Complete interruption of flow in the anterior cerebral artery is uncommon because the opposite artery has direct access to its distal territory through the anterior communicating artery. However, branch occlusions are well recognized:

- *Recurrent artery of Heubner:* the clinical picture resembles that of middle cerebral artery upper-division occlusion (see *Panel 27.2*), with motor weakness of the contralateral face and arm. A lacunar infarct high in the anterior limb of the internal capsule may disable fibers on their way from the lower part of the motor cortex to the pyramidal bundle in the posterior limb; the result here is known as 'dysarthria-clumsy hand syndrome.'
- *Callosomarginal:* the characteristic result is motor weakness and some cortical-type sensory loss in the contralateral lower limb, due to infarction within the paracentral lobule. Urinary incontinence may occur for

some days owing to interference with the bilateral 'social' control of the pontine bladder center (Chapter 19).* With dominant hemisphere lesions, initiation of speech may be difficult if the supplementary motor area is damaged.
- *Pericallosal:* infarction of the corpus callosum may produce 'split brain' effects (Chapter 24). In a right-handed patient a simple test is to ask the patient to feel an unseen object (e.g. a key) in the left hand and to name it. If the tactile information cannot be transferred from the right parietal lobe to the left, the object cannot be named ('tactile aphasia').

If the premotor cortex has been compromised, the patient may not be able to reach out with the contralateral arm on command (so-called 'sympathetic apraxia').

*Urinary incontinence may accompany clouding of consciousness following any large infarct in the hemisphere. Recovery of bladder control can be assisted by means of general sensory and cognitive stimulation of the patient.

MIDDLE CEREBRAL ARTERY OCCLUSION

Embolic and lacunar infarcts are frequent in late middle life and in the elderly. Hemorrhage from one of the striate branches is also a frequent event.

Embolism

An embolus may lodge in the stem of the artery, in the upper division, in the lower division, or in a cortical branch of either division.

Stem
Occlusion of the stem affects the central as well as the cortical branches. The picture is one of contralateral hemiplegia with severe sensory loss, together with contralateral homonymous hemianopia. Left-sided lesions are usually accompanied by global aphasia, right-sided ones with contralateral sensory neglect. Prognosis for significant recovery is poor. Many patients die in coma following midbrain compression by a swollen infarct.

Upper division
An embolus occluding the upper division gives rise to contralateral paresis (weakness) and cortical-type sensory loss in the face and arm, together with dysarthria arising from damage to supranuclear pathways involved in speech articulation. Left-sided lesions are usually accompanied by motor aphasia, right-sided lesions by contralateral neglect.

Lower division
Embolism of the lower division produces contralateral homonymous hemianopia, and sometimes a confused, agitated state attributed to involvement of limbic pathways in the temporal lobe. Left-sided lesions are also accompanied by Wernicke's aphasia, alexia, and sometimes by ideomotor apraxia.

Branch embolism
The following isolated deficits are attributable to an embolus lodged in one of the cortical branches:

- *Orbitofrontal:* elements of a dorsolateral prefrontal syndrome may be present (Chapter 24).
- *Precentral (prerolandic):* expressive aphasia (left lesion); monotone speech (right lesion).
- *Central (rolandic):* contralateral loss of motor and/or sensory function in the face and arm.
- *Anterior parietal (postrolandic):* contralateral astereognosis.
- *Posterior parietal:* contralateral visual defect (especially with right lesion).
- *Angular:* contralateral homonymous hemianopia; alexia with left lesion.
- *Posterior/middle temporal:* Wernicke's aphasia (left lesion); sensory aprosodia (right lesion).

Lacunar infarcts
In the presence of hypertension, lacunar infarction is suspected where the clinical evidence suggests a small lesion. Well recognized are:

- *Pure motor hemiplegia* signifies a lacune in the middle of the posterior limb of the internal capsule. With recovery of movement, the paretic limbs may show evidence of cerebellar ataxia because of entrapment of the cerebellocortical projection passing from the ventral lateral nucleus of the thalamus to the motor cortex (cf. *Figure 14.6*). This syndrome is known as *ataxic hemiparesis.*
- *Pure sensory syndrome* is produced by a lacune in the ventral posterior nucleus of the thalamus. There is severe impairment of tactile discrimination (Chapter 12) in the contralateral limbs, together with sensory ataxia.

Hemorrhage

The commonest source of a cerebral hemorrhage is one of the lateral striate branches of the middle cerebral. The commonest location is the putamen, with spread into the anterior and posterior limbs of the internal capsule. The usual cause is a pre-existing systemic hypertension. The hematoma may be as small as a pea or as big as a golf ball. Large hemorrhages rupture into the lateral ventricle and are usually fatal within 24 hours.

A typical clinical case is one in which a sudden, severe headache is followed by unconsciousness within a few minutes. The eyes tend to drift toward the side of the lesion, as noted in Chapter 19. With recovery of consciousness

CLINICAL PANEL 27.2 *Continued*

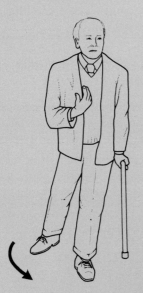

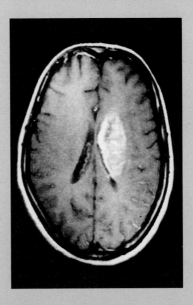

Figure CP 27.2.1   Hemiplegic gait. The patient's right side is affected.

Figure CP 27.2.2   Contrast-enhanced MR image taken from a patient 11 days after an embolic stroke (see text). (Reproduced from Sato *et al.*, (1991) *Neuroradiology* 178: 433-439 by kind permission of Dr S. Takahashi, Department of Radiology, Tohoku University School of Medicine, Sendai, Japan, and the editors.)

there is a complete, flaccid hemiplegia (apart from the upper part of the face). Tendon reflexes are absent on the hemiplegic side and a Babinski sign is present. Conjugate movement of the eyes toward the hemiplegic side may be impossible initially.

Following any kind of stroke involving the left internal capsule, righthanders often notice some initial clumsiness in the supposedly unaffected hand on the side of the lesion. fMRI studies indicate that in healthy righthanders the left motor cortex is more active during movements of the left hand than the right cortex is during movements of the right hand. In other words, the left motor cortex has a greater degree of bilateral control.

Considerable return of function is possible. During the first week, recovery is attributable to reduction of edema in the neighborhood of the infarct. Later improvement is due in part to increased activity in the ipsilateral motor cortex. The end result is often one of ambulatory spastic hemiparesis with hemihypesthesia (reduced sensation).

Figure CP 27.2.1 shows the typical posture during walking: the elbow and fingers are flexed and the leg has to be circumducted during the swing phase (unless an ankle brace is worn) because of the antigravity tone of the musculature. During the early rehabilitation

period an arm sling is required in order to protect the shoulder joint from downward subluxation; this is because the supraspinatus muscle is normally in continuous contraction when the body is upright, preventing slippage of the humeral head.

A lacunar infarct may select pyramidal tract fibers almost exclusively, giving rise to pure motor hemiplegia. A fascinating account of a personal case is that of the Norwegian neuroanatomist Alf Brodal (see Reference list). *Figure CP 27.2.2* is from an MR study of a patient who had suffered a right hemiplegia with sensory loss 11 days previously. The picture shows extensive infarction of the white matter on the left side, at the junctional region between the corona radiata and internal capsule, with compression of the lateral ventricle.

Internal carotid artery

As well as being a source of cerebral emboli, atheromatous plaques may cause partial or complete occlusion of the internal carotid artery itself (see *Panel 27.3*).

ally weeks or months. However, *hemorrhage into a tumor* may cause it to expand suddenly and to mimic the effects of a stroke. Very often the hemorrhage is into a *metastatic* tumor, notably from lung, breast, or prostate; in fact, a stroke may be the first manifestation of a cancer in one of these organs.

An unusual cause of vascular stroke is *rupture of a berry aneurysm into the brain*. As explained later, berry aneurysms usually bleed directly into the subarachnoid space because they originate in the circle of Willis, but they occasionally arise at an arterial bifurcation point within the brain. A ruptured aneurysm is always a prime suspect when a stroke comes 'out of the blue' in someone less than 40 years old.

ANTERIOR VERSUS POSTERIOR CIRCULATION

Clinicians refer to the internal carotid artery and its branches as the *anterior circulation* of the brain, and the vertebrobasilar system (including the posterior cerebral arteries) as the *posterior*

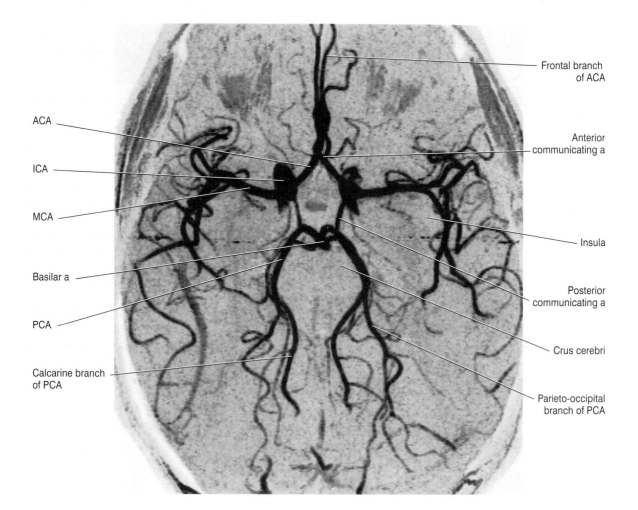

Fig. 27.1 Circle of Willis and its branches. This is an MR 'angiogram' based on the principle that flowing blood generates a different signal to stationary tissue, without injection of a contrast agent. Conventional angiograms, e.g. those in Figures 5.4 and 5.7, require arterial perfusion with a contrast agent. The vessels shown here are contained within a single thick MR 'slice;' some, e.g. the calcarine branch of the posterior cerebral artery could be followed further in adjacent slices. ACA, anterior cerebral artery; ICA, internal carotid artery; MCA, middle cerebral artery; PCA, posterior cerebral artery. (From a series kindly provided by Dr J. Paul Finn, Director, MR Research and Development, Siemens Medical Systems Inc., Iselin, New Jersey.)

CLINICAL PANEL 27.3

INTERNAL CAROTID ARTERY OCCLUSION

The lumen of the internal carotid artery may become progressively obstructed by atheromatous deposits. Common sites of obstruction are the point of commencement in the neck, and the cavernous sinus. A slowly progressive obstruction may be compensated for by the opposite internal carotid artery, through the circle of Willis. Additional blood may also be provided through the orbit from the facial artery. At the other extreme, sudden occlusion may cause death from infarction of the entire anterior and middle cerebral territories, and sometimes the posterior cerebral as well.

Warning signs of carotid occlusion take the form of *transient ischemic attacks* lasting for up to a few hours. As with TIAs elsewhere, the physician is unlikely to be present during an attack and must appreciate the import of the account given by the patient or relative. The territory of the middle cerebral artery is most often affected. Individual symptoms tend to occur in isolation and include any of the following: a feeling of heaviness or weakness or numbness or tingling in one arm/leg, halting or slurring of speech, disappearance of the left or right visual field. Disturbance of flow in the ophthalmic artery may cause dimness of vision or transient monocular blindness (one eye may be filled with 'white steam').

Occlusions within the posterior circulation

The clinical phrase 'long tract signs' is most often used in the context of brainstem lesions; it refers to evidence of a lesion in one or more of the three long tracts, namely the *pyramidal tract,* the *posterior column–medial lemniscal pathway,* and the *spinothalamic pathway.* All of the long tract signs occur in the limbs on the side opposite to the lesion.

Small brainstem infarcts may yield the following features, on the side of the lesion:

- *Midbrain:* Third nerve paralysis
- *Pons:* Facial +/- abducens +/- mandibular nerve paralysis +/- anesthesia of the face
- *Medulla oblongata:* Most characteristic is the *lateral medullary syndrome,* described in Chapter 16, caused by occlusion of the posterior inferior cerebellar artery. Occlusion of the labyrinthine branch of the anterior inferior cerebellar artery causes immediate destruction of the inner ear; *sudden deafness* in that ear is accompanied by *vertigo* with a tendency to fall to that side.

Large brainstem infarcts are usually fatal because of damage to the vital centers of the reticular formation.

Cerebellar ataxia of the limbs on one side, without brainstem damage, is more often due to occlusion of the top end of the vertebral artery on that side than to occlusion of one of the three cerebellar arteries.

The posterior cerebral arteries are usually perfused through the basilar bifurcation. Occlusion is more common in branches than in either main stem (*Panel 27.4*)

circulation. About 25% of CVAs (cerebrovascular accidents) originate in the posterior circulation.

The anterior and posterior circulations are connected by the posterior communicating arteries (*Figure 27.1*).

OCCLUSIONS WITHIN THE ANTERIOR CIRCULATION

The symptoms of vascular strokes in the territories of the anterior circulation are summarized in *Panels 27.1, 27.2* and *27.3*. In the Panels, the term 'occlusion' is used in a general sense to signify infarction however caused.

TRANSIENT ISCHEMIC ATTACKS

Transient ischemic attacks (TIAs) are episodes of vascular insufficiency that cause temporary loss of brain function, with total recovery within 24 hours. Most TIAs last for less than half an hour, with no residual signs at the time of clinical examination. Diagnosis is therefore usually based upon symptoms alone.

CLINICAL PANEL 27.4

POSTERIOR CEREBRAL ARTERY OCCLUSION

A variety of effects may follow occlusion of branches of the posterior cerebral artery. Usually the occlusion is limited to a branch to the midbrain, *or* to the thalamus, *or* to the subthalamic nucleus, *or* to the cerebral cortex.

Midbrain

The classical picture of a unilateral infarct of the midbrain is that of a *crossed third nerve palsy,* i.e. a complete oculomotor paralysis (Chapter 18) on one side with a hemiplegia on the other side (Weber's syndrome). The hemiplegia is due to infarction of the crus cerebri, which contains corticospinal and corticonuclear fibers in its mid-portion.

Thalamus

Occlusion of a thalamogeniculate branch may cause infarction of the posterior nucleus of the thalamus (which receives the lateral spinothalamic tract) and of the lateral geniculate nucleus. The rare and unpleasant *thalamic syndrome* (Chapter 22) may follow, together with contralateral homonymous hemianopia.

Subthalamic nucleus

Occlusion of a thalamoperforating branch may destroy the small subthalamic nucleus and give rise to *ballism* on the contralateral side, usually affecting the arm (Chapter 25).

Corpus callosum

Infarction of the splenium of the corpus callosum blocks transfer of written information from the right visual association cortex to the left. The result of infarction is *alexia* for written material presented to the left visual field.

Cortex

Occlusion of the stem of the posterior cerebral artery behind the midbrain gives rise to a *homonymous hemianopia* in the contralateral field. Macular vision may be spared. One view of 'macular sparing' is that it signifies bilateral representation of the fovea in the primary visual cortex. Another view is that the occipital pole is supplied by a long branch from the middle cerebral artery supplying the angular gyrus.

Occlusion of the *left* artery also produces *alexia*, the left visual field being the only area detectable by the patient.

A pure alexia, without agraphia, may follow a lesion of the left lingual gyrus.

Bilateral occlusion

Partial or complete *cortical blindness* may result from a thrombus arrested where the lumen of the basilar artery normally narrows below the basilar bifurcation, with consequent blockage of **both** posterior cerebral arteries. It has also been recorded following cardiac arrest with resuscitation.

Temporary cessation of flow in both posterior cerebral arteries sometimes affects only the the anterior parts of their territories. If damage is confined to the occipitotemporal junctions, *prosopagnosia* (inability to identify faces) may occur alone. (Prosopagnosia has been recorded with purely right-sided perfusion failure.) If the entorhinal cortex/hippocampus is compromised on both sides, *anterograde amnesia* may follow.

Most attacks follow lodgement of fibrin clots or detached atheromatous tissue at an arterial branch point, with subsequent dissolution.

■ Transient symptoms originating in the anterior circulation include: motor weakness (a 'heavy feeling') in an arm or leg, hemisensory deficit (a 'numb feeling'), dysphasia, and monocular blindness from occlusion of the central artery of the retina.

■ Transient symptoms originating in the posterior circulation include: vertigo, dipopia, ataxia, and amnesia.

Recognition of TIAs is important, because they serve notice of impending major illness. Without treatment, one case in four will die of a heart attack within 5 years, and one case in six will develop a stroke.

CLINICAL PANEL 27.5

SUBARACHNOID HEMORRHAGE

Blister-like *berry aneurysms* 5-10 mm in diameter are a routine autopsy finding in 2% of adults. Most are in the anterior half of the circle of Willis. *Spontaneous rupture* of an aneurysm into the interpeduncular cistern usually occurs in early or late middle age. The characteristic presentation is a sudden blinding headache, with collapse into semiconsciousness or coma within a few seconds. On physical examination, the only characteristic feature is neck rigidity; this is caused by movement of blood into the posterior cranial fossa, where the dura mater is supplied by the upper cervical nerves (Chapter 4).

The massive rise in intracranial pressure may be fatal within a few hours or days. Recovery may be impeded by a secondary elevation of intracranial pressure caused by *blood–clot obstruction* of cerebrospinal fluid circulation through the tentorial notch or even within the arachnoid granulations.

About a quarter of all cases develop a neurological deficit 4-12 days after the initial attack. The deficit is fatal in a quarter of those who get it. The immediate cause is *spasm* of the main, conducting segments of the cerebral arteries. The amount of spasm is proportionate to the size of the surrounding blood clot in the interpeduncular cistern.

It is usual practice to define the aneurysm by means of angiography, and to ligate it surgically. Without operation, most aneurysms will leak again at some future date.

ANEURYSMS

Subarachnoid hemorrhage may occur without warning, from a ruptured aneurysm at the base of the brain. About 25 000 cases occur annually in the United States. See *Panel 27.5* for details.

CORE INFORMATION

Thromboembolic infarctions originate from the lining of the internal carotid artery or the heart. Hypertensive infarctions may take the form of lacunes following small-artery closure, or major hemorrhage following arterial rupture. Three-quarters of infarctions occur in the anterior circulation, most commonly in the territory of one of the striate arteries. Contralateral motor weakness is the most frequent outcome. In the anterior circulation, a middle cerebral, striate, posterior capsular lesion yields contralateral hemiplegia including the lower face, with or without hemisensory loss and/or ataxia. An anterior cerebral striate (Heubner) lesion yields severe motor weakness of face and arm. Other lesions causing contralateral motor weakness are: prerolandic/rolandic occlusion → weakness of face and arm; callosomarginal → weakness of the leg; high anterior capsular lesion → dysarthria–clumsy hand. In the posterior circulation, the characteristic result is one of crossed paralysis, with a lower motor or sensory lesion on one side and limb paralysis on the other. The supranuclear supply to the facial musculature will escape if the lesion is midpontine or lower.

Occlusion of a perisylvian branch of the middle cerebral artery yields expressive/receptive aphasia if on the dominant side, aprosodia if on the minor side. A lesion of the angular gyrus may result in alexia with homonymous hemianopia. A contralateral homonymous hemianopia is especially characteristic of occlusion of the posterior cerebral artery. Bilateral posterior cerebral occlusion (or hypoperfusion) is rare; it may yield cortical blindness and/or anterograde amnesia.

SELF TEST

From the list of clinical features, select the parent artery (or branch thereof) that would come under suspicion:

1	Motor weakness in one leg	**A**	Anterior cerebral
2	Aphasia	**B**	Middle cerebral
3	Crossed third nerve paralysis	**C**	Posterior cerebral
4	Vertigo	**D**	Basilar
5	Crossed facial paralysis	**E**	Vertebral

From the list of clinical features, select the contralateral cerebral branch artery that would come under suspicion:

6	Ballism	**A**	Pericallosal (ACA)
7	Homonymous hemianopia	**B**	Anterior parietal (MCA)
8	Astereognosis	**C**	Posterior parietal (MCA)
9	Sensory neglect	**D**	Thalamoperforating (PCA)
10	Sympathetic apraxia	**E**	Calcarine (PCA)

REFERENCES

Adams, R.D. and Victor, M. (1989) *Principles of Neurology*, 4th edn. New York: McGraw-Hill.

Betz, A.L., Goldstein, G.W. and Katzman, R. (1989) Blood-brain-cerebrospinal fluid barriers. In *Basic Neurochemistry: Molecular, Cellular, and Medical Aspects*, 4th edn (Siegel, G.J. *et al.*, eds), pp. 591–605. New York: Raven Press.

Brodal, A.(1973) Self-observations and neuro-anatomical considerations after a stroke. *Brain* **96**: 675–694.

Brust, J.C.M. (1989) Cerebral infarction. In *Merritt's Textbook of Neurology*, 8th edn (Rowland, L.P., ed), pp. 206–214. Philadelphia: Lea & Febiger.

Duus, P. (1983) *Topical Diagnosis in Neurology*. New York: Thieme-Stratton, Inc.

Toole, J.F. (1990) *Cerebrovascular Disorders*, 4th edn. New York: Raven Press.

Yatsu, F.M., Grotta, J.C. and Pettigew, L.C. (1995) *Stroke: 100 Maxims*. London: Arnold.

Glossary of Neuroanatomical/ Neurological Terms

Abbreviations:
Ch. Chapter containing main reference; **Gr.** Signifies Greek origin; **L.** Signifies Latin origin.

Abducens L. 'leading away.' Abducens nerve stimulates lateral rectus muscle to abduct the direction of gaze (Ch. 18).

Afferent L. 'carrying toward.' Strictly, applies to nerve impulses traveling toward CNS along sensory fibers; is loosely applied within CNS, e.g. afferent connections of the cerebellum (Ch. 20).

Agnosia Gr. 'without knowledge.' Inability to interpret sensory information (Ch. 24).

Agraphia Gr. 'without writing.' Inability to express oneself in writing, due to a central lesion (Ch. 24).

Akinesia Gr. 'without movement.' Refers to immobility sometimes seen with Parkinson's disease (Ch. 25).

Allocortex Gr. 'other cortex.' Phylogenically old, three-layered cortex in the temporal lobe (Ch. 26).

Alveus Gr. 'trough.' Refers to the thin layer of white matter on the surface of the hippocampus (Ch. 26).

Amygdala Gr. 'almond.' Nucleus at the tip of the inferior horn of the lateral ventricle (Ch. 26).

Anopsia Gr. 'without vision.'

Antidromic Gr. 'running against.' Usually refers to nerve impulses which, traveling proximally along one branch of a Y-shaped sensory nerve fiber, arrive at the junction and travel distally along the other branch (Ch. 9).

Aphasia Gr. 'without speech,' eg. motor aphasia, sensory aphasia (Ch. 24).

Apraxia Gr. 'without movement.' Inability to carry out voluntary movements in the absence of paralysis (Ch. 24).

Arachnoid Gr. 'spiderlike.' Refers to the web-like delicacy of the arachnoid mater (Ch. 4).

Archi- (arche-) Gr. 'beginning,' referring to oldest areas, e.g. archicerebellum (Ch. 20).

Area postrema L. 'backend area,' referring to the posterior tip of the fourth ventricle (Ch. 21).

Astereognosis Gr. 'without knowledge of solid.' Refers to inability to identify common objects by touch alone (Ch. 24).

Astrocyte The 'starlike' neuroglial cell (Ch. 5).

Ataxia Gr. 'without order.' Describes the uncoordinated movements associated with posterior column (Ch. 12) or cerebellar (Ch. 20) disease.

Athetosis Gr. 'without stability.' Describes the continuous writhing movements sometimes associated with damage to the basal ganglia (Ch. 25).

Autonomic Gr. 'self-ruled' (Ch. 10).

Axolemma Gr. 'husk' covering the central part or 'axis' of a nerve fiber (Ch. 5).

Axoplasm Gr. 'substance' (i.e. cytoplasm) of the axon (Ch. 5).

Ballism Gr. 'throwing,' with reference to the flailing movements that follow damage to the subthalamic nucleus (Ch. 25).

Baroreceptor Gr. 'weight' receptor, refers to the blood pressure receptors of the carotid sinus and aortic arch (Ch 14).

Bradykinesia Gr. 'slow movement' characteristic of Parkinson's disease (Ch. 25).

Brain Intracranial CNS.

Brainstem Comprises midbrain, pons and medulla oblongata (Ch. 3). In the embryo, also includes the diencephalon (Ch. 1).

Bulbar L. 'bulb' of the brain, usually means medulla oblongata but 'corticobulbar' fibers project to pons as well (Ch.13).

Calcar avis L. 'spur of a bird,' refers to the elevation produced by the calcarine sulcus in the medial wall of the lateral ventricle (Ch. 2).

Cauda equina L. 'horse's tail,' refers to the leash of spinal nerve roots below the level of the spinal cord (Ch. 11).

Caudate L. having a tail (caudate nucleus, Ch. 2).

Cerebellum L. 'little brain.'

Cerebrum L. 'brain,' comprising cerebral hemispheres and diencephalon (Ch. 2).

Chiasma Gr., from letter resembling an X. Refers mainly to the optic chiasma (chiasm) Ch. 2.

Choroid plexus Gr. 'membranous network' of vessels within the ventricles of the brain (Ch. 2).

Chromatolysis Gr. 'dissolution of color' in the perikaryon, following axotomy (Ch. 7).

Cingulum L. the 'girdle' of white matter within the cingulate gyrus.(Ch. 2).

Claustrum L. the 'barrier' of gray matter between insula and lentiform nucleus (Ch. 2).

Colliculus L. 'little hill.' Four colliculi comprise the tectum of the midbrain (Ch. 3).

Commissure L. 'link' between the two sides of the nervous system, e.g. white c. of the spinal cord (Ch. 3), anterior c. of the brain (Ch. 2).

Contralateral L. refers to opposite side of the body (cf. ipsilateral, same side).

Convolution L. a gyrus (Ch. 2).

Corona radiata L. 'radiating crown' of white matter extending from cerebral cortex to internal capsule and vice versa (Ch. 2).

Corpus callosum L. 'hard body,' refers to the great transverse commissure connecting the cerebral hemispheres (Ch. 2).

Corpus striatum L. 'striated body' comprising caudate and lentiform nuclei (Ch. 2).

Cortex L. the 'bark' of gray matter at the surface of the cerebrum and cerebellum (Ch. 2).

Crus L. 'leg,' e.g. c. of fornix (Ch. 2), c. of midbrain (Ch. 2).

Cuneate L. 'wedge-like,' e.g. c. fasciculus (Ch. 11).

Cuneus L. 'wedge,' e.g. the gyrus of that shape (Ch. 2).

Decussation L. from Roman numeral X. Refers to X-shaped crossing of nerve bundles at junctional regions, e.g. pyramidal d. (brain-spinal cord, Ch. 3), d. of superior cerebellar peduncles (pons-midbrain, Ch. 3).

Dendrite(s) Gr. 'tree(s),' refers to the neuronal processes receiving the axons of other neurons (Ch. 6).

Dentate L. 'toothed,' e.g. d. nucleus of cerebellum (Ch. 2), d. gyrus in the temporal lobe (Ch. 26).

Denticulate L. 'little-toothed,' e.g. d. ligament anchoring the spinal cord (Ch. 4).

Diencephalon Gr. 'between-brain,' comprising epithalamus (Ch. 22), thalamus (Ch. 22), and hypothalamus (Ch. 21).

Diplopia Gr. 'double vision' (Ch. 18).

Dura mater L. 'hard cover.' Outermost meninx (Ch. 4).

Dys- Gr. 'difficult.'

Dysarthria Gr. 'difficult articulation,' e.g. cerebellar d. (Ch. 20).

Dysphagia Gr. 'difficult eating/swallowing,' e.g. following paralysis of pharyngeal constrictors (Ch. 15).

Dysmetria Gr. 'difficult measurement,' refers to reduced motor control in cerebellar disease (Ch. 20).

Ectoderm Gr. 'outer skin,' refers to the outer germ layer giving rise to the nervous system and to the epidermis of the skin (Ch. 1).

Emboliform Gr. 'pluglike,' e.g. e. nucleus of cerebellum (Ch. 20).

Embolus Gr. 'plug,' e.g. cerebral e. formed by a blood clot breaking away from the internal carotid artery (Ch. 27).

Endoneurium Gr. 'within nerve,' refers to the connective tissue sheath surrounding individual Schwann cells (Ch. 7).

Entorhinal Gr. 'in nose,' refers to e. cortex of temporal lobe (Ch. 26).

Ependyma Gr. 'upper garment,' refers to lining epithelium of ventricular system of brain (Ch. 2) and central canal of spinal cord (Ch. 3).

Epineurium Gr. 'on nerve,' refers to loose connective tissue investment of peripheral nerves (Ch. 7).

Epithalamus Gr. 'above thalamus,' includes pineal gland (Ch. 22).

Exteroception L. 'reception from outside,' refers to stimuli transduced at the body surface, rather than within the body wall/limbs (proprioception) or alimentary tract (enteroception).

Extrapyramidal L. outmoded term having reference to basal ganglia.

Falx L. 'sickle,' refers to shape, e.g. f. cerebri, f. cerebelli (Ch. 4).

Fasciculus L. 'small bundle' of nerve fibers within CNS, e.g. f. gracilis, f. cuneatus (Ch. 12).

Fastigial L. 'apex of a roof,' e.g. f. nucleus in roof of fourth ventricle (Ch. 20).

Fimbria L. 'fringe,' refers to the fringe of white fibers along the edge of the hippocampus (Ch. 26).

Foramen L. 'opening.'

Forceps L. 'pair of tongs,' e.g. f. minor, f. major (Ch. 2).

Fornix L. 'arch,' refers to the efferent projection of the hippocampal formation (Chs 2, 26).

Fovea L. 'pit, ditch,' e.g. f. centralis of the retina (Ch. 23).

Funiculus L. 'small cord.'

Ganglion Gr. 'knot.'

Geniculate L. 'knee-form,' meaning bent.

Genu L. 'knee,' meaning a bend.

Glia Gr. 'glue,' refers to the interstitial, neuroglial cells of the CNS (Ch. 5)

Globose L. 'ball-like,' refers to the g. nucleus of the cerebellum (Ch. 20)

Globus L. 'ball,' usually refers to g. pallidus in the cerebral white matter (Ch. 2).

Glomerulus L. 'little ball of yarn,' e.g. synaptic glomeruli in the cerebellum (Ch. 20) and olfactory bulb (Ch. 26).

Glossopharyngeal G. 'lingual-pharyngeal' with reference to the sensory distribution of the g. nerve (Ch. 15).

Gyrus L. convolution of the cerebral cortex (Ch. 2).

Gracilis L. 'slender,' e.g. gracile fasciculus in the spinal cord (Ch. 12).

Hemiplegia Gr. 'half-struck,' refers to paralysis of one half of the body following a major stroke (Ch. 27).

Hippocampus Gr. 'sea horse.' Part of the limbic system. (Chs 2, 26)

Hydrocephalus Gr. 'water-head,' meaning increased volume of cerebrospinal fluid (Ch. 4).

Hyper- Gr. 'excessive,' e.g. hyperacusis, excessive perception of sound (Ch. 17).

Hypo- Gr. 'below,' e.g. hypoglossal (Ch. 15), hypothalamus (Ch. 21).

Infundibulum L. 'funnel,' leading down to the hypophysis (Ch. 21).

Insula L. 'island' of cerebral cortex covered by the opercula (Ch. 2).

Internuncial L. 'messenger between,' refers to small connecting neurons (Ch. 5).

Intra- L. 'within,' e.g. intralaminar nucleus of thalamus (Ch. 22).

Ipsilateral L. 'on same side.'

Infarction L. 'stuffed into,' refers to blood-stuffed necrotic tissue resulting from vascular occlusion (Ch. 27).

Iso- Gr. 'equal,' e.g. isocortex, uniformly containing six layers of neurons (Ch. 24).

Kinesthesia Gr. 'perception of movement' (Ch. 12).

Lemniscus L. 'ribbon' of white matter.

Lentiform L. lens-shaped nucleus, part of the corpus striatum (Ch. 2).

Leptomeninges Gr. 'thin membranes' comprising the pia-arachnoid mater (Ch. 4).

Lesion L. 'wound,' refers to tissue damage of any kind.

Limbic L. 'marginal,' refers to limbic structures at the inner margin of the cerebral hemisphere (Ch. 26).

Locus ceruleus L. 'dark blue place' in the (fresh) floor of fourth ventricle (Ch. 19).

Macula L. 'spot,' e.g. macula of utricle (Ch. 16), macula lutea (yellow) of retina (Ch. 23).

Mamillary (mammillary) L. 'nipple-like,' refers to mamillary bodies (Ch. 21).

Medulla L. 'marrow,' refers to the marrow-like appearance of the fresh brain and spinal cord within their bony shells.

Mesencephalon Gr. 'midbrain.'

Mesoderm Gr. 'middle skin,' refers to the middle germ layer (Ch. 1).

Metencephalon Gr. 'after the brain,' comprises embryonic pons and cerebellum (Ch. 1).

Microglia Gr. small glial cells (Ch. 6).

Miosis Gr. 'constriction' of the pupil (Ch. 18).

Myasthenia Gr. 'muscle weakness' (Ch. 7).

Myelencephalon Gr. 'marrowbrain,' refers to the embryonic medulla oblongata (Ch. 2).

Myelin Gr. 'marrow,' refers to the myelin sheath of axons (Ch. 7).

Neo- Gr. 'new,' e.g. neocerebellum (Ch. 20), neocortex (Ch. 24).

Neurite Gr. process of a neuron, whether axon or dendrite (Ch. 6).

Neuroblast Gr. 'nerve germ,' refers to embryonic neuron (Ch.1).

Neurofibril L. refers to matted neurofilaments seen by light microscopy (Ch. 6).

Neurofilament L. the fine filaments seen in neurons by electron microscopy (Ch. 6).

Neurolemma Gr. 'nerve sheath,' comprising chains of Schwann cells (Ch. 7).

Neuron Gr. 'nerve,' refers to the complete nerve cell (Ch. 6).

Nociceptive L. 'taking injury.' Responsive to noxious stimulation (Ch. 9).

Nucleus L. 'nut.' Refers either to the trophic centre of a cell, or to a group of neurons within the CNS (Ch. 6).

Nystagmus Gr. 'nodding,' refers to involuntary oscillation of the eyes (Ch. 16).

Oculomotor L. 'eyemoving,' refers to the oculomotor nerve (Ch. 18).

Oligodendrocyte Gr. 'few tree cell.' A neuroglial cell with few processes (Ch. 6).

Operculum L. 'cover,' refers to any of the three opercula covering the insula (Ch. 2).

Ophthalmoplegia Gr. 'eye stroke,' signifies paralysis of extrinsic ocular muscles (Ch. 16).

Pachymeninx Gr. 'thick membrane,' the dura mater (Ch. 4).

Paleo- Gr. 'old,' e.g. paleocerebellum (mainly the anterior lobe, Ch. 20), paleocortex (olfactory, Ch. 26), paleostriatum (globus pallidus, Ch. 25).

Pallidum L. 'pale,' refers to globus pallidus (Ch. 25).

Pallium Gr. 'cloak.' Used interchangeably for Cerebral cortex.

Para- Gr. 'beside.'

Paralysis Gr. 'disablement.' Loss of voluntary movement.

Paraplegia Gr. 'paralysis,' refers to paralysis of both lower limbs (Ch. 12).

Paresis Gr. 'weakness.' Incomplete paralysis.

Peduncle L. 'little foot,' refers to stem, e.g. cerebral peduncle (Ch. 2).

Peri- Gr. 'around,' e.g. perikaryon, cytoplasm around the neuronal nucleus; perineurium, the epithelial and tight connective tissue investment of peripheral nerve (Ch. 7).

Pia mater Gr. 'soft cover,' the innermost layer of the meninges (Ch. 4).

Pineal L. 'pine cone.' Pineal gland is part of the epithalamus (Ch. 21).

Plexus L. 'interwoven.' Interwoven nerves or blood vessels.

Pons L. 'bridge.' Part of brainstem in the interval between midbrain and medulla oblongata (Ch. 2).

Projection L. 'forward throw.' Target of a neuronal pathway, e.g. spinothalamic tract projects to the thalamus (Ch. 12).

Proprioception Gr. 'self perception.' Conscious or unconscious reception by the brain, of information from muscles, tendons and joints (Ch. 12).

Pros- Gr. 'before,' e.g. prosencephalon, embryonic forebrain (Ch. 1).

Prosopagnosia Gr. 'face-no-knowledge.' Inability to recognize faces (Ch. 24).

Ptosis Gr. 'falling.' Drooping of the upper eyelid (Ch.18).

Pulvinar L. 'cushion,' refers to posterior bulge of thalamus above the midbrain (Ch. 2).

Putamen L. 'shell,' refers to outer part of lentiform nucleus (Ch. 2).

Quadriplegia L/Gr. 'four-stroke,' paralysis of all four limbs (Ch. 13).

Raphe Gr. 'seam,' refers to the midline. Gr. genitive case is used in nucleus raphes magnus (Ch. 19).

Receptor A term with two distinct meanings: (a) Sensory receptors eg. photoreceptors, neuromuscular spindles, transduce sensory stimuli; (b) Molecular receptors on or within cells are protein molecules acted upon by messenger molecules, e.g. hormones, neurotransmitters.

Reticular L. 'netlike,' e.g. reticular formation (Ch. 19).

Rhinencephalon Gr. 'nosebrain,' refers to olfactory areas (Ch. 26).

Rhombencephalon Gr. 'rhomboid-brain' containing the rhomboid fourth ventricle. Embryologically, the hindbrain vesicle (Ch. 1).

Rostrum L. 'beak.' R. of corpus callosum extends from genu to lamina terminalis (Ch. 2).

Rubro- L. 'red,' refers to projections from red nucleus (Ch. 14).

Satellite L. 'attendant,' e.g. satellite Schwann cells in spinal ganglia (Ch. 6).

Septal region L. 'partition,' related to septum pellucidum (Ch. 26).

Septum pellucidum L. 'transparent partition' separating the frontal horns of the lateral ventricles (Ch. 2).

Somatic Gr. 'body-related.' Implies body wall as distinct from viscera, e.g. somatotopic, containing a body map; **somesthetic,** perception of position/movement of trunk and limbs.

Splenium L. 'pad.' refers to posterior end of corpus callosum (Ch. 2).

Stellate 'starlike,' e.g. stellate ganglion (Ch. 10).

Strabismus Gr. 'squinting.'

Stria L. 'narrow band,' e.g. stria terminalis originating in the amygdala (Ch. 26).

Striatum L. 'furrowed,' refers to caudate nucleus and putamen taken together (Ch. 2).

Subiculum L. 'little layer,' refers to transitional zone between six-layered parahippocampal gyrus and three-layered hippocampus (Ch. 26).

Substantia L. 'substance,' e.g. **substantia gelatinosa** of spinal gray matter (Ch. 12), substantia nigra (L. 'black') of midbrain (Ch.14).

Subthalamus region below thalamus containing subthalamic nucleus (Ch. 25).

Sulcus L. 'groove.'

Sympathetic Gr. 'with-feeling,' i.e. responsive to emotional state.

Synapse Gr. 'contact,' refers to sites of contact between neurons (Ch. 6).

Syndrome Gr. 'running together.' A characteristic group of symptoms/signs.

Syringomyelia Gr. 'marrow-tube,' refers to central cavitation of the spinal cord (Ch. 12).

Tapetum L. 'carpet,' refers to sheet of callosal fibers above the lateral ventricles (Ch. 2).

Tegmentum L. 'covering,' refers to intermediate region of midbrain and pons (Ch. 14).

Tectum L. 'roof' (of midbrain, Ch. 14).

Tela choroidea L. 'membranous web,' consisting of vascular pia-ependyma (Ch. 2).

Telencephalon Gr. 'endbrain,' comprising the embryonic cerebral hemispheres (Ch. 1).

Tentorium L. 'tent.'

Tetraplegia Gr. 'four-paralysis,' synonymous with quadriplegia.

Thalamus Gr/L. 'bridal meetingplace.'

Thrombus Gr/L. 'clot' (of blood, Ch. 27).

Tract (L. tractus, 'district') A group of CNS axons having the same origin and destination.

Transduction L. 'leading across,' refers to conversion of sensory stimuli into trains of nerve impulses.

Trapezoid (L. 'diamond-shaped') **body** Collection of second-order auditory fibers in the pons (Ch. 15).

Trigeminal L. 'triplet,' refers to the three divisions of the trigeminal nerve (Ch. 16).

Trochlear L. 'pulley.' Transferred epithet: tendon of superior oblique muscle passes through a fascial pulley, and the name is applied to the nerve of supply (Ch. 18).

Trophic Gr. 'nourishing.'

Uncus L. 'hook' (Ch. 26).

Uvula L. 'little grape' (Ch. 20).

Vagus L. 'wandering' (Ch. 15).
Vallecula L. 'little valley' (Ch. 20).
Velum L. 'veil.'
Ventricle L. 'little belly.'
Vermis L. 'worm' (Ch. 20).

INDEX

Abdominal reflexes, 92, 124
Abducens nerve, 178
  development, 4
  paralysis, 181
Abducens nucleus, 135
Absence attacks, 259
Accessory cuneate nucleus, 114
Accessory olivary nucleus, 115, 133
Accommodation, 179, 184
Accommodation reflex, 86, 179
Acetylcholine (ACh) *see* Cholinergic neurons
Achilles tendon reflex, 101
Achromatopsia, 233
Acoustic neuroma, 173
Acoustic reflexes, brainstem, 161
Acupuncture, 193
Adamkiewicz artery, 128
Adrenal medulla, 85–8
Adrenalin *see* Epinephrine
Adrenergic neurons, 87
  see also Noradrenergic neurons
Adrenoceptors, 87–8
Afferents
  nociceptive, 78
  primary/secondary/tertiary, 108
  visceral, 91–2
Agonist drugs, 57
Agraphia, 243
Akinesia, 236, 251
Alar plate, 1, 95
Alcoholism, 202
Alexia, 243, 276
Alpha motoneurons, 74, 117–18, 121–2
Alvear path, 260
Alveus, 260
Alzheimer's disease, 262, 263

Amacrine cells, 220, 221, 222
Amine uptake pump, 88
Aminergic neurons, 181–9, 194, 200, 216
Aminergic pathways, 126, 200
Amines, biogenic, 126
  see also named amines
Γ-Aminobutyric acid (GABA) *see* GABAergic neurons
Ammon's horn, 260
  see also Hippocampus
Amnesia, 262
  anterograde, 276
Amphetamine, 89
Amputation neuroma, 65
Amygdala, 21, 265–6
Amyloid plaques, 263
Amyotrophic lateral sclerosis, 126
Analgesia
  antinociceptors, 192–3
  postcordotomy, 112
  stimulus-produced, 193
  stress-induced, 193
  see also Pain
Anesthesia
  caudal, 103
  epidural, 103
  spinal, 101, 103
Aneurysms, 274, 277
Angina pectoris, 91
Angular gyrus, 237, 243
  lesions, 243
Anhidrosis, 181, 182
Ankle clonus, 124, 127
Annulospiral nerve endings, 73
Anosmia, 258
Anosognosia, 241
Ansa lenticularis, 248
Anterior cerebral artery, 43
  occlusion, 43, 271

Anterior cingulate cortex, 262–3
Anterior cingulotomy, for pain, 263
Anterior circulation of the brain, 274
  vs posterior circulation, 274–5
Anterior commissure, 5, 9, 20
Anterior communicating artery, 42
Anterior corticospinal tract, 120
Anterior funiculus, 30
Anterior gray horn, 30, 117–19
Anterior inferior cerebellar artery, 118
Anterior nerve roots, 63
Anterior olfactory nucleus, 258
Anterior perforated substance, 43, 266
Anterior ramus, 63
Anterior spinal artery, 45, 128
Anterior spinocerebellar tract, 9
Anterograde amnesia, 262
Anterograde transport, 54
Anticholinergic drugs, 89
Antidiuretic hormone, 208–10
Aortic bodies, 149
Aphasias, 240
Appendicitis, 92
Appestat, 210
Apraxia, 242–4
Aprosodias, 237, 240
Aqueduct
  anatomy, 26, 27
  development, 3
Arachnoid granulations, 39
Arachnoid mater, 32, 34
Arachnoid trabeculae, 34
Arcuate fasciculus, 18, 237
Arcuate nucleus, 206
Areflexia, 126
Arnold–Chiari malformation, 38

Arteries, *see* named arteries
Artery of Adamkiewicz, 128
Ascending pathways (spinal cord), 105–16
Ascending reticular activating system, 114, 192, 215
Ascent of spinal cord, 96–7
Association fibers, 17, 230
Association nuclei of thalamus, 214–15
Astereognosis, 243
Astrocytes, 58–9
Astrocytoma, 60
Ataxia
    cerebellar, 110, 157, 202
    sensory, 110, 154
    truncal, 201
Athetosis, 252
Atonic bladder, 125, 127
Auditory association cortex, 234
Auditory comprehension, 237
Auditory cortex, 159, 162, 234
Auditory radiation, 161
Auditory receptors, 157–62
Auras, 259
Autogenetic inhibition, 74
Automatic bladder, 127
Autonomic nervous system, 83–94
    interaction with immune system, 91
    neurotransmission, 87–91
        see also Parasympathetic; Sympathetic nervous system
Autoreceptors, 87
Autoregulation, blood flow, 48–9
Axoaxonic synapses, 58
Axon
    defined, 51
    growth cones, 65–6
    degeneration/regeneration, 65–7
    structure, 55, 58–9
Axon reflex, 78, 79
Axotomy, 66

Babinski sign, 124, 129
Bainbridge reflex, 149
Balance *see* Vestibular reflexes
Ballism, 276
Baroreceptor (barosympathetic) reflex, 127, 191
Baroreceptor nucleus, 148, 149
Barovagal reflex, 191
Basal forebrain, 266–7
Basal forebrain nuclei, 266
Basal ganglia, 13, 14, 247–55

circuits, 247–53
    motor learning, 250
Basal nucleus of Meynert, 192, 216, 266
    neuron loss, 263
Basal plate, 95, 96
Basilar artery, 42, 118
Basilar membrane, 158
Basilar pons, 28
Basket cells
    cerebellar, 54, 198, 203
    cerebral, 53
Bell's palsy, 172
Beta blockers, 89
Betz cells, 120, 230
Biceps reflex, 101
Biogenic amines, 126
Bipolar cells, 230
Bladder *see* Urinary bladder
Blind spot, 220
Blinking reflex, 171
Blood supply, 42–51
    brainstem, 45–6
    forebrain, 42–5
    spinal cord, 128
Blood–brain barrier, 49–50
Blood–cerebrospinal fluid barrier, 49
Blood–extracellular fluid (ECF) barrier, 49
Body schema, 241
Boutons, 71
Brachioradialis reflex, 101
Bradykinesia, 251
Brain
    capillary bed, 49
    edema *see* Cerebral edema
    extracellular compartments, 49
    extracellular fluid (ECF), blood–ECF barrier, 49
    herniation, 271
    vesicles, 1–2, 3
Brain tumors, 60
Brainstem, 131–40
    aminergic neurons, 187–9
    anatomy, 25–8, 131–9
    blood supply, 45–6
    development, 2
    principal motor decussations, 136
    reflexes
        acoustic, 159, 161
        facial nerve, 171
Broca's area, 237
    see also Limbic
Broca's diagonal band, nucleus, 266
Brodmann's map, 231, 233, 239

Buffer nerves, 191

C fibers, 78, 192
Calcarine cortex, 226
Calcarine sulcus, 6, 10, 226
Caloric test, 156
Cardioinhibitory center, 135
Cardiovascular center, 191
Carotid arteries, 42
    accompanying fibers, 156–8
    occlusion, 273, 275
Carotid body, 149, 190
Carotid sinus, 149, 191
    function, 127
Catecholamines, 181
Cauda equina, 97, 99
    syndrome, 103
Caudal anesthesia, 103
Caudal cell mass, 96
Caudate nucleus, 6, 12, 13, 15
    cognitive loop, 252
Cavernous sinus, 33–4
Cavum of septum pellucidum, 20
Cellular laminae, cerebral cortex, 229
Central gray matter, 131, 134
Central reticular nucleus, 186
Central sulcus, 6
Central tegmental tract, 136
Cerebellopontine angle, lesions, 173
Cerebellum, 196–203
    afferent fibers, 198, 199–200
    anatomy, 28–9, 196–7
    blood supply, 45–6
    climbing fibers, 198, 200
    deep nuclei, 29
    development, 2, 3
    efferents, 200–1
    flocculonodular lobe, 29, 154
    folia, 29
    lesions, 201–3
    microscopic anatomy, 197–9
    mossy fibers, 197, 198–9, 203
    penducles, 135, 136, 160
    vermis, 29
Cerebral arteries, 42–6, 231
    embolism, 277
    occlusion, 272, 275, 276
    see also named arteries
Cerebral commissures, 18
Cerebral compression, 35
Cerebral cortex, 228–45
    association fibers, 17
    asymmetries of hemispheres, 236–8
    blood supply, 42–6, 231, 272–7
    cell types, 53, 230

Cerebral cortex (*continued*)
cellular laminae, 229
cytoarchitecture, 231
development, 4–6
entorhinal cortex, 258
histology, 229–199
isocortex, 229, 258
mesocortex, 258
modular structure, 229
motor areas, 234–5
neocortex, 228, 229
prefrontal, 236
premotor, 235–6
sensory, 231–2
supplementary motor area
(SMA), 249
Cerebral edema, 51
Cerebral hemispheres,
asymmetries, 236–8
Cerebral hemorrhage, 50, 271–4
Cerebral palsy, 252
Cerebral peduncle, 25–8
Cerebral veins, 46–8
Cerebrospinal fluid (CSF)
blood–ECF barrier, 49
circulation, 37–40
secretion, 39, 49
Cerebrovascular disease, 270–8
Ceruleospinal pathway, 193
Cervical enlargement, spinal
cord, 29
Cervical headache, 167
Cervical spondylosis, 102
Chemoreceptors
carotid, 149
medullary, 191–2
Cholinergic drugs, 89
Cholinergic neurons
aceytcholine release 88–90
autonomic, 87
hippocampus, 261, 262
motoneurons, 74
reticular formation, 191
septal nucleus, 261
Chorda tympani, 174
Choreoathetosis, 252
Choroid fissure, 5, 15
Choroid plexus, 5, 15, 21
Choroidal epithelium, 49
Chromaffin cells, 88
Chromatolysis, 66–7
Ciliary ganglion, 86, 177
Ciliary muscle, 176, 179
Cingulate cortex, 262–3
Cingulate gyrus, 114, 252, 264
Cingulate sulcus, 10
Cingulum, 18
Circle of Willis, 42, 43, 271
Circumduction (gait), 273

Cisterna ambiens, 36
Cisterna magna, 36
Clarke's nucleus dorsalis, 114
Claustrum, 15
Climbing fibers, 198, 200
Clonus, 124, 127
Coactivation, alpha–gamma
motoneurons, 121
Cochlea, 157–8
Cochlear nerve, 142, 159, 160,
162
Cochlear nucleus, 159
Cocontraction, 121
Cognitive loop, 252
Cognitive style, 238–9
Collicular commissure, 160
Colliculi, 26, 28
facial, 170, 174
inferior, 26, 27, 125, 159, 160
superior, 26, 27, 115, 125,
138, 183
Commissural nucleus, 148
Conductive deafness, 161
Coning, 60
Conjugate eye movement, 154,
182
Conscious proprioception, 108
Contralateral neglect, 243, 272
Convergence (ocular), 179
Cordotomy, 112
Corneal reflex, 173
Corona radiata, 13
Corpus callosum, 23
anatomy, 2, 5–6, 18–20
blood supply, 276
development, 6
Corpus striatum, 13, 15
development, 5–6
Corti, organ of, 158–9 ·
Cortical areas *see* Brodmann's
areas
Cortical blindness, 276
Cortical type sensory loss, 243
Corticobulbar fibers, 144
Corticomotoneuronal fibers, 121
Corticopontine fibers, 136
Corticopontocerebellar pathway,
136
Corticospinal tracts, 14–15, 74,
119–22, 125, 136
Cough reflex, 149
Coughing center, 189
Covert attention (orientation), 240
Cranial accessory nerve, 4, 144,
149
Cranial nerves
development, 4
general arrangement, 25–6,
141–2

see also individual nerves
Craniosacral outflow of
autonomic NS, 86
Cristae, 154
Crocodile tears, 172
Crossed hemiplegia, 173
Crossed third nerve palsy, 276
Crus cerebri, 13, 136
infarct, 276
CSF–blood barrier, 49
Cuneate fasciculus, 105, 110
Cuneate nucleus, 26, 28, 110,
114, 131, 132
Cuneate tubercles, 26
Cuneocerebellar tract, 114
Cuneus, 10
Cupula, 154

Deafness, conductive and
sensorineural, 161, 162
Declarative memory, 262
Decussation
of cerebellar peduncles, 136
of pyramids, 26, 28, 120, 124,
131
Deep nuclei of cerebellum, 29
Degeneration of nerve fibers,
65–7
Deiteroocular pathway, 154, 155
Deiterospinal tract, 154
see also Vestibulospinal tract
Deiters' (lateral vestibular)
nucleus, 154, 200
Déjà vu, 259
Dementia, 2–17, 253
Dendrites, 53–4
Dendritic spines, 53, 54, 58
Dendrodendritic excitation, 57
Denervation supersensitivity, 126
Dentate gyrus, 197, 260
Dentate nucleus, 29, 197
Dentatothalamic tract, 201
Dentatothalamocortical tract,
136
Denticulate ligament, 97
Depression, 92, 187, 189, 209
Depressor center, 191
Dermal plexus, 77
Dermatomes, 99–100, 100, 101
Descending motor pathways,
117–29
Diabetes insipidus, 208
Diabetes mellitus, 208
Diagonal band (of Broca), 266
Diaphragma sellae, 33
Diencephalic amnesia, 262
Diencephalon
anatomy, 11–12, 22
development, 2, 3

Diencephalon (*continued*)
see also Third ventricle
Diffuse noxious inhibitory
controls, 193
Dilator pupillae, 85, 180
Diplopia, 61, 181
Dissociated sensory loss, 112, 113
Dopaminergic receptors 248
Dopaminergic neurons
in hippocampus, 261
in hypothalamus, 208
in midbrain, 187–8
in sympathetic ganglia, 89
Dopaminergic pathway,
mesolimbic, 137
Dopaminergic receptors, 248
Dorsal nerve roots, 107
Down's syndrome, 263
Drugs
lock and key analogy, 57
and parasympathetic system, 90
and sympathetic system, 89
Dura mater
cranial, 32, 34, 38
innervation, 34
spinal, 37
Dyskinesias, 251
Dyslexia, 238, 241

Edinger–Westphal nucleus, 177, 178, 179
Ejaculation, 91
Electrotonus, 56–7, 220
Embolism, cerebral artery, 272
Embryology of the nervous
system, 1–7
Encapsulated nerve endings, 78–81
Endogenous depression, 92, 187, 189
Endolymph, 153
Endoneurium, 64
Endorphins, 193
Enkephalins, 192
Entorhinal cortex, 258
Ependymal cells, 60
Epidermis *see* Skin
Epidural anesthesia, 103
Epilepsy, 259
Epinephrine, 88, 187, 188
Epineurium, 63, 97
Epithalamus, 216–18
Expressive aphasia, 237, 240
Extensor plantar response, 124
Extensor thrust, 119
Exteroceptive sensations, 108
Extradural hematomas, 34

Extradural space, 103
Extradural venous plexus, 97
Extreme capsule, 15
Eye
eyerighting reflexes, 154
movement controls, 182–3
scanning and tracking, 182–3
sympathetic pathway, 180–2

Faces, recognition, 233
Facial colliculus, 170, 174
Facial nerve, 170–4
components, 170
lesions, 172–3
nervus intermedius, 171
reflexes, 171
Facial nucleus, 170
Facial pain, 167
Falx cerebri, 33
Far and near responses, 179–80
Fasciculation, muscular, 126
Fasciculus cuneatus, 105, 110
Fasciculus gracilis, 105, 110
Fasciculus retroflexus, 264
Fastigial nucleus, 197
Feeding center, 210
Fibrillation, muscular, 126
Filopodia, 65
Filum terminale, 96, 98
Fimbria, 260
Finger-to-nose test, 108
Fissures (cerebellum), 29
Fixation reflex, 179, 182
Flexor plantar response, 124
Flexor reflex, 119
Flocculonodular lobe, 29, 31, 154
Floppy infant syndrome, 252
Follicular nerve endings, 78
Forceps, major/minor, 18
Fornix, anatomy, 5, 15, 20, 261
Fourth ventricle
anatomy, 22
development, 3, 4
nuclei, 134
Fovea centralis, 220
Fractionation, 121
Frontal eye fields, 182–3, 236
Frontal forceps, 20
Frontal leukotomy, 237
Frontal lobe, 10
dysfunction, 237
see also Cerebral cortex
Fundus oculi, 38
Funiculus(i), 30

Gag reflex, 149
Gait, 202, 203
Gamma loop, 122

Gamma motoneurons, 74, 118
Ganglia *see under individual ganglia*
Ganglionic transmission, 87
Gasserian ganglion, 164, 167
Gate control, 192
Gaze centers, 182, 189
Geniculocalcarine tract, 224–6
Gennari, visual stria, 226
Giant cells of Betz, 120, 230
Giant motor unit potentials, 72
Glial scar, 68
Glioblasts, 95
Glioma, 60
Gliosis, 59
Globus pallidus *see* Pallidum
Glomerulus
of cerebellum, 200
of olfactory bulb, 257
Glomus cells, 191
Glossopharyngeal nerve, 4, 148–9
Golgi cells, 198–9, 203
Golgi complex, 54, 55
Golgi tendon organs, 74, 119
Gracile fasciculus, 105, 110
Gracile nucleus, 26, 28, 110, 131, 132
Gracile tubercles, 26
Granule cells
cerebral cortex, 229
dentate gyrus, 197, 257
Gray commissure, 30
Great cerebral vein of Galen, 47
Growth cones, axons, 65–6
Gustatory nucleus, 147
Gyri, 8, 10–12
see also under named gyri

Habenular commissure, 20, 22, 264
Habenular nucleus, 264
Hair cells
cochlea, 154
vestibule, 154
Handedness, hemispheric
asymmetries, 236–8
Head injuries, 35
eye signs, 181
Headache, 167, 169
Headrighting reflexes, 154
Heart, parasympathetic/sympathetic innervation, 88
Hemianopia, 225, 276
Hemiballism(us), 252
Hemineglect, 241, 243, 272
Hemiparesis, 124–5
Hemiplegia, 270
alternating, 173

Hemiplegia (continued)
    alternating/crossed, 157
    gait, 273
Hemispheric asymmetries,
        cerebral cortex, 236–8
Hering–Breuer reflex, 149
Herpes zoster oticus, 173
Herring bodies, 208
Heschl's gyrus, 161, 234, 239
Heubner, recurrent artery of, 43,
        277
Hippocampal formation, 260–2
    anatomy, 15–16
    development, 5, 15
    mnemonic function, 261–2
Histaminergic neurons, 211
Horizontal cells, 221–2
Horner's syndrome, 85, 146,
        181, 184
Huntington's chorea, 252
Hydrocephalus, causes and
        features, 39
5-Hydroxytryptamine see
        Serotonin
Hypercapnia, 48, 50, 51
Hyperhidrosis, 85
Hyperkinesia, 252
Hyperreflexia, 124–5
Hypertensive encephalopathy, 50
Hypogastric nerves, 85
Hypoglossal nerve, 134, 143–4,
        150
    development, 4, 5
Hypoglossal nucleus, 134, 142,
        144
Hypokinesia, 251, 253–17
Hypophysiotropic area, 207
Hypophysis, 205–12
Hypothalamic sulcus, 205
Hypothalamohypophyseal tract,
        207–8
Hypothalamus, 205–12
    anatomy, 12
    development, 5–6
    disorders, 208
    nuclei, 205
    subdivisions, 205–6

Ideomotor apraxia, 242–3
Idiopathic epilepsy, 259
Immune system, interaction with
        autonomic system, 91
Impotence, 85, 91
Incontinence see Urinary
        incontinence
Infarction, 271
Inferior brachium, 159
Inferior cerebellar peduncles,
        135, 136, 160

Inferior colliculi, 26, 27, 125,
        159, 160
Inferior longitudinal fasciculus,
        20
Inferior olivary nucleus, 28, 133
Inferior parietal lobule, and body
        schema, 241
Inferior sagittal sinus see Sinuses
Infranuclear palsy, 173
Infundibulum, 21, 205
Inhibition, autogenetic, 74
Insula, 8–9, 262
    development, 4
Intention tremor, 202
Internal capsule, 13–15
Internal carotid artery, occlusion,
        271, 273
Internal medullary lamina, 215
Internuncial neurons, 73–4,
        118–19
Interpeduncular fossa, 25
Interpeduncular nucleus, 264
Interthalamic adhesion, 12
Interventricular foramen, 4, 20
Intervertebral disc, prolapse, 102
Intralaminar nuclei, 215
Isthmus rhomboencephali, 136,
        137, 139

Jamais vu, 259
Jaw jerk, 169–70
Jaw opening/closing reflex, 169
Joint sense, 108
Joints, innervation, 75
Jugular foramen syndrome, 146
Junctional folds, 71
Junctional receptors, 87–9
Junctional transmission, 87

Kindling, 262
Kinesthetic sense, 108
Kinocilium(a), 153, 154
Kluver–Bucy syndrome, 266

Labor, 103
Labyrinth, 152–6
Lacrimal gland, 86
Lacunae, 39
Lacunar infarction, 271–2, 273
Lamina cribrosa, 177
Lamina terminalis, 21, 205
Laminae of Rexed, 106
Language, 237–8
    modular organization, 238
    see also Speech
Lateral corticospinal tract
        (LCST), 120–1
Lateral funiculus, 30
Lateral geniculate nucleus

        (LGN), 213, 214, 223–6
Lateral lemniscus, 136, 159,
        160, 162
Lateral medullary nucleus, 189
Lateral medullary syndrome, 157
Lateral reticular nucleus, 186
Lateral sulcus, 6, 8
Lateral ventricle, 3
    anatomy, 15, 20–2
    development, 37–9
Lateral vestibular nucleus, 154
Lateral vestibulospinal tract, 154
Left handedness, hemispheric
        asymmetries, 236–8
Lemniscus
    lateral, 136, 159, 160, 162
    medial, 110, 133
    spinal, 112, 136
    trigeminal, 110, 136
Lenticular fasciculus, 248
Lentiform nucleus, 5, 13, 15
Leprosy, 80
Leptomeninges, 32
Lesser petrosal nerve, 148
Levator palpebrae superioris,
        180, 184
Ligamentum denticulatum, 35
Limbic lobe, 11
Limbic loop, 252–3
Limbic system, 11, 258–67
Lingual gyrus, 10, 237
Lissauer's tract, 106, 107, 125,
        129, 193
Lock and key analogy of drugs,
        57
Locomotion, 123
    movement initiation, 241–3
    segmental control, 101
    see also Movement, voluntary
Locus ceruleus, 136, 188, 192,
        193
Long term potentiation, 262
Long-loop stretch reflex, 203
Low back pain, 102
Lower motor neuron disease,
        126
Lumbar cistern, 37
Lumbar enlargement, spinal
        cord, 29
Lumbar puncture, 37, 49, 101,
        103
Lumbar splanchnic nerves, 85
Lumbar sympathectomy, 85
Lumbosacral roots, compression,
        102
Luschka's joints, 82

Macula lutea, 220
Macula of saccule, 153, 154

Macula of utricle, 153, 154
Macular cortex, 225
Macular sparing, 225, 276
Magnetic resonance imaging, 231
Magnocellular reticular formation, 186, 208–10
Mamillary bodies, 22, 205, 211
Mamillothalamic tract, 211
Mastication, 169
Mechanoreceptors, 79
Medial forebrain bundle, 206
Medial geniculate nucleus, 159, 161, 213, 214
Medial lemniscus, 110, 133
Medial longitudinal fasciculus, 133, 182
Medial parabrachial nucleus, 191
Median eminence, 205
Medulla oblongata
  anatomy, 2, 3, 26, 28, 133
  cell columns, 141–2
  medullary chemoreceptor area, 190–2
  tractotomy, 165
Medullary reticulospinal tract, 122–3
Medullary syndromes, 157
Medulloblastoma, 201
Meissner's corpuscles, 79, 80–1
Melatonin, 217
Membranous labyrinth, 152
Memory, 210, 262
Meningeal arteries, 34
Meninges, 32–41
  cranial, 32–7
  CSF, 37–40
  spinal, 37–8
Meningioma, 258
Meningitis, 34, 38
Meningocele, 98
Meningomyelocele, 98
Merkel cell-neurite complexes, 77, 78, 78–81
Mesaxon, 64–5
Mesencephalic nucleus of trigeminal nerve, 136, 164–5
Mesencephalon, 1, 2, 3
Mesocortex, 258
Mesolimbic dopaminergic pathway, 137
Meyer's loop, 224, 225, 276
Meynert's nucleus, 192, 216, 263, 266
Microglia, 60, 95
Microtubules, 53–5
Micturition, 87, 189–90

Midbrain, 25–8
  infarction, 276
Middle cerebral artery occlusion, 272
Milk ejection reflex, 210
Mitral cells, 257
Modiolus, 162
Monoamine transmitters, 189
Monocular crescent, 220
Monosynaptic reflex, 73
Mossy fibers, 197, 198–9, 203
Motoneurons, 55–6, 73–4, 106, 117–22
  alpha, 73–4, 106, 117–19, 121–2
    tonic and phasic, 118
  gamma, 74, 106, 118, 121–2
Motor cell columns, 117–18
Motor cortex, 234–5
  blood supply, 42–6, 231
  plasticity, 235
Motor end plate, 71
Motor loop, basal ganglia, 247–52
Motor neuron disease, 124
Motor unit, 71–2
Multiple sclerosis, 59, 61, 180, 225
Muscle
  fiber types, 70–4, 118
  skeletal, innervation, 70–5
  smooth, innervation, 88
  spindles, 72–4, 114
Muscle stiffness, 125
Myasthenia gravis, 72
Myelin, deposition, 59
Myelination
  and conduction, 64–5
  demyelinating disease, 59–60, 61
  peripheral, 59–60
Myelocele, 98
Myoneural junction, 71

NANC neurons, 89–90
Near response, 179
Neck rigidity, 34
Neocerebellum, 201, 203
  lesions, 203
Neocortex, cellular laminae, 228, 229
Neostigmine, 72
Nerve(s)
  classification, 63
  microscopic anatomy, 63–5
  nervi erigentes, 90
  nervus intermedius, 171, 174
  peripheral, 63–9
Nerve endings

free, 74–5
  in joints, 75
  in muscle, 74–5
  in skin, 78–81
  in teeth, 167–8
Nerve fibers
  classification, 63, 63–4
  definition, 63
  degeneration, 67–8
  regeneration, 68
Nerve roots, 1, 63, 95–104, 174
  compression, 101, 102
Neural arches, 97, 98
Neural canal, 1, 95, 96
Neural crest, 1, 95
Neural folds, 1
Neural plate, 1
Neural tube, 1, 96
Neuraxial fibers, 230
Neuroeffector junctions, 87
Neuroendocrine cells, 206–7
Neurofibrillary tangles, 263
Neurofilaments, 53–4
Neurogenic inflammation, 75
Neuroglia, 53
  types, 58
Neurohumoral reflex, 210
Neurolemmal cells, 64
Neurolemmoma, 173
Neuroma, amputation, 65
Neuromelanin, 137
Neuromuscular spindles, 72–4, 118
  see also Muscle spindles
Neurons, 53–58
Neurophysin, 207
Neuropores, 1, 96
Neurotendinous spindles, 73–4
Neurotransmitters, 87–90
Neurulation, 1
Nicotinic receptors, 87
Nigrostriatal pathway, 137, 248
Nissl bodies, 54, 66–7
Nociceptive afferents, 78, 192
Nociceptors, 78
Nodes of Ranvier, 64
Noradrenalin see Norepinephrine
Noradrenergic fibers, 188, 261
Norepinephrine, 87, 88, 126, 187, 189, 216
  in depression, 189
Novelty detection, 200
Nuclei
  see under specific nuclei
Nystagmus
  cerebellar, 201
  vestibular, 156
Occipital lobe, anatomy, 10

Occipitotemporal gyri, 10
Ocular dominance columns, 226, 232, 234
Ocular motor nerves, 176–84
Ocular nerve palsies, 180, 182
Ocular sympathetic supply, 181
Oculomotor loop, 253
Oculomotor nerve, 25, 138, 176–8
  nucleus, 138
  paralysis, 180–1
Oculomotor (third nerve) palsy, 181, 276
Olfactory bulb, 10, 257
Olfactory epithelium, 256–7
Olfactory nerve, development, 4
Olfactory neurons, 256
Olfactory striae, 257
Olfactory system, 256–8
Olfactory tract, 10, 257–8
Oligodendrocytes, 59
Olive, 26, 28
Olivocerebellar tract, 133, 200
Olivocochlear bundle, 162
Opercula of insula, 9
Optic chiasm, 21, 205, 222, 225
  lesions, 225
Optic nerve, 222–4
  development, 2, 4
  lesions, 225
  sheath, 36–7
  see also Optic tract
Optic papilla, 37, 38
Optic radiation, 224
  tumors, 225, 276
Optic tract, 25, 222–4
  lesions of visual pathway, 224–6
  see also Eye
Organ of Corti, 158–9
Organum vasculosum, 209
Orientation columns, 229
Orthograde transneuronal atrophy, 68
Otic ganglion, 86, 148
Otoconia, 153
Otoliths, 153
Otosclerosis, 161

Pachymeninx, 32
Pacinian corpuscles, 75, 79–80, 81
Pain
  anterior cingulotomy, 263
  facial, 167
  gate control, 192–3
  low back, 102
  psychological, 92
  referred, 91, 167

  supraspinal controls, 193
  visceral, 91
  viscerosomatic, 91
Paleospinothalamic pathway, 114
Palisade nerve endings, 78
Pallidum
  development, 13
  internal/external, 247–9
  in Parkinson's disease, 251
  ventral, 266
Papez circuit, 262
Papilledema, 36–7, 38
Parabrachial nucleus, 189, 191
Parahippocampal gyrus, 11, 258–60
Paranodal pockets, 64
Paraplegia
  in extension, 127
  in flexion, 125, 127
Parasympathetic nervous system, 86–7
  and drugs, 90
Paraventricular nucleus, 206, 207, 208
Parietal lobe
  anatomy, 10, 239–41
  blood supply, 43
  Brodmann's areas, 239
  dysfunction, 243
  movement initiation, 241–3
  posterior parietal lobe, 239–41
Parkinson's disease, 171, 251
  treatment, 68
Partial seizures, 259
Parvocellular neurons, 186, 207–8
Patellar reflex, 73
Pattern generators, 123, 189
Peduncles
  see named peduncles
Pelvic ganglia, 85, 87
Percutaneous cordotomy, 112
Perforant path, 260
Periaqueductal gray matter, 27, 136, 193
Perigeniculate nucleus, 224
Periglomerular cells, 257
Perikaryon, 53–4, 55
Perineurium, 64, 97
Periodontal ligaments, 169
Peripheral nerves, 63–9
Peripheral neuropathies, 56, 80
Periventricular nucleus, 206
Petrosal nerves, 148
Petrosal sinuses, 32–4
Phonemic paraphrasia, 240
Photoreceptors, 219–21
Pia mater, 34–5, 37

Pia–glial membrane, 49
Pineal gland, 15, 22, 210–11, 216–17
Piriform cortex, 198
Piriform lobe, 258
Pituitary adenoma, 225
Pituitary gland, 22, 208–11
Plantar reflexes, 124
Planum temporale, 237, 238
Plasticity
  motor cortex, 235
  somatic sensory cortex, 232
  visual cortex, 234
Pleasure center, 264
Poles of cerebral hemispheres, 8
Polymodal receptors, 192
Pons
  anatomy, 26–8
  basilar, 135
  blood supply, 45–6
  development, 12
Pontine arteries, 46
Pontine center, 127
Pontine cistern, 36
Pontine nuclei, 136, 164–5
Pontine reticulospinal tract, 122–3
Pontocerebellar tract, 136, 198
Portal vessels, 208
Position sense, 108, 154
Positron emission tomography, 201, 231
Postcentral gyrus, 144
Posterior cerebral artery, 45, 46
  occlusion, 275, 276
Posterior circulation of brain, 274
Posterior columns, 28
  medial lemniscal pathway, 109–11
  nuclei, see Cuneate nucleus; Gracile nucleus
Posterior commissure, 20
Posterior communicating artery, 46
Posterior funiculus, 30
Posterior gray horn, 106
Posterior inferior cerebellar artery, 45
Posterior lobe of cerebellum, 29, 201
Posterior median septum, 30
Posterior nerve roots, 107
Posterior nucleus of thalamus, 213, 214
Posterior perforated substance, 43
Posterior rami, 63
Posterior spinal artery, 45, 128

Posterior spinocerebellar tract, 114, 114–15
Postjunctional receptors, 87, 88
Postrolandic artery, 272
Postsynaptic membrane, 55
Posture
 control, 127
 reflexes, 123, 203, 251
Posturography, 203
Precentral gyrus, 144
Precuneus, 10
Prefrontal cortex, 236
Prejunctional receptors, 87
Premotor cortex (PMC), 235–6
Preoccipital notch, 8
Preoptic nucleus, 206
Pressor center, 191
Presynaptic inhibition, 57–8, 58
Presynaptic membrane, 55
Pretectal nucleus, 178
Primary auditory cortex, 234
Primary somesthetic cortex, 243
Probst, tract of, 165
Procedural memory, 262
Progressive bulbar palsy, 126, 145
Progressive muscular atrophy, 126
Prolapsed intervertebral disc, 102
Proprioception, 108, 154
Propriospinal tract, 30, 105–6
Prosencephalon, 1, 2, 3
Prosopagnosia, 233, 276
Pseudobulbar palsy, 145
Pterygopalatine ganglion, 86
Ptosis of eyelid, 85
Pudendal nerve, 91
Pulvinar, 215
Pupillary light reflex, 178–9, 184
Purkinje cells, 154, 197–9, 200, 203
Putamen, 13
 executive area, 263
Pyramid, 28, 29
Pyramidal decussation, 26, 28, 120, 124, 131
Pyramidal neurons, targets, 230
Pyramidal tract, 14, 136
 see also Corticospinal tract

Quadriplegia, 127

Radicular arteries, 128
Radiculospinal arteries, 128
Rage attacks, 266
Rage and fear, 210
Ramsay Hunt syndrome, 173
Ranvier, nodes of, 64

Raphe (magnus), 125, 186, 191, 193
Raphespinal tract, 125–6, 193
Raynaud phenomenon, 85
Reading, 236
Receptive aphasia, 237, 240
Receptive fields, 77
Receptors
 receptor proteins, 56–7
 sensory receptors, 73
 stretch receptors, 73, 121
 see also under named receptors
Recurrent artery of Heubner, 43, 277
Red nucleus, 27, 136, 137, 201, 203
Reflexes
 see under named reflexes
Regeneration of nerve fibers, 68
Renshaw cells, 56, 106, 118, 119, 121
Respiratory centers, 149, 190
Reticular formation, 113, 186–94
 functional anatomy, 189–3
 organization, 186–9
 pattern generators, 123, 189
 topography, 27, 186–62
Reticular nucleus of thalamus, 215
Reticulocerebellar fibers, 200
Reticulospinal tracts, 113–14, 122–3
Retina, 219–22
 embryology, 219–20
 ganglionic cells, 219, 222
 lesions, 36–7
 structure, 220–1
Retinotopic map, 226
Retrograde transneuronal atrophy, 68
Retrograde transport, 54
Reward areas, 264
Rhizotomy, 107
Rhombencephalon, 1, 3
Ribbon synapse, 153, 158, 159
Rolandic fissure, 8
Romberg's sign, 111
Rostral interstitial nucleus, 182
Rostral spinocerebellar tract, 114–15
Rubrospinal tract, 128, 138
Ruffini endings, 75, 79, 80, 81

Saccades
 automatic, 182
 voluntary, 236
Saccule, 153, 154

Sacral parasympathetic system, 86–7
Sagittal sinus, 32–5, 39, 47
Salivatory nucleus
 inferior, 148, 189
 superior, 174, 189
Saltatory conduction, 65
Sarcomeres, 71, 73
Satellite cells, 64, 107
Satiety center, 210
Scanning movements, 182
Schaffer collaterals, 261, 262
Schizophrenia, 137, 238, 242
Schwann cells, 64–7
Scotoma, 61, 225
Secondary somatic sensory area, 231
Segmental antinociception, 192
Segmental gate control, 192
Seizures, 259
Semicircular ducts, 156
Sensation
 exteroceptive, 108
 modalities, 78
 nociceptive, 78, 192
 proprioceptive, 108, 110
 temperature, 210
 unconscious, 108
Sensorimotor loop, 248
Sensorineural deafness, 161
Sensory association cortex, 243
Sensory ataxia, 110
Sensory competition, 232
Sensory decussation, 110, 132
Sensory extinction, 243
Sensory neglect, 243
Sensory pathways, 105–16
Sensory testing, 108
Sensory units, 77
Septal area, 264–5
Septal nucleus, 264
Septal rage, 264
Septohippocampal pathway, 264
Septum pellucidum, 20
Serotonergic neurons, 216, 261
 and endogenous depression, 187, 189
 and pain, 193
 and sleep, 191
Sexual intercourse, 86
Sexuality, Kluver–Bucy syndrome, 266
Sigmoid sinus, 32–3, 33–4
Sigoma, 161
Sinuses of the brain, 32–5, 39
 see also under named sinuses
Skin innervation, 77–82
Sleep, 191, 210
Smell see Olfaction

Sneezing center, 189
Sole plate, 71
Soma of neuron, 53–4
Somatic sensory cortex, 229–30
  plasticity, 232
Somatic sensory pathways, 63,
  108–10, 141
Somatomotor cell columns, 117,
  118
Somesthetic cortex, 243
  association area, 232
Sound attenuation reflex, 171
Sound transduction, 159
Spasticity, 124–5
Speech centers, 202
Sphincter pupillae, 177
Spina bifida, 98
Spinal accessory nerve, 144, 150
  lesion, 146–7
Spinal arteries, 45, 128
Spinal cord
  anatomy, 29–30, 97–8,
    117–19
  ascending pathways, 105–16
  ascent, 96
  blood supply, 128
  caudal cell mass, 96
  cell columns, 141–2
  descending pathways, 119–28
  embryology, 4, 95–7, 141
  ganglia, 1, 66–7, 107
  injury, 127
  meninges, 37–8
  neurulation, 1
  sections, 105–6
Spinal lemniscus, 112, 136
Spinal nerves, 63–8
  distribution, 98–9
  enumeration, 97
Spinal reflexes, 114–15
Spinal tap, 37, 49, 101, 103
Spinocerebellar pathways,
  114–15, 199–200
Spinocerebellum, 197, 201
Spinocervical tract, 115
Spinomedullary junction, 132
Spinoolivary tract, 115, 200
Spinoreticular tract, 113–14
Spinotectal tract, 115
Spinothalamic pathway, 111–13
Spiral ganglion, 153, 159
Spiral ligament, 153
Splanchnic nerves, 85, 87, 90–1
Splenium, 9, 276
Split brain effects, 271
Spondylosis, vertebral, 102, 167
Startle reflex, 161
Stellate block, 85
Stellate cells

cerebellum, 198, 203
cerebrum, 230
Stellate ganglion, 84–5
Stereoacusis, 234
Stereocilia, 153, 159
Stereognosis, 81, 232
Stereopsis, 233
Sternomastoid muscle, 143
Straight sinus, 32, 48
Stretch receptors, 149
  muscle spindles, 73
  reflexes, 121
Stretch reflex, presynaptic
  inhibitory neurons, 121
Stria of Gennari, 226
Stria medullaris thalami, 264
Stria terminalis, 266
Striate cortex, 226
Striatum, 247, 252
Stroke, 124, 270, 274
  defined, 43, 271
  sites, 13, 182–3, 243
Strychnine poisoning, 119
Subarachnoid cisterns, 36
Subarachnoid hemorrhage, 274,
  277
Subarachnoid space, 34–5, 38–9
Subdural hematoma, 35
Subfalcal hernia, 60
Subiculum, 260
Submandibular ganglion, 174
Substantia gelatinosa, 192
Substantia nigra, 13, 27, 137
  pars compacta, 249–50
  pars reticulata, 247
Subsynaptic web, 57
Subthalamic nucleus (STN), 13,
  247, 248, 249, 276
Sucking reflex, 171
Sulci, 8
  see also named sulci
Superior colliculi, 26, 27, 115,
  125, 138, 183
Superior longitudinal fasciculus,
  17, 243
Superior olivary nucleus, 159,
  160
Supplementary motor area
  (SMA), 235–6, 249–50
Supplementary sensory area, 232
Suprachiasmatic nucleus, 206,
  210, 211
Supramarginal gyrus, 243
Supraoptic nucleus, 206, 208
Supraspinal antinociception, 193
Supraspinal nucleus, 144
Supratrigeminal nucleus, 164,
  165, 169
Sustentacular cells, 257

Swallowing center, 189
Swallowing reflex, 149
Sweat glands, 80, 87, 89, 90
Sylvian fissure, 8
Sympathectomy
  cervical, 84
  lumbar, 85
Sympathetic nervous system,
  84–6
  and drugs, 87–9
Synapse(s)
  axoaxonic, 58
  axodendritic/somatic, 53, 55–8
  chemical, 55–7
  electrical, 57–8
  excitatory, 57
  inhibitory, 57, 58
  ribbon, 153, 158, 159
  structure, 55–6
Synaptic cleft, 55–6
Synaptic vesicles, 55–6
Syringomyelia, 113

Tactile aphasia, 271
Tactile discrimination, 111
Tapetum, 18
Target cell recognition, 54
Taste buds, 149, 174
Taste pathway, 174
Tau protein, 263
Tectorial membrane, 158
Tectospinal tract, 125
Tectum, 37, 186
Teeth, innervation, 167–8
Tegmentum
  anatomy, 26–7, 205
  central tegmental tract, 136
  see also Reticular formation
Tela choroidea, 21
Telencephalon, 1, 3, 5
Teloglia, 64, 79
Temperature regulation, 210
Temporal lobe, anatomy, 10,
  11–12
Temporal lobe epilepsy, 259
Temporal plane, 237, 238
Tendon endings, 74
Tendon reflexes, 74, 101, 124
TENS (Transcutaneous electrical
  nerve stimulation), 192
Tentorium cerebelli, 33
Tetanus, 56
Tetraplegia, 127
Thalamic peduncles, 216
Thalamic syndrome, 276
Thalamocortical fibers, 230
Thalamostriate vein, 47
Thalamus, 213–17
  anatomy, 12, 12–13

Thalamus (*continued*)
  development, 5, 5–6
  nuclei, 213–15, 252
Thermosensitive units, 78, 210
Theta rhythm, 265
Third nerve palsy, 180–1, 276
Third ventricle, 20, 21–2
Thoracic nucleus, 114
Thoracolumbar outflow of
      autonomic system, 84
Tinnitus, 173
Toe the line test, 202
Tongue
  gustatory innervation, 147,
      148
  sensory innervation, 148, 174
  taste buds, 149, 174
Tonic motoneurons, 118
Tonsil (of cerebellum), 29
Tracheobronchial tree, 88
Tracking movements, 183
Tract
  definition, 14
  see also named tracts
Tractotomy, medulla, 165
Tractus solitarius, 147
Transcutaneous electrical nerve
      stimulation (TENS), 192
Transient ischemic attacks,
      275–6
Transmitter molecules, 55–6
Transneuronal atrophy, 68
Transverse sinus, 32–5, 47
Trapezius muscle, 143
Trapezoid body, nucleus, 159,
      160
Tremor
  intention, 202
  resting, 251
Triceps reflex, 101
Trigeminal afferents, 167
Trigeminal lemniscus, 110, 169
Trigeminal nerve, 25, 26,
      164–70
  development, 4, 5
  mesencephalic nucleus, 136,
      164
  motor nucleus, 164, 165, 167
  nucleus of spinal tract, 131,
      166–7
  sensory nucleus, 164–5
  spinal nucleus, 166–7
  supratrigeminal nucleus, 164
Trigeminal neuralgia, 165–7
Trigeminal sensory map, 165
Trigeminoreticular fibers, 164,
      168

Trigeminothalamic tract, 136,
      166, 169
Trigeminovascular neurons, 168
Trigger points, 167
Trigone, 20, 22
Triphasic response, 121
Triple response, 79
Trochlear nerve, 25–6, 177–8
  palsy, 181
Trophic factors, 68
Truncal ataxia, 201
Tsai's area, 188
Tuber cinereum, 21, 22, 205
Tuberoinfundibular tract, 207–8
Tuberomamillary nucleus, 192,
      211
Tympanic membrane and nerve,
      148

Uncal herniation, 60
Uncinate epilepsy, 258
Uncinate fasciculus, 18
Unconscious proprioception, 108
Upper motor neuron lesion,
      124–5
Urinary bladder
  atonic, 127
  automatic, 127
  control center, 189–90
  innervation, 87
Urinary incontinence, 271
Urinary retention, 61
Utricle, 153
Uvula (cerebellum), 29

Vagus nerve, 147, 149, 150
  branches, 149
  development, 4, 5
  dorsal nucleus, 134
  lesions, 145–7
Vallecula, 29
Vas deferens, 91
Vasoactive intestinal peptide, 48,
      90, 230
Veins
  cerebral, 46–8
  spinal, 128
  see also named veins; Sinuses
Velocity detectors, 183
Venous drainage of the brain,
      46–8
Ventral amygdalofugal pathway,
      266
Ventral nerve roots, 107
Ventral striatum, 266
Ventral tegmental area, 137
Ventral thalamus, 215–16

Ventricular system
  anatomy, 20–2
  development, 2–4
  hydrocephalus, 38, 39
  see also individual ventricles
Vergence, 179
Vermis, 29
  lesions, 201, 202
Vertebral artery, 118–19
Vertigo, 156, 173
Vestibular disease, 155–7
Vestibular ganglion, 153, 200–1
Vestibular hair cells, 154
Vestibular nerve, 152
Vestibular nucleus, 134, 154
Vestibulocerebellum, 200–1, 203
Vestibulocochlear nerve, 4,
      152–63
Vestibulocortical connections,
      156–7
Vestibuloocular reflexes, 156,
      182
Vestibulospinal tract, 125, 134,
      154
Vibration and vibration sense,
      79, 109
Visceral afferents, 91–3, 134,
      141–2
  nucleus, 148
Visceral efferents, 63, 142
Visceral pain, 91–2
Visual cortex, 183, 232–4
  association, 232–4
  lesions of visual pathway, 225
  plasticity, 234
  primary, 224–6
Visual fields, 220
  defects, 224–5
Visual neglect, 183, 241
Visual stria, 226
Visual system, 219–27
  see also Optic tract
Vomiting center, 189

Wallerian degeneration, 65–7,
      172
Weber's syndrome (crossed third
      nerve palsy), 276
Weight, sense, 231
Wernicke's area, 234, 237
Wheal and flare, 79
White commissure, 30
Willis, circle *see* Circle
Withdrawal reflex, 119

Zona incerta, 210

ANSWERS TO SELF TEST QUESTIONS

Chapter 1	1D	2D	3D	4B	5A	
	6C	7E	8B	9A		
Chapter 2	1C	2B	3E	4A	5A	
	6D					
Chapter 3	1E	2E	3D	4A	5E	
Chapter 4	1E	2B	3D	4D	5B	6E
Chapter 5	1D	2D	3C	4E	5E	6B
Chapter 6	1B	2A	3D	4C	5A	6B
	7D	8C	9C	10B	11D	12A
Chapter 7	1E	2C	3A	4C	5E	6E
Chapter 8	1D	2D	3B	4E	4C	6D
Chapter 9	1C	2B	3A	4B	5E	6D
Chapter 10	1B	2B	3A	4C	5A	6A
	7B	8D	9C	10B	11B	12A
	13B	14C	15D	16B	17A	18D
	19B	20B				
Chapter 11	1C	2D	3E	4B	5C	6A
Chapter 12	1E	2E	3A	4A	5E	6A

Chapter 13	1C	2D	3C	4A	5B	6C
	7B	8B	9A	10D	11C	12A
	13B	14B	15D			

| Chapter 14 | 1E | 2D | 3A | 4D | 5B | 6D |

| Chapter 15 | 1A | 2E | 3B | 4D | 5C | 6A |
| | 7C | 8B | 9D | 10E | 11B | |

| Chapter 16 | 1E | 2A | 3A | 4E | 5C | 6D |

| Chapter 17 | 1A | 2D | 3E | 4C | 5B | 6A |

Chapter 18	1C	2B	3A	4B	5D	6B
	7C	8C	9A	10B	11A	12C
	13D					

| Chapter 19 | 1B | 2A | 3C | 4D | 5E | 6C |
| | 7D | 8A | 9B | 10E | | |

| Chapter 20 | 1D | 2C | 3A | 4E | 5C | 6E |

| Chapter 21 | 1C | 2C | 3C | 4A | 5B | 6E |
| | 7B | 8C | 9D | 10A | | |

| Chapter 22 | 1B | 2A | 3D | 4E | 5C | |

| Chapter 23 | 1A | 2E | 3D | 4D | 5A | 6B |
| | 7C | 8E | | | | |

| Chapter 24 | 1B | 2B | 3C | 4E | 5B | 6B |
| | 7A | | | | | |

| Chapter 25 | 1A | 2C | 3A | 4B | 5C | 6C |
| | 7A | 8D | 9C | 10B | | |

| Chapter 26 | 1A | 2A | 3B | 4C | 5E | 6D |

| Chapter 27 | 1A | 2B | 3C | 4E | 5B | 6D |
| | 7E | 8B | 9C | 10A | | |